STEPHEN GASCOIGNE
M.B., Ch.B., C.Ac., Dip.C.H.M.

The MANUAL OF
CONVENTIONAL MEDICINE
for
ALTERNATIVE PRACTITIONERS

Volume I

RICHMOND

Jigme Press

First published in Great Britain by

JIGME PRESS
PO Box 217, Richmond, Surrey TW9 1TA

© Stephen Gascoigne, 1993

ISBN 0 9522189 0 9

First published 1993

Copies of this book can be obtained from

Jigme press, PO Box 20-26 SOUTH STREET DORKING, SURREY RH4 2HQ TEL: 0306 742150 1ond, Surrey TW9 1TA

To receive a copy please send a cheque for £22.00 (to include post and packing) made payable to Jigme Press

Printed by Antony Rowe, Chippenham, Wilts.
Cover design by Neal's Yard Desktop Publishing Studio.
Cat logo by Rob Hopkins

- CONTENTS -

Chapter

- ACKNOWLEDGEMENTS -

I owe my thanks to many people during the process of writing this book but especially to:

Sarah Cleverley, Dr Tim Duerden, Andrew Flower, Hilary Gascoigne, Andra Goldman, Stuart Gracie, Stephen Guy-Clarke, Rob Hopkins, Simon of Neal's Yard Desktop Publishing Studio, Nguyen Tinh Thong, Mark Tittle and all those students who have patiently allowed me to develop my ideas.

FOREWORD

Before I arrived in England, I thought that with such an advanced technology and prosperous life-style, the fortunate people who live here would be very peaceful, happy and healthy.

Now, the more I treat Western patients, the more I understand that the opposite is true. The society which has everything seems to be splintering and everything has to be approved by the cold eye of science as we forget how to call on our intuitive natures. Our advanced technology does not satisfy the voracious appetite of human desire for progress whilst simultaneously polluting the environment.

The common foundation of the family has been broken because mother and father have little time with their children. The majority of older people are lonely and lack self-esteem whilst many of the younger generation are dissolute. The generation gap widens. Understanding and co-operation between people decline whilst egotism, factionalism, selfishness, indulgence and irresponsibility are rife within our society.

True love and care, the desire for deep understanding and self-awareness have been supplanted by a spiralling consumption of materialism which leads to chronic mental disease and physical illness.

As an Oriental practitioner with a Buddhist perspective, I often ask myself after clinical days, "Have I done enough to express my gratitude to Great Britain, the country which was kind enough to grant me refuge? How can I best serve all beings that I encounter in this world?"

One fresh morning, Dr Stephen Gascoigne gave me a copy of his book and asked for my opinion.

I feel very touched by this work. In the Philosophy section he writes, "It depends as much on how medicine is practised as the method of practice." Yes, it is true that the patient's response depends on the attitude of the practitioner. It is like the relationship between the mother and baby. The old Vietnamese proverb says "Luong Y nhu tu mau". It means the good-hearted practitioner looks after their patients like the mother feeding her baby from the beginning of pregnancy throughout their childhood.

A wonderful thing about this book is the emphasis placed on understanding the essence of the relationship between the practitioner and the patient. It is as important as the relationship between mother and child and is called 'the consciousness of the Healing Tao' in the ancient texts. Practitioners should always relate to this and remember Stephen for setting it down in a modern idiom.

Nguyen Tinh Thong, London 1993.

1 INTRODUCTION

OBJECTIVES:

At the end of this book you will be able to:
State the terms used by conventional medicine
Link from anatomy and physiology to clinical medicine
Compare the philosophical bases of conventional and alternative medicine
Describe the disease processes of conventional medicine and relate them to the practice of alternative medicine
Explain how treatment by conventional medicine may affect treatment by alternative medicine
Apply this information in case management and explain how to manage clinical situations in an appropriate way

The aim of this book is to provide a suitable text for use by practitioners and students of alternative medicine. It is intended to provide support for practitioners who are not trained in conventional medicine and who on occasions may need access to information in a way that is clear and concise.

When I trained in conventional medicine, I always had the feeling that it did not "sound right". I found it hard to put my finger on the difficulty I had with the subject but I felt that the whole fabric of conventional medicine did not hang together in a logical way. I found that there are many discrepancies and contradictions that are not addressed and in most situations actively ignored. At the time, however, I thought that this was a problem that was mine and could not find a way to deal with my confusion. Sometimes it is said that to talk to a person who is insane can be very disconcerting since they may appear to be lucid, clear and rational. At the end of the conversation, you may realise that one of you is mad but you are not sure which one. This is the way I felt about conventional medicine.

When I was in general practice I had a crisis of confidence in that I began to see that many treatments of conventional medicine not only produce little benefit but may actually cause harm. This may not be obvious at first but over months and sometimes years, if you really listen to what people tell you, I came to see that drug-based treatment leads to effects that are worse than the original problem. Then I had to stop since I could no longer prescribe the drugs I felt were so harmful.

It is only with my subsequent training in Chinese medicine that I came to see conventional medicine in a different light. The actual information of conventional medicine is fine and may be useful in helping practitioners understand their patients. It is when these ideas are translated into clinical practice that the problems start. I remember having a conversation with an acupuncturist and herbalist who grew up and trained in the Orient who had also had some education in conventional medicine. He said that he had not really understood the connection in conventional medicine between diagnosis and treatment - how one led onto the other. Well, of course, there *is* no connection between these two things. The use of treatments is based on experience and "what works" rather than any sound connection with underlying physiological processes. This is particularly clear to those with an energetic understanding of the human being.

This book is the result of these years of trying to make sense of conventional information in a way that is useful in the practice of alternative medicine. In many respects this reflects the struggle we all have between the widely differing philosophies of alternative and conventional medicine. This is especially true for Westerners who have grown up with the belief that conventional medicine is the way to treat most disease states. I hope that the way I present information here will help alternative practitioners in their practice and enable them to view conventional medicine as a useful tool but not as an overwhelmingly, inevitable event.

The book follows the way in which conventional medicine outlines "systems" of the body. I have concentrated on describing processes in plain English. Many textbooks already in use are aimed at medical students, are very detailed and written in an obscure dialect of Graeco-Roman. Whilst a useful source of information, they are not always easy to follow and not always relevant to the needs of alternative practitioners. I have included all diseases which are commonly seen in clinical practice. I have omitted those diseases that are rare and unusual due to constraints of space. In each section I have arranged the information according to principles of *energetic* medicine and so the classifications may seem rather strange at first. They accord with principles derived from the medicine which we are using and so of much more benefit.

All the references in the book to alternative medicine apply to ideas gleaned mainly from Chinese medicine, my own chosen field of practice, or of homoeopathy. This is because I consider these to be complete medical systems in themselves and truly deserving of the title alternative medicine. There is much benefit to be derived from such therapies as osteopathy, massage, reflexology, aromatherapy, shiatsu and so on but perhaps not as primary treatments for severe medical conditions. I am aware, however, that such treatments can lead to fundamental changes in people's states of health so such a distinction is not always valid.

My other aim is to provide help and support to alternative practitioners so that the practice of such medicine in this country can be strengthened. I hope that in the future such medicine can be more available to people and the only way this will be provided in the long term is if we are competent and confident in our practice. Many practitioners I meet feel that they lack in confidence particularly regarding serious conditions. They often project this insecurity onto their lack of training in conventional medicine. It is true that my training in conventional medicine has given me experience in seeing and treating more serious disease. However, it is important to emphasise that faith in alternative medicine and its ability to help sickness comes from competence in our chosen field of alternative medicine. Therefore, any knowledge of conventional medicine must only be considered as an added extra to our main practice.

There is usefulness in all information. Knowledge about the methods of conventional medicine can be an adjunct to our practice. The person who comes for help will only recover by our skill and expertise in our therapy. This therapy is based upon the principles of alternative medicine. This must come first and all else follows. Therefore, to recycle a popular phrase of today - complementary medicine - this term would be better applied to what is commonly known as conventional medicine since alternative medicine is our chosen therapy and the one that is most appropriate to the needs of the individual because of its ability to lead towards "cure"[1]. Conventional medicine is complementary to this and would be better used either for structural problems incapable of any other help, e.g. trauma, or for life-threatening conditions.

Today, we see the opposite situation where alternative medicine is only used after a long time of conventional treatment. We live in a society that does not give much weight to non-physical ideas. Alternative medicine is criticised by those people who only see importance in material things. This, of course, is at the root of Western thought[2] - a division between mind and body coupled with the unfortunate association that mind is unimportant or even non-existent. This constant message of division and the undermining of people's belief in the non-physical affects us greatly. We lose faith in our ability to know ourselves and to heal ourselves. We then rely on "experts" who claim to know what is best for us. Consequently, women do not know how to give birth, people do not know how to die (not to mention live!), people do not know how to be well. This disconnection at very deep levels is, I think, partly responsible for the great dissatisfaction and angst that is felt by so many people in the West today. Spiritual matters are given little weight or dismissed completely. Methods of healing which are non-toxic and of great benefit in all areas of our lives are dismissed, made illegal or subtly opposed. It is no mistake when the sages of India and Tibet say we live in degenerate times.

---

[1] I use the term "cure" as it understood by homoeopathic medicine although the same principle can be applied to any method of healing of similar means. I discuss cure more fully in Chapter 2.
[2] There is a vitalistic tradition to Western philosophy as evidenced by the work of Paracelsus. Homoeopathy belongs to this tradition. When I use the term Western as applied to medicine or philosophy in this book, I am referring to the main strand of science which has become dominant in the Western world, i.e. materialistic, physical.

The hope is that there is definitely a change in consciousness occurring that is gathering pace. Even over the past 10 years in this country we see much more interest in alternative medicine, in self-help, in religious faith, in meditation, in matters that formerly were considered off-beat, non-scientific and of little or no value. Such practices can only accelerate as the momentum for change becomes irresistible. In this climate and that of the future, doctors will find themselves increasingly left behind as people embrace more holistic principles. Some medical practitioners have decided to change also and are moving over to alternative medicine. However, the profession as a rule is not noted for its innovation and radical views so my feeling is that any major change in health care and attitudes must come from the general public and alternative practitioners. It is time for us to reclaim those powers we have so carelessly given away to science, dogmatism and the denial of our deeper selves.

This process is not going to be easy as there are powerful groups who have vested interests in maintaining the status quo. However, the power of the individual cannot be denied and as people become more aware of issues to do with the environment, caring for others, growth and self-development, nothing will be able to stop these changes taking place.
I hope that this book may, in some small way, help in this process.

- LAYOUT OF THE BOOK -

There are two basic assumptions I make prior to you reading this book. The first is that you have a basic knowledge of anatomy and physiology. The second is that you have access to a medical dictionary. I have, as much as possible written in plain English, but there are terms which I have to introduce as I am dealing with a technical subject. A standard medical dictionary, of which there are many, will be useful reference for you.

As I mentioned previously, the Chapter headings correspond roughly to the 'systems' of conventional medicine, e.g. cardiovascular, respiratory and so on. Within each Chapter, I begin by giving a summary including relevant anatomy and physiology.

I discuss in detail the main diseases you will probably come across in the clinic. I have not included those conditions that are usually treated as an emergency in hospital or those which are unusual. After an account of the main clinical features, conventional investigations and treatment I spend some time giving an alternative viewpoint. This is important since the management of the person depends upon our having a different viewpoint from conventional practitioners. The basic information may be the same but it is how to use it that is the key factor. I include here some information about the Chinese medical viewpoint[3] of this disease. This will hopefully be of use to acupuncturists and shiatsu practitioners but also to anyone with an energetic understanding of the human body. Homoeopaths may see the energetic picture of remedies displayed in this account. I do not intend these sections to be exhaustive as this book is primarily about conventional medical knowledge. I hope it will enable you to see that it is indeed possible to view conventional information from the viewpoint of an alternative practitioner.

A warning is necessary at this point. Conventional disease labels are fixed entities and so many people with slightly differing clinical pictures and widely differing energetic remedies may have the same conventional label applied to them. Do not fall into the trap of thinking that conventional disease labels always correspond to a particular energetic picture. The whole point of alternative medicine is that it individualises the person. Fixing a label onto everyone will only lead to a weakening of alternative medicine and ultimately its destruction.

At the end of each Chapter is a discussion of symptoms found in that system and how to recognise serious disease. This is important to give you confidence that you are not treating someone who may have a potentially dangerous condition and to recognise when a person may require referral to another practitioner.

---

[3] I have not spent a long time in this book describing the theories of Chinese medicine since this is not my main aim and I do not want to overcomplicate matters. For anyone interested in the basic ideas of Chinese medicine I would recommend two books, "Between Heaven and Earth"by Beinfield and Korngold, (Ballantine, 1991) and "The Web Which Has No Weaver" by Kaptchuk (Congdon and Weed, 1983).

NOTE: Nothing in this book should be construed as medical advice on an individual basis. Although many disorders can and are treated safely individually, I would urge anyone with a health problem that is chronic or severe to seek out appropriate advice and help from a competent practitioner - orthodox or alternative. It is your choice.

2 PHILOSOPHY

OBJECTIVES:

At the end of this section you will be able to:
State the philosophical basis of conventional medicine.
Compare the philosophical bases of conventional and alternative medicine.
State the meaning of symptoms to a conventional and alternative practitioner.
Define the 3 levels - mental, emotional and physical.
Define the terms cure and suppression.
Describe the effect on symptoms and levels of curative and suppressive treatment.
List the criteria for deciding whether a symptom indicates a serious problem.

- INTRODUCTION -

When I studied medicine there was no mention of philosophy and no discussion of the theories underpinning the practice of conventional medicine. There was talk of the "medical model" referring to a particular view of human beings. However, this did not extend to debate concerning its origin or whether alternative views existed - only that this was the way to do it.

I hear many alternative practitioners say that there is no philosophy of conventional medicine. There is always a philosophical view that drives our actions. We cannot act if we have no belief system. In Tibetan Buddhism this sequence of events is described as 'View, meditation and action.' To have an action, there must be preceding thought and for this to occur there must be preceding belief. In modern society people think that an action is a spontaneous event. The cause is rarely considered if even acknowledged. Many people believe that conventional medicine as practised today appeared, perhaps with little association with the past. This first section will consider its driving philosophical force.

- PHILOSOPHICAL VIEW OF CONVENTIONAL MEDICINE -

Conventional medicine, in common with the prevailing scientific view in the West, believes there is only a physical body which can be measured, weighed and analysed by physical methods. This leads to the available treatments of surgery, radiotherapy and material chemical substances (drugs) which are purely physical in their application. Although there is occasionally mention of mind, indicating an entity other than the physical body, this is seen as being coexistent with the brain. It is not viewed as non-material in nature. A consequence of this view is that anything which is not physical is seen as being unimportant. These ideas enter the language as 'immaterial', 'it does not matter'.

The materialistic ideas behind Western science and conventional medicine have gained ground over the past 2000 years with a division between spirit and matter, doctor and priest, science and art, between man and woman. It has pervaded all aspects of society and since medicine reflects the views of the society in which it is practised we also see such a polarisation in conventional medicine. This can be described as a flourishing of the Yang principle[1] as that term is understood by Chinese medicine. Unfortunately, it has not been balanced or grounded by Yin. Unchecked it leads to aggression rather than assertiveness, Fire which flares up easily and dissipates quickly, a dryness and rigidity which is not balanced by aspects of nurturing and flexibility. This process is changing as all things must change. Definitely there is a change in consciousness as people begin to embrace more holistic principles.

In Western society we have usually divided the spirit from the body. We have people who deal with the body - doctors - who assume the role of mechanics. They "fix" the physical machine by manipulating physical parts with drugs or inserting "new" parts. Annual "health checks" similar to MOT's are advocated to persuade people that these brief encounters with a qualified mechanic will guarantee health for another year.

The spirit is dealt with by priests who traditionally had a healing role but since the early centuries AD have been less and less involved with what became to be considered the realm of doctors. It is only in recent years that a more holistic view has arisen in science. This is revealed in the new theories of quantum physics. Their ideas formerly seemed to be the province of Buddhism or Hinduism but now have been mirrored in theories of physics and the nature of existence of matter.[2] Whilst these are the source of much debate amongst scientists, they have not filtered through into the practice of medicine. Conventional thought is still involved with physicality. Anything else is seen as being non-existent or of no importance.

There are new specialities such as psychoneuroimmunology which try to make some sense of the whole person and bring together ideas from different areas. In the reality of everyday medicine, however, the treatments remain the same. I believe that people are best judged by their actions and the actions of most conventional practitioners are to treat the patient as a machine. This leads to the treatments which primarily act on the physical level of surgery, chemical drugs and radiation.

- PHILOSOPHICAL VIEWS OF ALTERNATIVE MEDICINE[3] -

Alternative medicine believes there are other parts of the human being - non-physical - and that these are at least as important. These ideas have always been found in society. The acknowledgement of other levels leads to the treatments which utilise energetic methods such as homoeopathy, herbal medicine, acupuncture and so on.

The human being is more than a mere collection of physical parts. In recent years there has been a resurgence in healing ministry as people become disillusioned with conventional medicine and seek other methods of help which incorporate ideas of wholeness. At the same time there has been a strong interest in Oriental philosophies and religions which connect body and mind into a single unit.

The essence of alternative medical thought is that there is a vitalistic[4] principle behind and encompassing any physical object. For the human body this means that the physical body is merely the outer manifestation of an inner energetic state. Any changes in that inner state are reflected in the physical body and changes of the physical body can affect the inner energetic state. However, since the whole person is a manifestation of their innermost energetic condition, the only way in which true balance can be achieved is by change in that energetic condition. The cause must be dealt with not the result. Conventional medicine sees the outer physical aspect of the person and so can only attempt to

---

[1] Yang, in Chinese medicine, is applied to aspects which are active, going upwards and outward, external, hot, masculine, intellectual and so forth. Yin, in Chinese medicine, is applied to aspects which are passive, going downwards and inwards, internal, cold, feminine, intuitive and so forth.
[2] "The Tao of Physics" by Fritjof Capra (Flamingo, 1981) and "The Turning Point" by Fritjof Capra (Flamingo, 1982)
[3] Throughout this book I make reference to the term 'alternative medicine'. I know that this is used in many situations to mean widely differing things. When I use this term I am referring primarily to the philosophical views as espoused by Chinese medicine and homoeopathy. They are exceedingly similar in their beliefs despite differences in use of language.
[4] Vitalism is the term which is applied to energetic systems of thought. Its use indicates that there are existent objects which are non-physical in part or whole.

'treat' the physical body. This will naturally also affect the inner energies but this approach cannot possibly lead to balance.

The foregoing is not to say that there is no benefit, when appropriate, in conventional medicine and its methods. Certainly in acute life-threatening situations there may be nothing better than such medicine. In a crisis, treatment in hospital with the use of powerful drugs may be the only thing which is available for certain disease states. Once this is over it would clearly be inappropriate to use such methods but to turn to more gentle, balancing treatments. The drugs used in an emergency such as corticosteroids, bronchodilators, antihistamines, antibiotics and the like are given to patients for years and years. This can only lead to severe depletion of the patient's energy. With Chinese medicine it would be like using an emergency Rescue Yang formula for years instead of for the usual 2-3 weeks and then changing to a more gentle, balanced treatment.

Since the essence of alternative medicine is vitalistic many levels of a human being can be recognised. These are not just physical, but emotional, mental, spiritual. The spiritual level is of great importance. Attention to spiritual health needs to be made by each individual in their own way and there are qualified spiritual teachers who can help with these. Meditation, ritual, prayer, discussions of teachings and so on are of inestimable value in achieving increased awareness and movement to higher states of consciousness. Each individual makes their own choice of path. It is one of the reasons why the Western world is prone to mental and emotional anguish and agitation. We have lost contact with these deeper spiritual levels.

The important things to consider with relation to health and disease from our perspective of practitioners are to do with physical, emotional and mental levels. I want to consider them each in turn and then draw them together. In this way it is possible to develop a model which can be used in understanding disease and monitoring response to treatment. It is possible by such methods to order these levels into a hierarchy of importance. This can help in assessing the severity of disease since if it primarily affects the deeper level then that patient would be severely affected.

The narrow view of conventional medicine sees health as absence of symptoms.[5] I prefer to use a more positive definition. I would define health as freedom from limitation of activity. Symptoms are a limitation of the individual's function. On the physical level this would mean that there is no restriction of physical activity, on the emotional level it would mean that the person is happy and well-balanced emotionally and on the mental level it would mean that thoughts are clear and awareness is unrestricted. This is clearly a state of perfection but the point is that it is something to aim for - a direction or a path as well as a state to ultimately attain. On the physical level, there are restrictions placed on us by the nature of physical matter and the inescapable fact that our physical body will not last forever.[6]

With medical practice it is possible to help people to achieve more freedom. I like to think that such freedom will be used to benefit others and to allow more self-realisation and self-development. This is the essence of Chinese medicine - that there is no separation between spiritual health and our health in this physical body in this life-time. There is no separation between religion and science. These things are not separately and inherently existent. One will affect another with the innermost levels being the root. Deal with the root and all else will fall into place. This is why in the East mental and emotional levels are given much more weight than the physical. It is only in the West that the physical assumes overwhelming importance.

---

[5] It is difficult to find a formal definition of health which is used by conventional medicine. There is a significant absence of such terms in medical dictionaries. However, in general usage a person would be considered healthy if they had no symptoms.

[6] From the time of conception we are involved in the ageing process leading to our eventual physical death so there is only so much that is achievable with our physical bodies. There is a completely different situation with our mental and emotional health and there are no limitations on the states we can achieve with the motivation and the use of meditation or other techniques to purify the mind. Enlightenment, as the term is understood in Buddhist thought, is possible and meditation practices exist to attain this state. This is the realm of spiritual teachers and teachings but it is clear that our health on a mundane level cannot be separated from our health on a supramundane or spiritual level.

- SYMPTOMS -

These may be defined as manifestations of ill-health which are reported by the patient or observed by the practitioner. Conventionally there is a separation into symptoms which are reported by the patient (subjective) and signs which are observed by the doctor (objective). This merely serves to underline the division in conventional medicine between physical and non-physical and the difference in status between doctor and patient.

For the purposes of this book I shall include every manifestation in the term 'symptoms'. For the conventional practitioner the symptom is a manifestation of a physical problem - this may be at the biochemical level but nevertheless is physical. For the alternative practitioner this is a manifestation of an imbalance at the level of energy - Qi (sometimes spelt *chi*), vital force - and so on. Therefore, symptoms may exist before physical changes are manifest.

Symptoms can be divided according to the level[7] at which they manifest - physical, emotional or mental. By manifestation I mean at which level in the patient does the imbalance appear? I am not referring here to the cause. For example, if a person suffers a bereavement which could be said to be an emotional factor, the result may be pneumonia or grief (emotional) or confusion (mental). The level at which the imbalance manifests is determined by the particular tendency of that person and the strength of their energy. The weaker we are then the deeper will the problem manifest. This is why disease in the West is more serious since our energies are more disturbed at deeper levels.[8]

Symptoms, therefore, mean very different things to different practitioners. A conventional doctor will see symptoms as being caused by a disease. Disease is perceived as an inherently existent entity which can be discovered by the doctor. Removal of the disease will lead to cessation of the symptoms. The emphasis is on the physical nature of disease and symptoms. They are negative, unpleasant and to be removed if health is to be achieved. Health is the absence of symptoms and this is a conventional practitioner's definition of cure.

In alternative medicine, symptoms are the result of an internal imbalance. In addition, the symptoms are a direct manifestation of the inner energetic state.[9] They point directly to the state of Qi[10] and Blood as understood by Chinese medicine. Removal of the symptoms without attending to the underlying imbalance will lead to removal of Qi and Blood and this is the concept of suppression. If the symptoms only disappear because they are not allowed to be expressed then the energetic imbalance has been suppressed deeper into the body. If the symptoms disappear because the energetic imbalance has been rectified then true cure is the result. The alternative practitioner views symptoms as positive and helpful. They are pointing to the inner imbalance and are an opportunity to regain balance and for self-awareness.

In addition, symptoms may be seen as the body's best attempt at self-healing. In any situation, there are homeostatic mechanisms which try to maintain health. If there is an imbalance then they try to maintain the next best state. Symptoms are only serious and deep when there is no other option for the person. This has consequences for treatment since if the symptom is removed without balancing the inner energetic disharmony, that avenue of expression is denied to the person. The only place now

---

[7] An excellent account of the principles of alternative medicine, in this case homoeopathy, and theories of levels can be found in "The Science of Homoeopathy" by George Vithoulkas (Thorson's, 1980).

[8] Chronic degenerative disease is more common in the West as our immune systems become weaker. There are real increases each year in the incidence of diseases such as cancer, heart disease, stroke and so forth. According to the National Cancer Institute in the US, the incidence of cancer has risen by 11% in the last 40 years. In traditional cultures diseases manifests more superficially although this is changing as 'civilisation' develops. Homoeopaths use more remedies now which are indicated to treat mental and emotional disease than were used in the last century. Disease has passed into the interior.

[9] It may be helpful to consider symptoms as metaphors. Why does a person place a certain pathology in a particular place? What is the meaning of symptoms? For example, the person who is 'pissed off' may get cystitis, the person who has too much of a load to bear may get back pain, the person with a difficult relationship may get a pain in the neck. I shall explore such ideas as I discuss disease states in this book.

[10] Qi in Chinese medicine is difficult to translate but corresponds to vital force or energy of the Western vitalistic tradition of homoeopathy.

for a symptom to manifest is on a deeper, more internal level.[11] This is potentially extremely dangerous and is one of the reasons why conventional medical treatment is often followed by other, more severe disease. Conventionally, these are called side-effects but from an energetic viewpoint they are the results of suppressive treatment.

You can see why these two contrasting philosophies have such problems with each other. If conventional medicine tends to be suppressive and alternative medicine tends to be curative it is difficult to imagine how they can work together to any great extent. They are doing opposite things. Alternative medicine is moving in one direction and conventional medicine is moving in the other. These ideas are summarised in Table 2.1.

ALTERNATIVE MEDICINE	CONVENTIONAL MEDICINE
Energetic	Physical
All symptoms considered	Emphasis on physical symptoms
Useful for chronic condition although in the correct context is very helpful in acute disease also	Useful for crisis intervention, life-threatening situations
Holistic	Separatist
Connectedness	Disconnectedness
Transformative	Eliminative
Labour intensive, uses natural remedies	Reliant on technology, chemicals
Curative	Suppressive
Gives responsibility to the patient	Gives responsibility to the disease (and hence to the doctor)
Not state supported (UK)	State supported
Cheap (this is distorted by the fact that state support is not available here)	Expensive (in the UK, due to the National Health Service, we have the mistaken idea that health care is free)
Disease is merely a term applied to a group of symptoms	Disease is independently existent entity
Disease will change if symptoms change	Disease is fixed state - you have it or you do not
Symptoms are result of energetic imbalance	Symptoms are caused by disease
Symptoms are useful, positive, force for change	Symptoms are unpleasant, negative, to be got rid of
Health is balance of energies and freedom from limitation	Health is absence of symptoms
Cure is balance of energetic disharmony	Cure is removal of symptoms

TABLE 2.1: COMPARISON OF ALTERNATIVE AND CONVENTIONAL MEDICAL PHILOSOPHIES

It is important to remember that the lists in Table 2.1 are comparisons of philosophies not of practitioners. In the end, the practice of medicine depends upon the view of the practitioner. I know some conventional practitioners whose practice is more in line with the terms on the left. I also know of some alternative practitioners whose practice is more in line with the terms on the right. It depends as much on the how medicine is practised as the method of practice.

PHYSICAL LEVEL

This is the outermost layer of existence and is the one most easily seen. It corresponds to those parts which we can see, touch and perceive with our physical senses. The organs and structures of this level can be ordered according to a hierarchy. That is, some organs are relatively superficial and some are relatively deep. The organs which are more essential for life are more internal and more vital for health. These tend to be the single organs or those with important functions such as the heart, liver, kidneys and so on. These ideas are summarised in Table 2.2.

---

[11] "Chronic Disease" by Samuel Hahnemann (Jain, 1982) contains many accounts of the results of suppressive treatment.

```
┌─────────────────────────────────────────────┐
│                 OUTER LEVELS                  │
│                                               │
│ Energy                                        │
│ Skin                                          │
│ Muscles                                       │
│ Joints                                        │
│ Intestines                                    │
│ Digestive system, lungs                       │
│ Liver                                         │
│ Kidney                                        │
│ Heart                                         │
│ Endocrine system                              │
│ Blood - red blood cells                       │
│ Blood - white blood cells[12]                 │
│                                               │
│                 INNER LEVELS                  │
└─────────────────────────────────────────────┘
```

TABLE 2.2: HIERARCHY OF ORGANS WITHIN THE PHYSICAL LEVEL

You can see that more superficial organs are placed at the top and the deeper organs at the bottom. If pathology manifests at a particular level it is possible to reach a conclusion as to its severity. Disease of the heart is clearly more serious than disease of the large intestine, disease of the stomach is not as serious as disease of the liver. This is usually true and it is important to take into account the picture presented by each patient. Short duration, acute disease is more superficial than long-lasting chronic disease although the acute nature of the symptoms may, in themselves, be hazardous. This distinction between acute and chronic disease is important because they have different meanings regarding the patient's energy.

The list in Table 2.2 corresponds with ideas in Chinese medicine which are known as the 6 levels. Each stage corresponds to a particular organ or organs. Although it is often used to explain the passage of acute pathogenic influences into the body, there is value in considering this with all disease including chronic conditions. The 6 levels are shown in Table 2.3.

Acute disease may be defined as a disease of rapid onset, short duration which ends in recovery or death and usually has strong symptoms. People who have an acute disease know that they are ill! It is clear cut and indicates that the person is of relatively strong energy. For an acute manifestation to take place there must be strong energy in the system. This is why children tend to have acute illnesses. Occasionally, in patients with energy which is intermediate in type, a chronic illness may result.

Chronic disease can be defined as a disease of slow onset, long duration which ends in gradual deterioration of health. The symptoms are much vaguer than those of an acute problem. This picture indicates that the patient's energy is much weaker. There are examples of few symptoms despite serious chronic disease, e.g. elderly patients with bronchopneumonia may have mild or no cough or fever. They may only present with breathlessness or perhaps confusion. There are however some patients with chronic disease who do recover maybe because the cause has subsided or their lifestyle has altered. The only therapeutic way of course for recovery to occur is by means of methods available to alternative medicine given the comments on Page 22 regarding healing and placebo effect.

---

[12] In conventional medicine, it is this level which is to do with antibodies, white cell changes in immune system disease and so forth. I use the term immune system in a much wider sense to include all defensive levels from the most superficial energetic layers to the deepest internal organs. Conventional medicine manipulates the blood by means of vaccination, corticosteroids which reduce lymphocyte levels, cancer chemotherapy which reduces all the cells in the blood. Throughout this book, all references I make to the immune system are in the wider energetic sense.

NAME OF LEVEL[13]	ORGANS[14] INCLUDED
Taiyang	Exterior level of body, Urinary bladder, Small Intestine
Yangming	Stomach, Large Intestine
Shaoyang	Gall Bladder, San Jiao - half interior half exterior
Taiyin	Lung, Spleen - now disease is internal in nature
Shaoyin	Kidney, Heart
Jueyin	Pericardium, Liver

TABLE 2.3: THE 6 STAGES OF DISEASE ACCORDING TO PRINCIPLES OF CHINESE MEDICINE

There are diseases which do not fit easily into either category and these are usually the acute manifestations of a chronic illness. I would argue that virtually all acute disease is a manifestation of a chronic imbalance and to only treat the acute manifestation will not lead to removal of the chronic problem. However there are some diseases which are clearly acute in nature and I would put the childhood infectious diseases in that category.

SUPERFICIAL, RELATIVELY LESS SEVERE DISEASE

ACUTE CHILDHOOD ILLNESSES OF MEASLES, MUMPS, CHICKENPOX, RUBELLA
COMMON COLD
INFLUENZA
ACUTE UPPER RESPIRATORY TRACT INFECTIONS
TONSILLITIS
ECZEMA, PSORIASIS
IRRITABLE BOWEL SYNDROME
ULCERATIVE COLITIS
CROHN'S DISEASE
DIVERTICULITIS
ASTHMA
CHRONIC BRONCHITIS, EMPHYSEMA
MYALGIC ENCEPHALOMYELITIS
TUBERCULOSIS
SARCOIDOSIS
CANCER
ACQUIRED IMMUNE DEFICIENCY SYNDROME

INTERNAL, RELATIVELY MORE SEVERE DISEASE

TABLE 2.4: HIERARCHY OF DISEASE ACCORDING TO PRINCIPLES OF ALTERNATIVE MEDICINE

So, when developing a hierarchy, if you combine ideas of acuteness/chronicity with ideas of depth it is possible to list diseases according to how deeply they affect the person. The list in Table 2.4, therefore, is of diseases according to depth. It is important to be careful with this since conventional medical labels are fixed entities and so I have used them in the sense of how they are *generally* understood. When faced with an individual patient it is important to decide in that case the actual characteristics presenting rather than the precise name given by conventional medicine. The infectious diseases I have included should be considered together with the discussions in Chapter 5 about the nature of infection according to principles of alternative medicine.

---

[13] These terms refer to the stages of Yin and Yang in the body. I mention them here to allow a connection to be made with books on Chinese medical theory.
[14] The names of organs here refer to organ systems as they are understood by Chinese medicine. They include energetic functions and are not the merely physical organs of conventional medicine. By common usage these are always referred to by using an initial capital letter. For example, the spleen in conventional medicine is an organ of the lymphatic system which has a function in red blood cell destruction and the manufacture of lymphocytes. By contrast, the Spleen of Chinese medicine is concerned with transformation and transportation of food amongst other functions.

The placing of a disease in Table 2.4 depends upon the degree of acuteness and the organ involved. Therefore, cancer is placed at the bottom since it is a serious degenerative condition whilst tonsillitis is placed near the top since it is an acute condition (albeit usually the result of a chronic imbalance in a relatively superficial site. All disease can be placed in such a way. Although it is difficult to precisely order all diseases into the same list it is helpful to think of different diseases and decide on relative severities. This is what I do throughout the book to give you a clear idea as to what is serious, what is not and how to recognise improvement and worsening.

EMOTIONAL LEVEL

This is the next level inward and is to do with feeling, emotion or to use the technical word, affect. Mild degrees of disturbance on this level are manifest as mild irritability or anxiety. More severe imbalance would be shown as depression and the most severe symptoms are those of suicidal depression and complete absence of feeling. These are summarised in Table 2.5. The emotional level is discussed in detail in the Chapter dealing with psychological disorders.

SUPERFICIAL, MILD DISTURBANCES

IRRITABILITY
ANXIETY
SADNESS
FEAR
DEPRESSION
HOMICIDAL FEELINGS
SUICIDAL FEELINGS
COMPLETE ABSENCE OF FEELING

DEEP, SEVERE DISTURBANCES

TABLE 2.5: SUMMARY OF EMOTIONAL STATES LISTED ACCORDING TO DEPTH

MENTAL LEVEL

This is even deeper into the person and is the most difficult to see and treat. It is to do with thought, perception, cognition. Mild abnormalities may be revealed as lack of concentration or poor memory whilst the most severe appear as hallucinations, confusion or eventually complete disintegration of the personality. These ideas are summarised in Table 2.6. The mental level is discussed in detail in Chapter 6 - Psychological disorders.

SUPERFICIAL, MILD DISTURBANCE

LACK OF CONCENTRATION
POOR MEMORY
THOUGHT DISORDERS
HALLUCINATIONS
DELUSIONS
CONFUSION
DISINTEGRATION OF THE PERSONALITY AS IN SOME CASES OF
SCHIZOPHRENIA

DEEP, MORE SEVERE DISTURBANCE

TABLE 2.6: SUMMARY OF MENTAL STATES LISTED ACCORDING TO DEPTH

INTEGRATION OF MENTAL, EMOTIONAL AND PHYSICAL LEVELS

In a person, these three levels are interconnected and so you see symptoms on all levels. The main point for the practitioner is to decide the emphasis of the pathology. Where is the main manifestation of the imbalance? If this is in the physical level then we call it a physical disease, if it is in the emotional level then we call it an emotional disease and if it is in the mental level then we call it a mental disease. This explains the common observation that schizophrenics have a much lower rate of cancer than the general population. If most of the energy is in the mental level then there is not enough to manifest symptoms on the physical. People with cancer tend not to suffer from acute problems such as the common cold or allergic reactions. The pathology is too deep into the physical level for these to occur.

In conventional medicine, diseases are perceived as being discrete, fixed entities. In reality they change according to the energetic state of the patient. It is important not just to consider the present state but also what preceded this condition. In this way a complete picture may be built up of the patient's state of health. Table 2.7 illustrates a patient's medical history revealing disease states over a number of years.

AGE	SYMPTOMS/DISEASE MANIFEST
6 months	Eczema
2 years	Whooping cough
5 years	Mucus collection in the middle ear, partial deafness, chronic bowel problems
12 years	Recurrent tonsillitis
19 years	Depression
22 years	Hay fever
25 years	Inflammatory bowel disease diagnosed as ulcerative colitis
35 years	Episodes of indigestion diagnosed as duodenal ulcer
55 years	Onset of tremor, stiffness and rigidity diagnosed as Parkinson's disease

TABLE 2.7: PAST MEDICAL HISTORY OF A PATIENT REVEALING INTERCONNECTIONS OF LEVELS

The information in Table 2.7 may seem that the person is particularly unfortunate but when you discuss medical history with patients it is common to find similar events. The main factor determining the next event is whether the treatment given at the time is curative, i.e. the pathology moves to the exterior or suppressive, i.e. the pathology moves to the inside. Conventional medicine tends to be suppressive since it does not address the underlying energetic imbalance. It is symptomatic in the true sense of the word.

When a patient with eczema is given corticosteroid creams the rash may well disappear. Some months later a deeper problem may appear such as asthma. To a conventional doctor, trained to see people as a collection of separate parts, this is perceived as 'cure' of the eczema and the appearance of asthma. Now drugs are given which suppress the asthma and may lead to symptoms such anxiety, apprehension or perhaps more serious pathology.

In terms of alternative medicine the pathology is passing into the deeper levels of the patient. The patient is now more ill than they were previously. Treatment with alternative medicine tends to move the pathology out of the body and so treatment of the asthma may well lead to reappearance of the eczema. If the eczema is then treated correctly and disappears, this can be truly called cure. The internal levels are balanced and the symptoms have resolved.[15]

Not all patients who have conventional treatment, however, end up with a disease worse than the original and some people seem to do very well, on all levels. It may be useful to discuss the possible consequences of treatment. These ideas are summarised in Table 2.8.

---

[15] This is one of the basic tenets of Hering's Law of Cure as stated in homoeopathic philosophy. Cure is the movement of pathology from inside to out, from above to down, from most important organs to least important and symptoms disappear in reverse order of their appearance.

EFFECT ON SYMPTOMS	INTERPRETATION
No change	No effect by treatment
Worsen	1. Treatment is curative and this is a short-term phenomenon - an aggravation[16] 2. No effect by treatment and condition is worsening 3. Treatment is making the condition worse
Improvement	1. Cure a) Appropriate energetic remedy b) 'Placebo' effect - healing c) Would have improved anyway perhaps because of natural movement towards cure or removal of exciting cause 2. Suppression - inappropriate energetic remedy

TABLE 2.8: INTERPRETATION OF THE EFFECT OF TREATMENT ON SYMPTOMS

The difficulty here is to decide why symptoms have disappeared. Is it due to cure or to suppression? With cure, the energetic imbalance is moving out of the person and so inner levels will clear first. Patients report improved energy, feeling better in themselves, improved mental and emotional states before changes in the physical level. This is what patients describe who receive alternative medical treatment. In the short term their presenting symptoms may get worse since the treatment is increasing their energy levels. The strength of symptoms is directly related to the strength of the patient's energy. In alternative medicine aggravation occurs first followed by amelioration.

Suppressive treatment also means that the symptoms disappear but the key here is that internal levels are more disordered. The patient may feel tired, lethargic, depressed or anxious and symptoms may now be present on deeper physical levels. This is what happens with antibiotic treatment. The patient has a sore throat, for example, and the administration of antibiotics leads to disappearance of the main complaint. Now the patient complains of tiredness, depression, diarrhoea, 'thrush' symptoms and so on. The problem has been suppressed into the interior. In conventional medicine there is amelioration followed by aggravation.

Cure can be attained by a practitioner in two ways. The first is the application of the appropriate energetic remedy which must be given according to the principles of the therapy practised. In terms of Chinese medicine this is by diagnosing the condition of the Qi and Blood and giving a treatment to balance these two substances. In terms of homoeopathic medicine it is by deciding upon the simillimum - the most similar remedy.

The energetic remedy is the key. Conventional medicine may occasionally give the appropriate energetic remedy and examples of this would be the use of platinum[17] for ovarian tumours, digitalis[18] for heart failure, carbenoxolone[19] for peptic ulcers, aspirin[20] for acute fevers. There are very few other examples and the refining of substances as well as the administration of large doses leads to toxicity. The difference is that in Chinese medicine and homoeopathy these substances are used as the result of careful observation, enquiry and the application of a self-consistent theoretical base. In conventional medicine they are the result of chance.

I have put 'placebo' effect and healing together because I think that they are essentially the same phenomena. The term placebo is used pejoratively by the medical profession today but it has a long

---

[16] An aggravation is a short-lasting exacerbation of the presenting symptoms. It is due to a resonance between the energy of the person and the energy of the applied remedy. It can be recognised by its short duration (hours or days) and the clearing of internal levels first to be followed by improvement of the physical. It is distinguished from a 'healing crisis' which occurs during the course of treatment. This takes place when the person's energy is strong enough to throw out more symptoms. A healing crisis, particularly in the case of serious disease such as cancer can be difficult to distinguish from a worsening of the illness. Again you have to pay attention to inner levels and assess according to the treatment applied and its results over a length of time.

[17] Platina is the homoeopathic remedy derived from platinum. Tumours of the ovary are included in the materia medica entry of platina.

[18] Digitalis was originally extracted from foxglove which is a herbal remedy for dropsy (heart failure).

[19] This is a derivative of licorice which tonifies the energy of the stomach and is commonly used in herbalism.

[20] Originally extracted from willow bark, this has the effect of relieving acute fevers by releasing the exterior energy of the body and causing a sweat. Its energy is warm and dispersing in nature.

and honourable history. The word[21] is generally applied to a substance which has no known (conventional) medical effect. It has always been known the mere suggestion that something has healing powers is enough to lead to health in some cases and in some people. The power of placebo is increased by ritual, suggestion and by the perceived ability of the person giving the placebo. Do not underestimate the power of placebo in conventional medicine. This is the reason most heart tablets are red and tranquillisers are green or blue - they are more effective. The ability of doctors to suggest that patients can and will get better may be a powerful factor in some people's recovery. It may not be much to do with the treatment but with the relationship people have with the doctor. This is true healing and is very effective. People get better *despite* the treatment they receive rather than *because* of it. Many conventional treatments have no proven efficacy or are effective for no known reason. The power of a doctor to heal is an important factor to be considered particularly in those cases where strong faith is present.

Of course, this power may be used in the other direction and some patients are told they have no hope, e.g. patients with multiple sclerosis may be told that they have a degenerative condition which will lead in a short time to inability to walk and reliance on a wheelchair. Such statements, made by someone in authority, can lead to their eventual fulfilment even in people with no disease.

As to suppression, it is possible to do this by any method of treatment. It is commonly stated that alternative medicine is safe and cannot do harm. This is not true and it is possible to suppress disease and symptoms by means of Chinese medicine, homoeopathy and so on. It is not easy and suggests a failure to reach a correct diagnosis and treatment. The most powerful suppressant today is conventional medicine, however, and causes many difficulties for alternative practitioners. This, combined with pollution of water, air, food and increased levels of stress and worry are responsible for the increasing rates of chronic disease.

The hope for the future is to offer patients an alternative to heavily suppressive forms of treatment with information about how to live as healthy a life as possible. In this way the general health of people will be improved as well as allowing all of us to achieve our true potential.

- HOW TO RECOGNISE SERIOUS SYMPTOMS -

Which symptoms indicate 'serious' disease[22]? What is serious in orthodox medicine is also serious in alternative medicine - after all the patient is the same! I believe that anyone can understand pathology based upon an understanding of symptoms and symptom pictures. It is not necessary for a conventional medical diagnosis to be made. It may be useful for some people and in certain circumstances but I do not think it is essential.

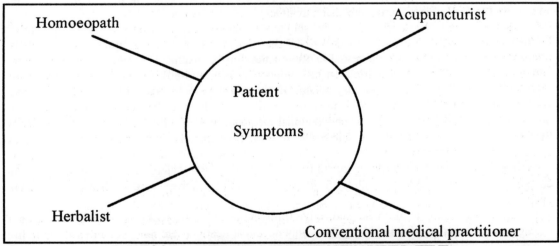

TABLE 2.9: PRACTITIONERS AND THEIR VIEW OF THE PATIENT

Table 2.9 is a diagrammatic representation that the patient is the same but different practitioners take a different view because of the angle at which they observe the patient. The point to emphasise here is that conventional practitioners tend not to see the whole patient - they only see the

---

[21] The root is the Latin, "I please".

[22] 'Serious' in this context indicates a situation which is potentially life-threatening. This may due to the immediate situation or a progressive underlying process. This latter case would include cancer.

physical. Therefore, conventional medical terms are restrictive in nature and cannot be directly translated into the terms used by alternative practitioners. There is some correlation but they are not the same thing. Hence it is valid for any alternative practitioner to only take account of their particular diagnosis and treatment since that, by definition, encompasses the whole person. The only thing to add to this is that it is important to be able to recognise symptoms indicating a severe imbalance. Some patients need closer observation or they may require emergency treatment and so on. However, it is possible for *any* practitioner to determine this by close observation of the patient and their symptoms.

The seriousness of a symptom is dependent upon the degree of limitation of the patient's activity or functioning. If health can be defined as freedom from limitation then disease or a symptom is a limiting factor.

The indicators of a serious situation would be:

- severe symptom
- life-threatening situation (ultimate limitation)
- moving into deeper levels - either physical or into the emotional/mental levels
- acute - this indicates sudden change
- progressive - more symptoms appearing indicating a worsening situation

Throughout this book I shall be summarising the symptoms which indicate serious imbalances. A summary is included at the end of each Chapter.

- CONVENTIONAL RESEARCH -

There is an emphasis in conventional medicine of gathering information and trying to decide if certain treatments are effective or not. The criteria for effectiveness are those I have already discussed, namely, removal of the primary physical symptom. The placebo response has always been recognised as having great power yet conventional medicine seeks to negate or neutralise it in order to determine the 'real' action of the medicine or treatment applied. This is an attempt to discover objective truth by removing the subjective element.

The gold standard of conventional research is the double blind controlled trial.[23] In such a trial neither the patient nor the doctor knows whether a 'real' treatment is being applied or a 'sham' treatment. For example, if a drug is being studied, some patients will be given the drug and others will be given tablets containing no active substance. In this way, differences in the outcome of the two patient groups can be attributed to the effects of the drug. This would, at first sight, seem to be an effective method of discovering whether a treatment is effective or not.

The question to ask is whether the subjective element can ever be removed completely? Perhaps it is possible to affect the outcome of the trial merely by mental attitude. A consultant rheumatologist I know became interested in acupuncture for the treatment of arthritis. He was always being asked to perform clinical trials on his patients for new anti-arthritis medication. His senior registrar was in charge of the day-to-day conduct of the trials and many pieces of research were done. As the consultant became more and more involved in acupuncture, he became more and more disillusioned with the efficacy of the conventional medication. As a reflection of this, the results of the trials became less and less favourable for the drugs until eventually the pharmaceutical companies stopped using his unit for research. It was almost as if his mental attitude were affecting the trials even though he was not personally involved in them. This is clearly understood if you subscribe to an energetic view of the universe. It is tendencies and possibilities which exist rather than solid, concrete events.

It is not possible to eliminate subjective truth and detach it from objective truth. This is as if saying you can separate Yin and Yang. This only occurs at death. There must be both aspects in life to achieve movement. For alternative medicine, it means that these conventional methods of research are of no help since the subjective element is the very factor we aim to utilise in our treatments. It is

---

[23] See "The Controlled Clinical Trial: An Analysis" by Harris L Coulter (Centre for Empirical Medicine and Project Care, 1991). This is a critique of their usefulness and is especially relevant to the needs of alternative practitioners.

the unseen, the vitalistic principle[24] which pervades us all. It is possible to perhaps analyse cases and treatments people have received but double blind trials[25] are not applicable.

Some groups are working towards developing research methods and this is all to the good. As the case of the consultant showed it is important to be in charge of the research yourself if optimum results are to be obtained. If I did a study on the effectiveness of acupuncture in disease X, I am sure that acupuncture would be shown as being very effective. This would not be true if I did research about a drug used in the same condition or if a conventional doctor did research on the usefulness of acupuncture.

It is clear from the above that it is our view which changes the results. We create our own reality and this is the essence of treatment. How can patients change their mind so that they change their symptom picture? If we believe something to be true then it becomes true for us and this principle is behind methods of visualisation and meditation used in spiritual practice and medical treatments.[26]

Sadly, the search for more information in conventional medicine means that there are some practices which may not be helpful or beneficial. If the patient does not know whether they are receiving treatment or not, this does not allow them to make a decision based on information. The principle of informed consent is, I believe, a vital part of medical practice. All patients must decide for themselves whether to accept any form of treatment and this is process is particularly hazardous if they lack certain pieces of information about their treatment.

The other point to consider is that animal experimentation is widely used in conventional medical research. In my opinion this is unethical since it involves inducing suffering to a sentient being. There has never been a case of a medical advance which has resulted from the use of animals and I would hope that the practice may soon cease. The pronouncements that animal experimentation is essential to discover the 'cure' for this disease or that disease are, I am afraid, the results of confusion, lack of rigorous thought and desperation. Unfortunately, some groups in alternative medicine and I am thinking here particularly about the research carried out in China with regard to acupuncture and herbs, use animals in their experiments. As concerned practitioners, it is important to consider these aspects and oppose them. It is our responsibility to relieve suffering, not to inflict it.

- DOCTORS AND PATIENTS -

It is not my intention to increase conflict between someone and their conventional medical advisor. In my dealings with people, I do not wish them to be in the middle of a philosophical discussion between conventional and alternative medicine. It is often true though, that people find difficulty in obtaining information[27] about medical procedures and treatments. You have a role to play here since education and information can be given by any practitioner and I would hope that the information in this book may be useful for you to explain options to people.

Any form of medical practice is, at least at the beginning of treatment, a power imbalance between therapist and the person consulting them. The therapist is the one with the knowledge and skills whilst the other is unwell, somewhat vulnerable and requesting assistance. Such discrepancies in power mean that the therapist has responsibility not to abuse it and to facilitate the process whereby they allow people to contact and utilise their own strength. This is the essence of a truly holistic medicine.

The key factor is health and well-being. My aim is to support people to allow them to regain their health and independence.

---

[24] "The Presence of the Past: Morphic Resonance and the Habits of Nature" by Rupert Sheldrake (Collins, 1988). The vitalistic principle here is called morphic resonance by Sheldrake. It explains the observation that if a rat in one part of the world learns how to get through a maze then very soon all the rats in the world, despite no physical connection with this rat, will know how to get through the same maze. There is an energetic field effect behind the physical events and this explains how connections can occur and effects experienced without any physical contact.
[25] Some people receive no treatment although they do not know this. As a practitioner, I feel it is unethical to provide no treatment to people when I have skills and information which may be helpful. I often think that such trials are for the benefit of the researcher rather than the patient.
[26] These are outlined in Chapter 6 with regard to alternative treatments of cancer.
[27] "How To Survive Medical Treatment" by Stephen Fulder (Century, 1987) is an excellent account of the issues around people receiving conventional treatment. It is out of print now but useful if you can get hold of a copy.

The following pieces of advice may be useful for anyone who has dealings with conventional practitioners[28]:

- go with a friend or advocate who can support you - never go alone.
- ask about effects, side-effects and other options available.
- why is a particular investigation being performed and how will the information be used?
- your body is your property and no-one has the right to do anything without your full, informed consent.
- search out alternative choices.
- whatever you decide - be happy!
- seek out sympathetic sources of conventional advice. There are some doctors now who are moving over to holistic views and can offer support and help to people searching for treatment appropriate to their needs.

- SUMMARY -

Conventional medicine only sees the physical and applies physical treatments.

Alternative medicine is vitalistic in nature and accepts the existence of energies within people.

Treatment needs to encompass all levels of the individual to ensure cure.

Treatment of only the outer, physical level may lead to suppression and the appearance of more serious disease later.

Symptoms manifest in those with strong energy as strong symptoms, acute picture, in less important organs, relatively superficial.

Symptoms manifest in those with weak energy as weak symptoms, chronic picture, in more important organs, relatively deep.

The most important things to remember are:
- where is the pathology - at which level?
- where is it going - into the interior or to the exterior?
- is the condition worsening or improving?

---

[28] It is wise to check out all practitioners and in the end it is the practitioner we have to feel comfortable with whether they are alternative or conventional.

3 BASIC PATHOLOGICAL PROCESSES

OBJECTIVES:
At the end of this Chapter you will be able to:
State the symptoms of inflammation.
List the causes of inflammation.
Describe the importance of inflammation to the practice of conventional medicine.

- INTRODUCTION -

I tend towards the view that clinical medicine can be understood by considering symptoms. I do not, therefore, give much weight to the processes which conventional medicine considers as underlying disease. Having said that, it may be helpful to consider a few pathological processes to shed some light on the practice of conventional medicine.

As I discussed in Chapter 2, the underlying tenet of conventional thought is that a physical abnormality is the cause of disease. A search is always made for such an event. Even in those diseases where an abnormality is absent or difficult to find such as schizophrenia, anxiety or depression and so on, the assumption is that one day science will discover a physical cause.

The primary process of conventional medicine is inflammation. This is seen as the basis of many diseases. Other processes such as thrombosis, embolism, haemorrhage, demyelination of nervous tissue and so on are considered in their relevant Chapters.

- INFLAMMATION -

In conventional medicine, the emphasis is on physical pathological processes which are held to be at the root of disease. The main process which is seen as the cause of many disorders is inflammation. It may be the result of a wide range of different processes but it is seen as the problem to be treated.
The cardinal symptoms of inflammation are redness, swelling, pain, heat and loss of function. These are due to an increased blood supply locally for the provision of nutrients and immunological defences. Inflammation is a beneficial reaction of the body and suppression of such a response may be dangerous. There are many commonly used drugs which do just this. They include antibiotics, anti-inflammatory agents, corticosteroids and anti-histamines.

The labelling of disease reflects this emphasis on inflammation. The suffix '-itis' indicates that inflammation is present. The majority of conventional disease labels can be seen to be inflammatory in nature - tonsillitis, gastritis, vaginitis, bronchitis, colitis, dermatitis. The Latin term for an organ is attached to the -itis to form a label. This means, of course, that these are merely descriptive terms. Patients are reassured by such diagnoses whereas it is merely technical language to describe the symptoms of the patient. For example, if a person has a pain in the ear with redness and swelling of the eardrum and difficulty in hearing, they will be told they have otitis media (inflammation of the middle ear). The patient will then go away feeling greatly reassured that a diagnosis has made without perhaps realising that the name only describes their symptoms in another language.

Inflammation has several causes according to conventional medicine and these are summarised in Figure 3.1.

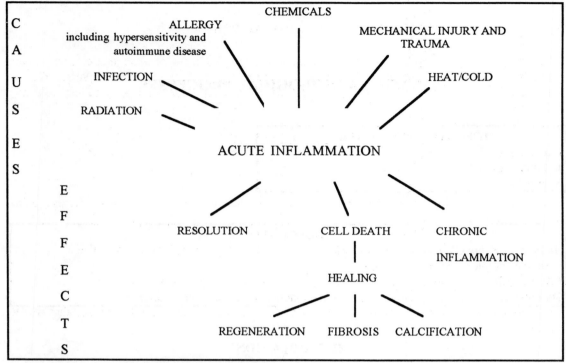

FIGURE 3.1: CAUSES AND EFFECTS OF INFLAMMATION.

The essence of Figure 3.1 is that damage to the cell results in acute inflammation. The causes of cell damage are recognised by conventional medicine as being physical in nature. If an external agent comes into contact with the cell, the result will be inflammation. There is no room here for mental or emotional factors. Anyone who has a child will know that psychological factors are a potent producer of fevers and inflammation. This is more clear in children due to their strong energy and its tendency to flare up into heat. I remember one occasion when my son was disturbed at the thought of having to eat something he did not like. Within a few minutes he was hot, flushed and feverish. On being told that he did not have to eat the offending item he settled down and the fever disappeared as rapidly as it had appeared. This was a graphic illustration of the effect of emotional factors and the speed with which symptoms may change.

In general, the causes of inflammation can be divided into two types - those due to infection and those not due to infection. The first group are treated with antibiotics or other drugs to combat organisms. Patients may also be given antibiotics frequently for inflammation in the assumption of an infective cause. In situations where this is clearly not the case or later on after labelling of an -itis, anti-inflammatory drugs of varying kinds will be prescribed. These may be fairly simple remedies such as aspirin through to powerful drugs such as corticosteroids. The underlying aim is to reduce inflammation. Any physical changes are approached by physical means - abnormal cells are removed surgically, e.g. dysplasia cells in the cervix by laser therapy, inflammation is suppressed by means of chemicals, e.g. anti-histamines in allergic disease. Although this summary is somewhat simplistic, it is commonly encountered in conventional clinical practice.

This practice is dangerous since the inflammation serves a protective function - as indeed do all symptoms. Removal of the inflammation leads to a worsened state since the original cause - which as I have said before must be on an energetic level - is allowed to continue unhindered. This is the reason for people developing problems after the suppression of an inflammation.

In conventional medicine it is realised that the use of corticosteroids in inflammation associated with infection is harmful. Removal or reduction of the inflammation leads to rapid spread of the infection.

The correct way to deal with an inflammation is to consider the total picture including any exciting or maintaining cause. Then, and only then, deal with the totality in an appropriate way. This may mean, in occasional life-threatening situations where the inflammation is severe, that an emergency treatment has to be used. However, to use powerful anti-inflammatory drugs, and I would include antibiotics in this category, for the vast majority of minor inflammatory symptoms is excessive and hazardous.

- OTHER PATHOLOGICAL PROCESSES -

There are pathological processes which are seen as often being the result of inflammation or due to an underlying metabolic abnormality. I shall deal only those which are clinically important. These include thrombosis, atheroma, embolism, haemorrhage. I discuss them individually in their relevant Chapters.

- SUMMARY -

Pathological processes in conventional medicine are physical in nature and origin.

The primary process is inflammation which gives rise to characteristic symptoms of redness, pain, swelling, heat and loss of function.

Most diseases in conventional medicine are merely descriptions of an inflammatory process.

There are many prescribed drugs available which have an anti-inflammatory effect.

In general, inflammation may be divided into that which is associated with infection and that which is not.

4 INVESTIGATIONS

OBJECTIVES:
At the end of this chapter you will be able to:
Describe the pros and cons of undergoing investigations
State the criteria for deciding on the degree of invasiveness of an investigation
Describe the main investigations used in conventional medical practice

- INTRODUCTION -

Investigations are those tests carried out after a case has been taken and a physical examination made of the person. There are many different types used in many different situations. It is possible to try to categorise them according to their effect on the person. I think it is useful to think of them in terms of their degree of invasiveness. Then a patient may decide that perhaps a less invasive test may be requested to minimise the potential harm.

CATEGORY OF INVESTIGATION	MEANING
1	Relatively non-invasive with little or no risk of illness
2	Invasive and carry a significant risk of morbidity
3	Invasive and may, in some circumstances, cause death.

TABLE 4.1: INVASIVE OF INVESTIGATIONS - GENERAL CATEGORIES

- REASONS FOR INVESTIGATIONS -

Doctors perform investigations for several reasons and these may be different to those which others consider important. Such tests aim to detect pathological changes within the body not discernible to the ordinary senses. It is important to realise that no method of perception is infallible and so all investigations must be considered in the light of other evidence. I would never recommend a course of action solely on the basis of an investigation. This is particularly true if the person feels healthy.

An investigation may enable the doctor to make a diagnosis or to confirm a clinical diagnosis. It may be possible to decide on the degree of pathological change. The disease may be staged as to its severity. This is invariably done in the case of cancer. Do not confuse this with prognosis. Prognosis can only be judged on the basis of an assessment of the person's energy. It is notoriously difficult to assess prognosis on the basis of the nature of physical disease and there are many people alive today who were told they only had several months to live.

In general, the degree of structural change has a very poor relationship with symptoms. Some people with severe symptoms of pain and stiffness in the cervical spine may have minimal change on X-ray whereas some people with gross radiological evidence of degeneration may have little or no symptoms. The person must be treated, not the X-ray. Symptoms are an indication of the energetic imbalance and so are related to function more than structure. What something looks like is not so important as how it works.

Fear of a particular disease or process may lead to investigations. This is particularly true for infectious diseases even where there is no conventional treatment. HIV infection is a case in point here where the conventional treatment available makes no difference to the state of HIV infection and yet people may be advised to discover their HIV antibody status.

Regarding the person, there are several reasons why someone may choose to have investigations. I would suggest it is primarily for reassurance since there is a great sense of relief when they are done. This is before any result is obtained. It may be why such great disappointment is felt when the test comes back revealing some abnormality. Investigations are seen as 'something being done' and so are regarded as positive in themselves. They are seen as treatment or at least the initiation of treatment. This is potentially dangerous in the sense that investigations lead only to the gathering of information and, usually at least, have nothing to do with treatment. In addition, the almost blind faith in the power of investigations to reassure can lead to despair and depression if they do not live up to this expectation.

So, many people seek to be reassured that they are well. The medical profession undertakes investigations for the exact opposite reason - to detect abnormality! It is not possible to diagnose normality by investigation, only abnormality and even then not all abnormality. Therefore, it must only be regarded as an aid and not, as is so often the case, an end in itself.

There may be morbidity associated with an investigation. There is a significant degree of illness after investigations and the degree of risk is directly related to their invasiveness. There may be mortality - some investigations may actually kill the person.

The more routine an investigation, i.e. the more automatically it is done then the less revealing it is. Routine X-rays of the lumbar spine, for example, which are used in cases of low back pain reveal an abnormality in 1 in 4000 cases.

A recent survey studied 595 people who attended a clinic in Switzerland. They had a total of 2,378 tests performed of which 65% were considered to be routine. In only 0.3% of cases did the results of such tests lead to a change in management. Over the next 15 months it was noticed that 60% of the blood change abnormalities returned to normal. The conclusion of the report was that 30% of these blood tests were unnecessary.[1]

Not only is this a large expenditure in terms of money and time for the health services, it is unnecessary for health, may damage the person and leads to increased levels of anxiety.

Screening procedures are the use of investigations in people with no complaints or known health problems. They serve to provide employment for a large number of medical and paramedical staff. There has never been a recorded instance of mass screening campaigns changing the course of a disease. Why is this? The degree of invasion and anxiety production seems to be counterproductive.[2] Although some problems will be revealed others will be caused. In addition, conventional medical treatment may make no difference to the course of a detectable abnormality.

---

[1] Annals of Internal Medicine, Mar 1st, 1991; 114(5): 432.

[2] There have been several studies which cast doubt on the oft-stated belief that screening leads to reduction in disease. Breast cancer investigations using mammography are a case in point where the incidence may be *increased* in the study group. This may be due to several factors such as trauma to the breast by mammography where the breast is squeezed between X-ray plates and the anxiety generated by the test, waiting for the result, recall for further investigation, false positive results. The Journal of Clinical Epidemiology 1990; 43(3): 215-25 states that ".... for each woman who can derive a direct benefit in terms of a prevented breast cancer death, hundreds of women have to suffer the anxiety of a positive screening mammography. Moreover, it is possible that adverse effects of breast cancer screening may contribute to mortality from other causes."

The foregoing discussion does not mean that an individual investigation done in an individual case for an individual problem is without benefit. A person may decide that they would benefit from the knowledge such an investigation may give them. The widespread, indiscriminate use of investigations, however, supported by large amounts of time, money and energy is of no benefit.

The golden rule of all investigations is: *only perform an investigation if the result will change the management of the case.* For example, if a woman is not going to take female sex hormones for a gynaecological condition there is no point in ascertaining levels of oestrogen and progesterone. If a person is not going to have a coronary bypass operation, there is no point in an angiogram to determine the state of the coronary arteries. If the person is not going to have chemotherapy or radiotherapy for cancer treatment, there is no point in removing lymph glands or other structures to make a conventional decision about staging.[3]

- TYPES OF INVESTIGATIONS -

- BLOOD TESTS -

Invasiveness of category 1.

FULL BLOOD COUNT

This is a general investigation of the blood. The tests available, their results and meaning are shown in Table 4.2. Normal values are shown against each although different laboratories may differ slightly. Where only one figure is shown then this is the upper limit of normal. There is always a degree of error and so minor deviations from the normal can usually be safely ignored. If a result is abnormal then repetition may reveal "return to normal". This could indicate an initial error or a minor problem which has now subsided.

TEST	NORMAL[4] RANGE	MEANING
Haemoglobin (Hb)	Male - 13.5-18G/100ml Female - 11.5-16.5G/100ml Pregnancy - 6.8-9.3G/100ml New-born - 17-22G/100ml Infant - 6.8-7.8G/100ml Child 12-14G/100ml	Anaemia - low in all types.
Mean corpuscular volume (MCV) - size of red blood cells	80-96 cubic microns	Anaemia - low in iron deficiency, chronic blood loss, pregnancy, chronic disease. High in pernicious anaemia, folate deficiency, malabsorption, malnutrition, aplastic anaemia.
Mean corpuscular haemoglobin (MCH) - amount of haemoglobin in red blood cells	27-31 pcg	Anaemia - low in iron deficiency, chronic blood loss, malabsorption, pregnancy, low levels of gastric acid. High in pernicious anaemia, folate deficiency, malnutrition, hypothyroidism, aplastic anaemia.
Mean corpuscular haemoglobin concentration (MCHC)	18.6-21.1mmol/l	Anaemia - low in iron deficiency, pregnancy, chronic disease.

---

[3] The staging of malignant disease is discussed in Chapter 6.
[4] Normal here refers to the *usual* result. This explains why some people may have results slightly outside of the quoted range with no problems.

Haematocrit or packed cell volume (PCV) - volume when red blood cells are packed together	Male - 40-54% Female - 32-42% Child - 32-42%	Blood disease - low in anaemia. High in polycythaemia, dehydration.
Red blood cell count	Male - $4.5\text{-}6.5\times10^{12}$/l Female - $3.9\text{-}5.6\times10^{12}$/l	Blood disease - low in haemolytic anaemia, aplastic anaemia. High in polycythaemia.
White cell count (WCC)	Adult - 4000-10000/mm^3 Child - 10000-20000/mm^3	Infection and blood disorders - low in leukaemia, viraemia, elderly. High in bacterial infection, leukaemia.
Neutrophils	2500-6500/mm^3 (40-60%)	Infection - low in viral infection, overwhelming bacterial infection, vitamin B12 deficiency, folate deficiency, leukaemia, aplastic anaemia, SLE. High in bacterial infection, herpes zoster. Very high in pneumococcal pneumonia.
Basophils	10-100/mm^3 (0-1%)	Blood disorders - high in chronic inflammation, hypothyroidism. Very high in chronic myelocytic leukaemia, polycythaemia.
Eosinophils	50-400/mm^3 (1-3%)	Inflammation - low in acute bacterial infection, corticosteroid treatment. High in allergy, hay fever, polyarteritis nodosa, Hodgkin's disease, parasitic infestation. Very high in malignancy, eosinophilic leukaemia.
Monocytes	200-800/mm^3 (4-8%)	Low in chronic infection, Hodgkin's disease.
Lymphocytes	1500-3500/mm^3 (20-40%)	Blood disorders, infection - low in stress, injury, haemorrhage, overwhelming infection, Hodgkin's disease, elderly. High in chronic infection, acute viral infection, acute lymphatic leukaemia.
Platelet count	150000-350000/mm^3	Bleeding disorders - low in thrombocytopenia. High in chronic leukaemia, polycythaemia.
Erythrocyte sedimentation rate (ESR)	Male - 0-10mm/hour Female 0-20mm/hour Child 0-20mm/hour	Non-specific test of inflammation - high in pregnancy, infections, some malignancies. Very high (50mm or more) in autoimmune disease.

TABLE 4.2: FULL BLOOD COUNT - COMPONENTS, RESULTS AND INTERPRETATION

SERUM TESTS

These have an invasiveness of category 1. They are investigations carried out on the blood but relating to the presence of substances such as nutrients, waste materials and the like.

TEST	NORMAL RANGE	MEANING
Acid phosphatase	0-13iu/l	High in malignant disease of the prostate, acute myelocytic leukaemia
Glutamic pyruvic transaminase	3-60iu/l	Liver or heart disease - high in obstructive jaundice, , chronic hepatitis, malignant disease of the liver, myocardial infarction, glandular fever. Very high in acute hepatitis.
Albumin	3.5-55G/100ml	Liver disease - low in liver cell death, cirrhosis, malnutrition, malabsorption, some types of glomerulonephritis, leukaemia. High in shock, dehydration.
Alkaline phosphatase	10-95iu/l	Bone and liver disease - low in hypothyroidism. High in malignant disease of bone, rickets, Paget's disease of bone, secondary malignancy of liver.

Amylase	70-300iu/l	Pancreatic disease - low in hepatitis, toxaemia of pregnancy. High in acute pancreatitis, cancer of the pancreas, mumps, salpingitis, perforated duodenal ulcer, liver disease, ruptured ectopic pregnancy.
Glutamic oxaloacetic transaminase	8-40iu/l	Liver disease - high in obstructive jaundice, acute hepatitis, cirrhosis, heart attack, liver cancer, haemolytic jaundice, injury.
Bicarbonate	22-31mmol/l	Acid-base imbalance - low in hyperventilation, diabetes mellitus, severe kidney disease. High in potassium depletion, vomiting, Cushing's syndrome.
Bilirubin	Total - -20mcmol/l Direct - 1.6mcmol/l Indirect 2-13 mcmol/l	Liver disease and anaemia - high indirect in haemolysis. High both in hepatitis, biliary obstruction, toxaemia.
Calcium	2.2-2.7mmol/l	Kidneybonedisease - low in Vitamin D deficiency, renal failure, nephrotic syndrome. High in osteoporosis, cancer, sarcoidosis, excess calcium intake, Hodgkin's disease, Paget's disease of bone, thiazide diuretics.
Carbon dioxide	4.8-6.1 kPa	Repeated measurements taken in severe respiratory disease give a reliable guide to lung function.
Chloride	97-108mmol/l	Water and electrolyte imbalance, kidney disease - low in dehydration, diuretics. High in excess intake, dehydration.
Cholesterol	1.2-7.0mmol/l	Obesity, hypertension, heart disease - low in acute hepatitis, hyperthyroidism, acute infections, uraemia, malnutrition. High in hypothyroidism, diabetes mellitus, nephrotic syndrome, chronic hepatitis, cirrhosis, elderly, familial hypercholesterolaemias.
Creatine phosphokinase	50-100iu/l	Muscle death - high in myocardial infarction, muscle injury, dystrophy, polymyositis.
Creatinine	0.06-0.11mmol/l	Kidney disease - low in pregnancy. High in renal failure, urinary tract obstruction.
Cyanocobalamin	200-900pcg/100ml	Anaemia - low in pernicious anaemia.
Free thyroxine index (FTI)	1.3-5.1u	Thyroid disease - low in hypothyroidism. High in hyperthyroidism.
Globulin	Total - 20-35G/l Alpha 1 - 2-4G/l Alpha 2 - 4-8G/l Beta - 6-10G/l Gamma - 6-15G/l	Liver disease - low Total in malnutrition, lymphatic leukaemia. Low Alpha 1 in nephrotic syndrome. Low Gamma in nephrotic syndrome, leukaemia, corticosteroid treatment. High Total in cirrhosis, chronic hepatitis, SLE. High Alpha 1 in oestrogen treatment. High Alpha 2 in acute infections, myocardial infarction, injury, nephrotic syndrome. Beta high in hypercholesterolaemia, cirrhosis, nephrotic syndrome, pregnancy, hypothyroidism. Gamma high in infection, autoimmune disease, cirrhosis
Glucose	3.5-6.0mmol/l	Carbohydrate metabolism - high in diabetes mellitus, hyperthyroidism, overactivity of adrenal cortex (includes treatment with corticosteroids), liver disease.

Iron	Male - 15-30mcmol/l Female - 14-28mcmol/l	Anaemia - low in iron deficiency anaemia, dietary lack, malabsorption, chronic blood loss, Hodgkin's disease, elderly. High in other anaemias.
Lactic dehydrogenase	120-280iu/l	Cell death - high in myocardial infarction, kidney damage, acute hepatitis, polycythaemia, pernicious anaemia.
Lipids (including cholesterol and triglycerides)	400-600mg/100ml (after no food for 12 hours)	Lipid metabolism - high in diabetes mellitus, hypothyroidism.
Luteinising hormone	Female - 5-22mu/ml (30-250mu/ml whilst ovulating)	Menstrual disorders and infertility - low in infertility. High at ovulation.
Magnesium	0.7-0.9mmol/l	Kidney disease - low in alcohol abuse, cirrhosis, malabsorption, cancer chemotherapy, diuretic use.
Oestradiol (oestrogen)	Female 500-1100 pmol/l - mid-cycle	Low in post-menopausal women (< 150 pmol/l) - this is normal since the menopause is not a disease state.
Oxygen	10-13.3 kPa	Repeated measurements taken in severe respiratory disease. Give a reliable guide to lung function.
Paul-Bunnell test	up to 1:128	High in glandular fever
Phosphorus	0.9-1.5 mmol/l	Bone and kidney disease - low in rickets, osteomalacia, insulin treatment, after meals. High in kidney disease.
Potassium	3.5-5.2 mmol/l	Electrolyte imbalance - low in fluid loss, diuretic use, malabsorption, purgative use, diabetes mellitus, corticosteroid use. High in acute renal failure, uraemia.
Progesterone	>30 nmol/l - second half of cycle	Reduced in progesterone deficiency states which may be found in irregular menstruation, infertility, habitual miscarriage, heavy menses (most cases are normal).
Prolactin	Female - 3-25mcg/l Male - 2-15mcg/l	Female infertility. High in pituitary tumours and overactivity, brain injury, unknown causes.
Protein	60-80G/l	Low in nephrotic syndrome, chronic renal failure, malnutrition.
Rheumatoid factor	Absent	Positive in 75% of people with rheumatoid arthritis and many normal people.
Sodium	137-150mmol/l	Electrolyte imbalance - low in dehydration, oedema, Addison's disease, acute renal failure. High in dehydration.
Thyroxine	64-160nmol/l	Thyroid disease - low in hypothyroidism, nephrotic syndrome, phenytoin use. High in hyperthyroidism, pregnancy, female sex hormone use.
Triglycerides	<1.9mmol/l after 12 hour fast	High in nephrotic syndrome, chronic renal failure.
Urea	3.2-6.6mmol/l	Kidney function - low in liver failure, severe weight loss, diabetes insipidus, pregnancy. High in nephritis, urinary tract obstruction, dehydration, gastrointestinal bleeding, shock, underactivity of adrenal cortex, elderly.

TABLE 4.3: SERUM INVESTIGATIONS - SUBSTANCES TESTED, RESULTS AND MEANING

- ELECTROCARDIOGRAPHY (ECG) -

This is non-invasive and so would be in category 1 unless done whilst exercising (see below). It merely records electrical activity of the heart during the cardiac cycle. From this information, it is possible to infer certain structural changes. Abnormalities detected include cardiac arrhythmias, enlargement of certain areas of the heart, myocardial infarction, angina pectoris (usually only if an exercise ECG is abnormal), pulmonary embolism. In the case of myocardial infarction, it may take 24 hours for the ECG to become abnormal.

An exercise ECG is used to diagnose the angina pectoris and is of category 3 invasiveness. The resting ECG is usually normal in this condition and so measurement whilst exercising may provide evidence of ischaemia. An exercise ECG leads to myocardial infarction in 0.05% of cases and has a death rate of 0.01%.

- ELECTROENCEPHALOGRAPHY (EEG) -

This is the cerebral equivalent of the ECG and is non-invasive - category 1. It measures the electrical activity of the brain. The primary use is to diagnose epilepsy but abnormalities are also seen in encephalitis, dementia and hypoglycaemia. It may be normal between epileptic attacks. Some people with epileptics have normal EEGs and some 'normal' people have abnormal EEGs.

- ELECTROMYOGRAPHY (EMG) -

This has an invasiveness of category 2. It is a measurement of the electrical activity of muscle by inserting a needle electrode into the muscle. Abnormalities detected include myopathy, myasthenia gravis, nerve entrapment syndromes and neuropathy.

- PULMONARY FUNCTION TESTS -

These have an invasiveness of category 1 unless drugs are used to check their effect in which case category 2. They are performed as an outpatient and involve breathing into various instruments to measure force of expiration and lung volume. They give a quantitative measure of lung function and can be repeated to check on changes in response to treatment. They may have a role to play for the alternative practitioner who would like objective evidence of improvement. Abnormalities detected include obstructive airways disease such as asthma, chronic bronchitis and emphysema.

- SKIN TESTS -

These have an invasiveness of category 2. They are used to test for allergic responses to a variety of substances. A scratch is made on the skin and the test substance placed on the wound. Some days later the area is tested for evidence of an allergic response. In my experience they are of minimal help since there is virtually no relationship between the results of the tests and the symptom picture. They also serve to reinforce people's ideas that manipulation of the external environment can lead to health. In some cases the removal of an offending allergen may markedly affect symptoms but what usually happens is that the pathology moves somewhere else or the person then develops an allergy to something else.

- X-RAYS -

These have an invasiveness of category 2 since medical sources of radiation are the commonest cause of exposure to radiation over and above natural sources. The risk obviously increases in line with any increase to exposure to the amount of radiation. Such radiation leads to increases in rate of malignant disease such as cancer and leukaemia. Radiologists and radiographers have a higher incidence than the general population. Although there is little risk with one X-ray investigation, care needs to exercised in the case of repeated usage. It has been estimated that the effects on health of one barium examination of the intestines is the equivalent of smoking 20 cigarettes for a year. The effects are much greater on children and babies.

PLAIN

These are the simplest X-rays since they use a relatively low dose and are taken without the aid of radio-opaque substances. Their use in summarised in Table 4.4.

ORGAN/STRUCTURE STUDIED	ABNORMALITY DETECTED
Chest	Structural defects
Lungs (via chest X-ray)	Collapse, pleural effusion, pneumonia, fibrosis, infections such as tuberculosis, sarcoidosis, cancer, lymphatic gland enlargement, increased or decreased pulmonary blood flow
Heart (via chest X-ray)	Enlarged heart, abnormal heart shape, pericardial effusion (large), calcification
Abdomen (gall bladder)	Gall stones (10%)
Abdomen (pancreas)	Calcification
Abdomen (kidney)	Kidney stones (90%), bladder stones, calcification
Abdomen (peritoneal cavity)	Air in the peritoneal cavity due to perforated ulcer
Skull	Fractures, erosion of bony structures by tumour, calcification
Spine	Fractures, degenerative changes, vertebral collapse, tumours
Bones	Fractures, osteoporosis, rickets, osteomalacia, tumours
Joints	Arthritis

TABLE 4.4: PLAIN X-RAYS

COMPUTERISED AXIAL TOMOGRAPHY

This is also an X-ray examination which uses increased doses of radiation in order to give more detailed information about the tissue examined. This investigation can also be known as a CAT scan or an EMI scan (after the company which makes the equipment). The use of this type of scan is summarised in Table 4.5.

ORGAN/STRUCTURE STUDIED	ABNORMALITY DETECTED
Lung	Cancer, sarcoidosis, lymphoma, dust diseases (in each case more detail than can be detected by plain X-rays)
Abdomen	Lymphatic gland enlargement
Liver	Tumours
Gall bladder	Gall stones
Pancreas	Tumours
Brain (misses lesions <1cm diameter or close to the skull)	Tumours, haemorrhage, haematoma, atrophy, pituitary disease
Spine	Tumours, disc prolapse
Kidney and urinary tract	Tumours of kidney, bladder and prostate
Adrenal	Tumours

TABLE 4.5: COMPUTERISED AXIAL TOMOGRAPHY

BARIUM STUDIES

Barium is radio-opaque and such studies can reveal information about organs of the gastrointestinal tract which are not easily displayed on plain films. They can diagnose a wide range of disorders such as carcinoma, ulcers, polyps, strictures, diverticulitis and the inflammatory bowel diseases.

Screening is carried out at the same time which is observation of the movement of the intestine during the investigation. This necessitates the exposure to more radiation than would be the case if only static pictures were taken.

People are given these tests as an out-patient. People who are to have barium meals have nothing to eat or drink from the previous night. They have a low fibre diet for 3 days and laxatives for 1 day before the investigation. A colon washout is performed immediately prior to the X-ray. This is why people who have this test can feel so tired. The use of laxatives and a colonic washout lead to the loss of energy and fluid from the body. In a depleted person this can cause marked feelings of fatigue.

BARIUM MEAL

This is used to examine the upper gastrointestinal tract of oesophagus, stomach, duodenum and jejunum. If the passage of the barium into the small intestine is observed then abnormalities of the ileum can be diagnosed. People are X-rayed with their head down to try to demonstrate reflux from the stomach to the oesophagus or the existence of a hiatus hernia. As I discuss in the Chapter dealing with the gastrointestinal system, these appearances may occur in people with no symptoms and may be a direct result of the posture attained in this investigation. Abnormalities detected include reflux into the oesophagus, hiatus hernia, oesophageal cancer, gastric ulcer, gastric cancer, duodenal ulcer, Crohn's disease.

BARIUM ENEMA

This is used to examine the large intestine and terminal ileum. The lowest part of the rectum must be examined by other means such as rectal examination or sigmoidoscopy. Abnormalities detected include cancer of the large intestine, ulcerative colitis and diverticulitis.

CHOLECYSTOGRAM

Gallstones can be detected merely by a plain X-ray of the abdomen in only 10% of cases. Because of this, dye studies are the norm. It is not used in jaundiced people. This investigation has, in many situations, been replaced by ultrasound examination.

Oral cholecystograms involve taking a dye in tablet form which is concentrated in the gall bladder. Some hours later, X-rays of the gall bladder are taken before and after the ingestion of fat. Abnormalities detected include gall stones.

PERCUTANEOUS TRANSHEPATIC CHOLANGIOGRAPHY

This has an invasiveness of category 3. It is used to obtain information about the biliary system. A needle is passed through the skin and superficial tissues into the liver, after injection of a local anaesthetic, to allow the injection of dye into the biliary system. X-rays are taken subsequently. Abnormalities detected include obstruction of the biliary system. Complications include bleeding, infection of the biliary system, septicaemia.

INTRAVENOUS PYELOGRAPHY (UROGRAPHY)

This is the injection of dye which is excreted by the kidney and allows X-ray examination of the kidney and urinary tract. This has an invasiveness of Category 2 since some people are severely allergic to the dye leading to anaphylactic shock and occasionally convulsions.

It is used to define the size and shape of the kidneys as well as urine flow out of the urinary tract. Abnormalities detected include stones, obstruction to urine flow, long-term kidney disease such as pyelonephritis or glomerulonephritis, tumours of the kidney and bladder. Studies of bladder function and emptying can be made by taking films whilst the person is urinating.

MYELOGRAPHY

This has an invasiveness of category 2. It is the injection of dye into the subarachnoid space, usually in the lumbar (occasionally cervical) area, to allow X-ray or computerised axial tomography of the structures around the spinal cord. Lumbar puncture is performed first and then dye injected. I would refer you to Page 45 for information about lumbar puncture.

Recently a newer type of dye has been used which is water soluble. In the past, a heavy oily dye was used which remained in the area for a long time and has been implicated as leading to arachnoiditis. This is an unusual inflammation which causes headaches and nerve problems including tingling and weakness. It may be severe in its manifestations. Abnormalities detected by myelography include spinal tumours and prolapsed disc.

- CARDIAC CATHETERISATION -

This has an invasiveness of category 3. There are several uses of this procedure which is the passage of a tube (catheter) into the heart or to allow the injection of dye (cardiac angiography). The right side of the heart is accessed via a vein, usually in the neck. The left side of the heart is accessed via an artery, usually the femoral artery in the groin. Blood samples may be obtained, pressures measured or dye injected (angiography) depending upon the actual clinical situation. Abnormalities detected are included in Table 4.6 with regard to angiography.

ANGIOGRAPHY

This is the injection of dye into the vascular system and can give information about the blood supply. It is used to investigate structures such as the heart or the circulation of any organ or area of the body. Its use is summarised in Table 4.6.

ORGAN/STRUCTURE STUDIED	ABNORMALITY DETECTED
Heart	Aneurysm, cardiomyopathy
Coronary arteries	Atherosclerosis
Liver	Tumours
Brain	Vascular abnormalities such as thrombosis or aneurysms
Carotid artery	Narrowing, atherosclerosis
Vertebral artery	Narrowing, atherosclerosis
Kidney	Tumours, renal artery disease in e.g. hypertension

TABLE 4.6: ANGIOGRAPHY

- SCANS -

This is a general term used to describe methods of obtaining an idea of internal structure without needing to resort to surgery. They utilise various means including radiation, magnetic fields and ultrasound. Invasiveness depends upon the particular type. Each is indicated separately. Computerised axial tomography (CAT) described above may be designated as a scan.

ULTRASOUND SCANS

These are described in conventional textbooks as being non-invasive. This is not true and I would rate their invasiveness as being category 1 unless applied to pregnant women where the effect on the baby will be in category 2.

Such scans involve the use of sound waves to bounce off tissue of differing depths and types. A cross sectional image of the organ or area, e.g. the abdomen, is obtained. They are commonly used in obstetric practice and increasingly so.[5] [6]

---

[5] Doubts are occasionally expressed about the wisdom of routine ultrasound testing. The degree of anxiety generated is an important factor to consider particularly if the investigation reveals an

ORGAN/STRUCTURE STUDIED	ABNORMALITY DETECTED
Heart (echocardiography)	Valve disease, infective endocarditis, cardiomyopathy, pericardial effusion, congenital heart disease
Liver	Tumours (over 1 cm. in diameter), cirrhosis
Gall bladder	Gall stones (98% accuracy)
Pancreas	Tumours
Abdomen	Tumours
Kidney and urinary tract	Tumours, cystic kidney disease, kidney size and urine obstruction in kidney failure, prostate tumours
Pelvic organs	Uterine fibroids, ectopic pregnancy, foetal abnormality, tumours, abnormal placental site

TABLE 4.7: ULTRASOUND EXAMINATION

There is no hard evidence that such procedures are harmful to the foetus[7] but there is no evidence that it is not harmful. This is yet another example of the medical profession experimenting on large sections of the population with no long-term follow-up of possible effects and with no *informed* consent obtained from pregnant mothers. There have been numerous articles in the professional journals about the uselessness of mass ultrasound screening and yet it is continued. Such behaviour can only lead to problems in the future. If you observe a foetus who is undergoing ultrasound examination, he/she will hold their hands up to their ears and move away from the source of the sound. Whilst it may be reasonable in some circumstances to perform ultrasound in pregnancy, it is unreasonable to subject every mother regardless of her personal situation.[8]

Ultrasound provides information about the foetus such as gestational age, stage of development and the normality of internal organs as well as the site of the placenta. They are usually performed at around 10-12 weeks and later in pregnancy at around 36 weeks. The other uses of ultrasound scans are summarised in Table 4.7.

RADIONUCLIDE SCANS

These have an invasiveness of category 2. I have read conventional medical textbooks where these procedures are described as being 'safe and non-invasive'. This reveals, at the least, an interesting use of the English language.

The scans are performed by injecting radio-active materials (isotopes) and a radiation monitor is used to determine the uptake into the relevant organ. They are performed in many conditions. People may feel unwell for several weeks after this procedure as would be expected from the injection of radiation into the body. Their uses are summarised in Table 4.8.

---

abnormality of little significance, an abnormality for which there is no treatment, an abnormality which cannot be addressed until after delivery or an image which is difficult to interpret (this is becoming increasingly common as equipment is more sensitive). See Journal of Family Practice Dec 1989; 9(6): 660-4 for a discussion of the routine use of ultrasound scans in pregnancy.
[6] Report of the Royal College of Obstetricians and Gynaecology Working Party on Routine Ultrasound Examination in Pregnancy 1984 discusses the indications and risks of ultrasound.
[7] Diagnostic Ultrasound Equipment Federal Register, Part III, 2 Feb. 1979. Animal studies of ultrasound examination reveal that there may be altered emotional behaviour, delayed muscle and nerve development, increased death rates and changes to the electroencephalogram.
[8] "The American Way of Birth" by Jessica Mitford (Gollancz, 1992). This is a thorough description of the medicalisation of the birth process as has occurred over the past 30-40 years. Ultrasound is discussed in clear detail on pages 103-106. This book is recommended reading for every pregnant couple and every practitioner dealing with pregnancy.

ORGAN STUDIED	ISOTOPE	ABNORMALITY DETECTED
Heart	Thallium^{201} or technetium^{99}	Myocardial infarction, angina pectoris
Lung	Technetium^{99} or xenon^{133}	Pulmonary embolus (may not give definitive result)
Liver	Technetium^{99}	Cirrhosis, alcoholic hepatitis
Gall bladder	Technetium^{99}	Acute cholecystitis
Oesophagus	Technetium^{99}	Oesophageal reflux
Stomach	Technetium^{99}	Slow gastric emptying
Small and large intestine	Radioactive white blood cells	Inflammatory bowel disease
Brain	Technetium^{99}	Tumours, haematoma, infarction
Kidney	Technetium^{99}, iodine^{123} or gallium^{67}	Renal artery disease, obstruction to urine flow, bladder emptying, kidney size and shape, inflammation

TABLE 4.8: RADIONUCLIDE SCANS

MAGNETIC RESONANCE IMAGING

This is a newly developed investigation and uses magnetic fields to give detailed information of internal organs in greater detail than some other tests. It has an invasiveness of category 2. The use of magnetic fields in this way may lead to health problems but they are too new for any conclusions to be drawn. However, magnetic fields in other situations such as those formed by overhead electricity pylons have been implicated in the several disorders including suicide, psychological disturbances, leukaemia and cancer.[9] Magnetic resonance imaging may not have such a deleterious effect on health but you would expect some problems to be revealed as we know more about them.

ORGAN/STRUCTURE STUDIED	ABNORMALITY DETECTED
Heart	Structural defects
Lungs	Tumours, lymphatic gland enlargement
Liver	Tumours
Brain	Tumours, multiple sclerosis (not definitive)
Spine	Tumours, spinal cord compression

TABLE 4.9: MAGNETIC RESONANCE IMAGING

- ENDOSCOPY -

In general these have an invasiveness of category 3 since perforation of the organ is a risk. If a general anaesthetic is required this would entail increased risk.. In the latter case especially, careful thought has to be given to whether similar information may be obtained by other means. Some endoscopy procedures also allow treatment to be performed and so are not just for investigative purposes.

Endoscopes are instruments which allow the operator to directly see the internal structure of the body. They provide access to internal organs for biopsy, sampling of secretions or cells, injection of other investigative media such as dyes and may allow the application of treatment for some conditions. They are usually performed in the outpatient department but some require a general anaesthetic.

BRONCHOSCOPY

This is performed under local anaesthesia to the throat and intravenous sedation with diazepam due to its unpleasantness. It allows the direct examination of the larger airways. Sputum and biopsies may

---

[9] "Subtle Energy" by John Davidson (C.W.Daniel, 1987). This is a clear account of energies as described by various medical systems as well as discussing planetary energy. The problems caused by pollution due to radiation of all types including electromagnetic are described in Chapter 4. Also see "Electromagnetic Man" by Cyril Smith and Simon Best (J.M.Dent, 1990)

be obtained at the same time. It is a useful method to remove aspirated objects. Abnormalities detected include cancer, tuberculosis, a variety of other lung infections.

UPPER GASTROINTESTINAL TRACT ENDOSCOPY

An oesophagoscope, gastroscope or duodenoscope is used to examine the upper gastrointestinal tract. The same instrument may be used to examine all organs. The person has nothing by mouth overnight and is examined as an outpatient. Intravenous sedation, usually with diazepam, is given as well as local anaesthetic spray on the throat. Intravenous diazepam is used partly since it induces sedation but also because amnesia is a common effect. Abnormalities detected include reflux oesophagitis, oesophageal cancer, gastritis, gastric ulcer, gastric cancer, duodenitis, duodenal ulcer.

An additional procedure is endoscopic retrograde cholangiopancreatography (ERCP) where a tube is passed in to the common bile duct or pancreatic duct. Secretions can be obtained for analysis as well as dye injected for X-ray studies. Risks of this procedure include infection of the biliary system and pancreatitis.

COLONOSCOPY

A colonoscope can allow examination of the large intestine and terminal ileum. There is some preparation involved as with a barium enema. People have only fluids the day prior to the test and are given a stimulant laxative. On the day of the investigation they are given sedation, usually diazepam, and an opiate analgesic, e.g. pethidine. The terminal ileum is reached in 80% of cases. There is a mortality rate of 1 in 100000. Abnormalities detected include cancer of the large intestine, Crohn's disease, ulcerative colitis, diverticulitis, polyps.

LARGE INTESTINE ENDOSCOPY

A proctoscope and sigmoidoscope are short instruments used for direct visualisation of the rectum and lower sigmoid colon used in an outpatient setting. Both are relatively painless and require no preparation or sedation. Abnormalities detected include haemorrhoids, polyps, ulcerative colitis, fissures, cancer of the rectum and anal margin. A longer sigmoidoscope is available which is used after an enema. This allows more of the colon to be examined and 70% of colonic tumours can be reached.

LAPAROSCOPY

A laparoscope is an instrument which is used to examine the abdominal cavity. It is necessary to pump air into the abdomen to separate the organs and allow clear access. The presence of air forces the diaphragm up and so respiration is impaired. A general anaesthetic is administered to prevent respiratory difficulties.

It is mainly used in gynaecological conditions to allow examination of the pelvic organs. Treatment can be administered at the same time. Abnormalities detected include ovarian disease, endometriosis, pelvic inflammatory disease, uterine fibroids, tumours.

- death rate of 1 in 5000 but this risk is increased for the young and the elderly.
- heart attack especially in those with a previous one and particularly if it was in the preceding 6 months.
- injury whilst unconsciousness during transfer off and on the operating table
- psychological reactions - lack of concentration, poor memory, disordered mental function. These can last for at least 6-8 weeks after an anaesthetic
- babies - if delivered by Caesarian Section - breathing difficulties, slowness and dullness
- epidural - less dangerous than general anaesthesia. Headaches and back pain are common. These may last many months. Babies delivered by Caesarian Section suffer from slowness and dullness for at least 6 weeks. They are twice as likely to develop jaundice.

TABLE 4.10: RISKS OF ANAESTHESIA

At this stage, it may be useful to consider the risks of general anaesthesia (Table 4.10) and surgery (Table 4.11). No-one knows the incidence of problems due to anaesthesia since complications may be described as being due to the original disease. Death due to anaesthesia may be labelled as being caused by the condition requiring treatment. During my medical education I was told by an anaesthetist that there are three stages of anaesthesia - awake, asleep and dead. Although this was an attempt at a medical joke, the reality may not be far away. Severe problems with anaesthesia are clearly uncommon but minor degrees of illness may be more frequently encountered.

- infection - 3000 people die from post-operative infections in the UK each year. Over 30% of women who have a hysterectomy develop post-operative infections.
- blood transfusion - may result in HIV infection, hepatitis, mismatching, reactions to the transfused blood - one death in 9000
- haemorrhage
- embolism
- shock
- injury from error during the operation
- scars and cosmetic considerations
- pain
- psychological reactions
- wrong operation

TABLE 4.11: RISKS OF SURGERY

- BIOPSY -

This is the examination of pieces of tissue obtained by various means. It is the only way in which many diseases such as cancer can be definitively diagnosed and treated by conventional medicine. This is because the exact cell type and structure needs to be known. I have included in this section all types of tissue and body fluid sampling.

SPUTUM ANALYSIS

This has an invasiveness of category 1. Naked eye inspection may reveal the presence of blood if red or of inflammation if yellow or green. Further studies of culture are performed to detect bacterial infection. The antibiotics which are most effective can then be determined. The presence of cells can be checked and if they are abnormal. This may be used to diagnose cancer of the lung. It is of variable reliability.

URINE ANALYSIS

There are several tests which can be performed on a fresh urine sample. They are cheap, non-invasive and easy to perform.

DIPSTICK TESTING

This has an invasiveness of category 1. The urine can be examined by the naked eye and more detailed information obtained by testing by various dipsticks easily available from the chemist. This may be of help to the alternative practitioner especially in monitoring people with diabetes mellitus or checking for abnormalities in people with symptoms of kidney disease. Substances which can be detected include blood, protein, ketones and sugar.

Blood in the urine (haematuria) can be seen with the naked eye if severe, imparts a smoky appearance if not so much and is invisible in many cases. It may be in urine as a contaminant in women who are menstruating. In other cases it may be further studied by urine microscopy (see below). Diseases which may cause haematuria include cystitis, pyelonephritis, bladder tumours, kidney tumours, kidney and bladder stones. Trauma can also result in haematuria.

Protein in the urine (proteinuria) is often mistakenly viewed as being synonymous with infection and people are given antibiotics. Further study by culture is necessary to confirm or exclude infection. There are several causes of proteinuria and they include infection of the urinary tract, contamination by skin/hair and so on, inflammatory diseases of the kidney of which there are many. Blood in the urine will test positive for protein. It is reasonable to check two or three times if protein is detected before thinking about further investigation especially if there are no symptoms.

Sugar in the urine (glycosuria) is almost always indicative of diabetes mellitus. It is more likely to be present in urine passed some time after a large carbohydrate intake.

Ketones in the urine (ketonuria) indicate that the body is obtaining energy from supplies of fat rather than sugar. Ketones are a breakdown product of fat metabolism. They are seen in diabetes mellitus when hyperglycaemia is present and in fasting.

Bacteria may be tested for using special dipsticks. They rely upon detecting nitrites but are unreliable indicators of infection.

MICROSCOPY

This is the next investigation to be performed and has an invasiveness of category 1. It aims to detect several abnormal constituents. White cells in the urine indicate inflammatory disease which may or may not be infective in origin. Red cells will be seen in those people with haematuria.

Casts are collections of cells which have the shape of the tubules of the kidney. The types and their meaning are summarised in Table 4.12.

CAST	MEANING
Hyaline	Normal especially after exercise
Fine	Normal especially after exercise
Granular	Kidney disease
Red cell	Kidney disease
White cell	Pyelonephritis
Tubular cell	Acute tubular necrosis

TABLE 4.12: URINARY CASTS AND THEIR MEANING

Bacteria may occasionally be seen and would suggest infection but it is important to be guided by the symptom picture. This is true, of course, for all investigations.

URINE CULTURE

This has an invasiveness of Category 1. Urine is cultured under various conditions to see if bacteria can be grown. This would suggest that infection is present but I would refer you to Chapter 5 - Infectious Disease - for a discussion of the relevance of such a finding especially in the asymptomatic. Subsequently, tests are performed on the bacteria to discover which antibiotics(s) are effective. This investigation would be the preferable way to manage all urinary infections to prevent overuse of antibiotics or their inappropriate use. It takes 2-3 days for results to return from the laboratory.

SEMEN EXAMINATION

This is a non-invasive examination. There may be difficulties for some religious groups where masturbation is not permitted. In this case, the only way in which semen may be obtained for investigation in cases of impaired fertility is by means of a post-coital examination on the woman. Normal values are:

*   Volume 3.5ml
*   ph 7.4
*   Sperm count 60,000,000 to 200,000,000
*   Motility - 90% at 45 minutes and 65% at 3 hours
*   Abnormal forms 10-20%

LUMBAR PUNCTURE

This has an invasiveness of Category 3. Cerebrospinal fluid is obtained by inserting a needle through an intervertebral space in the lower lumbar spine. Common problems after this procedure are severe throbbing headache and lower back ache. These may last for many months. It must be used with great care if there is evidence of a cerebral tumour. In such cases the increased pressure in the skull can force the brain stem down into the cervical spine with possible fatal consequences. Abnormalities detected include meningitis, encephalitis, multiple sclerosis (not definitive), subarachnoid haemorrhage, tumours.

CERVICAL SMEAR

This has an invasiveness of Category 2. It is a sample of cells taken from the uterine cervix. A wooden spatula is used to scrape cells from around the cervix and they are smeared onto a slide for examination under a microscope. There are various grades of abnormality and the issues around smears are fully discussed in Chapter 18 - Gynaecology.

Smears frequently lead to a small amount of vaginal bleeding and some women develop irregular periods or heavy periods for a short time. In Chinese medical terms, they stagnate the energy of the Liver and so drinking lemon juice before and after may prevent any adverse reactions.

AMNIOCENTESIS[10]

This has an invasiveness of Category 3 due to the risk to the baby. It is a procedure to obtain samples of amniotic fluid - the fluid surrounding the foetus in the uterus. It is performed at about 15-20 weeks. The sample is examined to detect foetal cells for determination of sex, chromosomal abnormalities and serious abnormalities such as spina bifida. It is offered mainly to women in their 30's and older when foetal abnormalities tend to be more common. It is only of use to those who are considering termination of pregnancy since there are risks to the life of the baby.

It is performed under ultrasound control so that the risk of damage by the needle to the foetus, placenta or maternal organ is minimised.

The procedure can involve discomfort as the needle is inserted into the uterus. Complications include miscarriage (1%), neonatal respiratory difficulties, postural deformities and Rhesus sensitisation. The combined losses of pregnancy due to amniocentesis are 5.7% and due to miscarriage, termination of pregnancy, stillbirth and neonatal death.

CHORIONIC VILLUS SAMPLING[11]

This has an invasiveness of Category 3 due to the risk to the baby. This is performed for the same reasons as amniocentesis. Samples of the chorion are obtained for examination. It is done by either a transabdominal approach which is similar to the method of amniocentesis or by a transcervical approach.

The risks of transcervical sampling are greater than those of the transabdominal approach. Whichever is performed, it is essential to determine that the operator is skilled in its use. Some experience is obtained by training on women undergoing termination of pregnancy.

Complications of this procedure include miscarriage (1-5% for the transabdominal approach and 2.5-10% for the transcervical), intrauterine infection, septic shock, Rhesus sensitisation, foetal abnormalities. Vaginal bleeding as evidenced by spotting is common and is seen in 35-60% of women. There may be associated lower abdominal discomfort. If the bleeding is heavy then miscarriage occurs in 25-50% of these. If mild vaginal bleeding occurs then there must be abstinence from sexual intercourse and for one week after sampling in any case. The combined losses of pregnancy due to chorionic villus sampling are 7.2% and due to miscarriage, termination of pregnancy, stillbirth and neonatal death.

---

[10] "Prenatal Diagnosis in Obstetric Practice", Edited by MJ Whittle and JM Connor (Blackwell, 1989).
[11] "Prenatal Diagnosis in Obstetric Practice", Edited by MJ Whittle and JM Connor (Blackwell, 1989). "A Practical Guide to Chorionic Villus Sampling" by David Liu (OUP, 1991)

JOINT ASPIRATION

This has an invasiveness of Category 2. Fluid is removed from joints in cases of joint swelling. This may diagnose infective arthritis and gout. Treatment may also be given at the same time by allowing drugs, e.g. corticosteroids to be injected into the joint. Removal of the fluid may also constitute treatment to relieve swelling or discomfort. Complications include infection (1 in 10000), inflammation and increased risk of joint deterioration.

PLEURAL ASPIRATION

This has an invasiveness of Category 2. Fluid is removed from the pleural cavity in cases of pleural effusion for examination and culture. Causes of pleural effusion include cancer, tuberculosis and mesothelioma. Removal of fluid in this way may lead to cough and severe breathlessness particularly if a large amount is extracted.

PLEURAL BIOPSY

This has an invasiveness of Category 2. It is performed through the chest wall under local anaesthesia. It is positive in 60% of cases of mesothelioma and 80% of cases of tuberculosis.

LIVER BIOPSY

This has an invasiveness of Category 3. Liver cells are obtained by needle biopsy through the abdominal wall. Local anaesthesia is used. Abnormalities detected include hepatitis, cirrhosis, tumours, metabolic disease.

Complications include bleeding into the peritoneal cavity (common) or biliary system, infection including septicaemia, pleurisy, peritonitis. Death occurs in 2 per 100000.

RENAL BIOPSY

This has an investigation of Category 3. It is performed by needle through the loin whilst viewing with ultrasound. Abnormalities detected include glomerulonephritis and the causes of kidney failure.

Complications include pain in the loin and shoulder tip, infection, haematuria (20%), haematuria requiring blood transfusion (3%), haematuria requiring surgical intervention or removal of kidney (0.5%), death (0.1%).

- SUMMARY -

Investigations are commonly used in many situations.

In some cases, investigations and treatment may be combined.

There are different levels of invasiveness and some investigations may lead to illness or death.

Everyone has the right to request a different investigation to obtain the same or similar information.

No investigations must be performed if their results will not change the management of a case. The only exception to this may be the use of completely non-invasive tests which carry no risk of damage to the person.

5 INFECTIOUS DISEASE

I have only included a few specific infectious diseases in this Chapter. I have placed most in their corresponding Chapter according to their main symptoms. For example, acute bronchitis is in Chapter 8 - Respiratory System, skin infections are in Chapter 11 - Dermatology and so on.

OBJECTIVES:

At the end of this chapter you will be able to:

State the philosophical differences of alternative and conventional medicine with regard to infectious disease.

Describe the 'normal' diseases of childhood and state the symptoms which would indicate the presence of complications.

Describe the clinical appearances of glandular fever, myalgic encephalitis and AIDS.

Discuss how to manage people with such chronic disease.

Discuss the pros and cons of vaccination.

List the vaccination schedule for vaccination in the UK.

- INTRODUCTION -

This is a classification of disease which conventional medicine considers to be of essential importance. Through various stages of its history, such ideas have attained almost supernormal significance. Today is no exception and large amounts of energy and time are spent in studying tiny organisms and inventing new ways to kill them. Infection and its control holds the Western world in a mystical spell.

It has been a recurrent view through the ages that there are external morbific influences which lead to the development of disease and even to death. The search for these external factors has been one of the main driving forces behind medical research over relatively recent years. This, of course, continues right up to the present day with conditions such as A.I.D.S.

Lucretius who lived 99-55 BC said, "Invisible animals enter via the nose and mouth and cause difficult diseases." Even before the discovery of bacteria it was known that removing pump handles from contaminated wells during a cholera epidemic could stop the spread of the disease.

With the discovery of organisms in the latter half of the 19th century, there seemed to be incontrovertible evidence that these cause disease. This has led to the development of pasteurisation, antibiotics and vaccination.

The above is not the only conclusion to be drawn. Antoine Bechamp[1], a contemporary of Pasteur, suggested that organisms already exist in tissues and are not a problem until there is a change in the immune system[2] which would allow such organisms to cause disease. This counter argument has been suppressed with time and is dismissed by conventional medicine as being of no value. For the practitioner of alternative medicine, such ideas are of great interest since they support the view that it is the immune system, the energy of the person, which is the important factor.

However, Pasteur's theories were generally accepted and conventional medicine holds the views that infectious disease is caused by agents known as bacteria (later viruses and other organisms were added as they were discovered) and that destruction of these bacteria will lead to recovery. This has led to the development of antibiotics and a whole system of medicine which is geared to the detection of external agents.

Koch, who discovered the TB bacterium postulated four things which should always be true in an infectious disease:

1.) The organism must always be present in all cases of the disease.
2.) The organism should be obtainable and grown in a culture.
3.) Organisms from such cultures must produce the disease when injected into a healthy person.
4.) The organism must be recoverable from that person.

Even if these four statements were always true[3], there is one vital component which is not given any importance and that is the person themselves. Why is it that in any epidemic there are certain people who are exposed but who do not contract the disease? Why is it that if people do contract the disease, it takes different forms with each of them? The answer is that each person's condition is different and it is this which is of overriding importance in the discussion of infectious diseases. It is from this basis that there should be consideration of such things as treatment by antibiotics, the relevance and safety of vaccination and the occurrence of complications of the illness. It was this very thought which led even Pasteur, for so long an advocate of the importance of the bacterium in the cause of disease, to say later in life, "The condition is everything, the germ is nothing."

It is a common observation that organisms, of the exact type associated with disease, are found in normal, healthy individuals. People only become ill when some other factor occurs. Susceptibility, therefore, is the preceding state which leads to the appearance of disease which is called infectious. The organism is very much the secondary phenomenon.

The original work of Bechamp included the observation that there are tiny organisms present in all tissues as well as supposed inanimate matter such as chalk. He called them microzymas or small

---

[1] "Pasteur Exposed" by Ethel Douglas Hume (Bookreal, 1989). This book, originally published in 1923, clearly delineates the rival theories pursued by Bechamp and Pasteur and their attempts to find the truth by experimental methods. Pasteur was very much the seeker of fame and is the one who has been recognised by history. Bechamp, whose main work was blatantly plagiarised, worked away quietly and diligently to support the theory that it is the 'soil' - the immune system - which is the key, not the organism.

[2] I would remind you of my comments in Chapter 2 about the immune system. I use this term throughout the book to refer to a wide, energetic view which includes superficial energetic levels, skin, mucous membranes, muscles and joints, bowels, internal organs and finally blood.

[3] The existence of organisms and their appearance are interesting to consider. Diseases of similar appearance may or may not have the same organisms associated with them. Many organisms associated with disease are present in the environment and ourselves all the time. Symptoms appear, i.e. disease is diagnosed, only when the conditions are right. There is no relationship with the organism itself as an external entity.

bodies. Subsequently, other workers have described such bodies including Rife[4] who invented a microscope capable of observing living tissue at many times the usual magnification and Gaston Naessens.[5]

Naessens, a French biologist, has found that there are tiny particles in living tissue which have a life-cycle and can be observed. These are almost certainly the microzymas of Bechamp. By careful observation, they can be discovered in tissues of healthy people but in people with disease states they can be observed to undergo an abnormal life-cycle. In this case, they can take on the appearances of bacteria, viruses or fungi depending upon the stage of their development. The prerequisite for this is a disordered state of the immune system. Recovery is associated with the disappearance of the abnormal forms.

This is completely opposite to the conventional view which states that bacteria, viruses and fungi cannot change from one into the other. They are considered to be of fixed form. This is in line with the philosophical ideas I discussed in Chapter 2 where conventional medicine thinks of phenomena as being inherently existent and unchanging. The discoveries of Bechamp, Rife and Naessens reveal that this is not true. Organisms arise from material in the body, as well as existing in many other places, and are capable of dynamic change. This is understandable only if you subscribe to an energetic view of existence.

The consequence of this misunderstanding of the origin of 'infection' is that chemicals are given to kill organisms and vaccination is given in an attempt to prevent their existence. In reality, it is not the organism which is the problem. It is only the result of a prior imbalance. The true cause is a disturbance in the energetic state of the person followed by the appearance of symptoms. If a doctor discovers an organism in that person then this is regarded as the cause to be attacked. If not, then some other reason is suggested for the cause of the inflammation and other drugs are given such as corticosteroids, anti-inflammatory agents, antihistamines and so on. Conventional medicine has been diverted down a blind alley.

In energetic medicine, for example, traditional Chinese medicine, it *is* possible to talk about external pathogenic factors such as WindHeat or WindCold or DampHeat invading the body and causing disease. These are not the same as bacteria or viruses. They implicitly involve the condition of the person and the two factors are not separated as in conventional medicine. The most beneficial way to view such theories is that the conditions of external attack are manifest on the surface of the body. This does not mean that the problem has come from the outside only that the person's energy has manifest the disturbance on the exterior of the body. It is the balance of the relative strengths of pathogenic factor and the Qi or vital energy of the body which is the important question.

These ideas are clearly illustrated by the following quotation[6]:

"Shao Yu replied: The wind generated by the heaven is fair and square to all the people without discrimination, but those who offend it will be under attack and those who avoid it will be free from attack. Therefore, people become sick, not because of the vicious energy of the wind comes to attack, but rather because they themselves offend the wind."

This is why drugs such as antibiotics can be such a problem because they actually lead to continuance of the pathogenic factor in the body. Vaccination is the deliberate introduction of the pathogenic factor into the body and at a deeper level than would naturally occur and so we can see how problems can be expected with this procedure.

A further example of Chinese thought may help to illustrate these ideas.[7]

"Chi Po replied: Wind, rain, cold, and heat cannot harm the human body unless the latter is already in deficiency. Some people do not become sick in the face of sudden gale and rainstorm, because they are not in deficiency so that the vicious energies cannot do them any harm. When people become sick

---

[4] Royal Raymond Rife, inventor of the Rife microscope in the 1920's, used this instrument to study tissue at magnifications far in excess of any equipment then available. However, his discoveries were so at variance with medical thought, then and now, that they have been difficult to even hear about. See "What Has Become of the Rife Microscope" by Christopher Bird, New Age Journal, March 1976.
[5] "The Persecution and Trial of Gaston Naessens" by Christopher Bird (Kramer, 1991).
[6] The Yellow Emperor's Classic of Internal Medicine (known as the Neijing). Translation by Henry Lu. Volume IV, 46.1.
[7] The Yellow Emperor's Classic of Internal Medicine (known as the Neijing). Translation by Henry Lu. Volume IV, 66.2.

due to external energies, it is because their bodies are already in deficiency so that they are susceptible to the attack of deficiency energies which come to reside in their bodies as guests."

There may be several sequelae of "exposure to infecting organisms" and the same holds true for the consequences of vaccination. This is shown in Table 5.1.

NOT SUSCEPTIBLE	SUSCEPTIBLE
No disease - so no symptoms	Strong symptoms - defence system is strong and is likely to have successfully thrown off the invasion. Mild illness: weak reaction by defence system so organism is not thrown off. Likelihood of chronic disease. Mild symptoms can also indicate mild problem. Differentiation is by careful questioning and determining the general state of health.[8] Complications such as meningitis, otitis media: weak defence system which is somewhat overwhelmed. If death does not intervene then health may be affected chronically.

TABLE 5.1.: ENERGETIC VIEW OF CONSEQUENCES OF CONTACT WITH 'INFECTING ORGANISM'

In energetic medicine, because the person is seen to be an interconnected whole, there are different levels at which disease may manifest and to which it may descend. These were described in detail in Chapter 2. As we are practising energetic medicine, it would seem to be more important to emphasise climatic factors and their influence on health. I shall return to these ideas later when dealing with specific diseases such as the common cold. The six climatic factors are heat, cold, damp, wind, dryness and summer heat.

- ACUTE AND CHRONIC DISEASE -

It is useful at this point to consider again the difference between acute and chronic disease since the former may be associated with infection, whilst the latter is the type of problem commonly encountered in outpatient clinical practice.

Acute disease may be defined as a disease of rapid onset, short duration which ends in recovery or death and usually has strong symptoms. People who have an acute disease know that they are ill. It is clear cut and indicates that the person is of relatively strong energy. For an acute manifestation to take place there must be strong energy in the system. This is why children tend to have acute illnesses since their energy is strong. Occasionally, in people with energy which is intermediate in type, a chronic illness may result.

Chronic disease can be defined as a disease of slow onset, long duration which ends in gradual deterioration of health. The symptoms are much vaguer than those of an acute problem. This picture indicates that the person's energy is much weaker and in fact there are some instances of very few symptoms despite serious chronic disease, e.g. elderly people with bronchopneumonia may have very little in the way of cough or fever. They may only present with breathlessness or perhaps confusion. There are some people with chronic disease who do recover perhaps because the cause has subsided or their lifestyle has altered. The only therapeutic way for recovery to occur is by means of methods available to alternative medicine.

There are diseases which do not fit easily into either category and these are usually the acute manifestations of a chronic illness. I would argue that in fact virtually all acute disease is a manifestation of a chronic imbalance and to only treat the acute manifestation will not lead to removal of the chronic problem. However there are some diseases which are clearly acute in nature and I would put the childhood infectious diseases in that category.

- CONVENTIONAL VIEWS OF INFECTION -

Conventional medical textbooks classify infectious disease according to the causative organism. This is in accordance with the belief that such organisms are fixed, unchanging entities. For the alternative practitioner this is not a helpful method since you are not going to treat the organism. In this section, for completion, I shall describe this conventional classification to enable a link to be made with other

---

[8] Do not confuse no disease which has no symptoms with mild disease which has weak symptoms.

texts.

ORGANISMS

There are several which are considered to be able to cause infection.

- bacteria - cocci, e.g. staphylococci, streptococci, pneumococci (pneumonia), gonococci (gonorrhoea), meningococci (meningitis); bacilli, e.g. tetanus, spirochaetes; e.g. syphilis; vibrio, e.g. cholera.
- viruses, e.g. measles, mumps, rubella, chickenpox, influenza, polio.
- fungus, e.g. Candida ('thrush'), tinea (ringworm).
- protozoa, e.g. trichomonas, giardia, amoeba, malaria.
- parasites, e.g. worms. These is technically an infestation but it is useful for our purposes to consider this with the above.

MODE OF TRANSMISSION

Certain diseases are considered to be spread in particular ways. These depend primarily upon the site of the disease. For example, respiratory disease will be mainly spread through sneezing or coughing, bowel disease through contact with faeces.

- Droplet spread, e.g. sneezing, coughing, dust. Diseases include influenza, whooping cough, pulmonary tuberculosis, common cold.
- Contamination of food/water. Diseases include gastroenteritis, dysentery, cholera, typhoid, polio.
- Implantation including wound contamination. Diseases include skin conditions caused by streptococci and staphylococci, tetanus,
- Direct contact. Diseases include scabies and the sexually transmitted diseases of syphilis and gonorrhoea.
- Injection into the body, e.g. injections, insects. Diseases include HIV infection, hepatitis, malaria, yellow fever. I would include transplacental spread here since the mode of transmission is similar, i.e. via the blood. Diseases include rubella, syphilis, HIV infection.

INCUBATION PERIOD

The incubation period is the time between invasion of the organism and the development of symptoms. It may be of importance in informing people of the natural history of an infectious disease. They are often variable and you will see times such as 7-10 days. This would seem to confirm that it is the person rather than the organism which is the important factor.

NOTIFICATION OF INFECTIOUS DISEASE

There are certain infectious diseases which are notified to the Department of Health. This only applies to registered medical practitioners and so does not affect alternative practitioners. The reason for notification is to compile the incidence of infectious disease as well as instituting specific public health measures, if necessary.

Public health legislation and its observance is an important factor in the prevention of these diseases since it stops the contamination of water and food as well as laying down standards for living and working conditions.

- ALTERNATIVE CLASSIFICATION OF INFECTIOUS DISEASE -

The important factors in deciding upon a classification are the underlying state of health and the site of manifestation of the symptoms. Both of these are interconnected and result in the appearance of the disease at a particular level in the individual.

There are several diseases of childhood which are almost universal and I would take the view that they are necessary for normal development. The immune system requires exposure to experiences to aid maturation just as we need other kinds of experience to help our mental and emotional development. The diseases of measles, mumps, rubella and chickenpox are essential for the healthy development of our immunity. This naturally has great consequences for the practice of mass vaccination because if measures are actively taken to prevent these conditions the immune system will necessarily be weakened. It will lay ourselves open to the development of other disease, perhaps more serious, at a later date. This is in line with the observation that disease is becoming more chronic and deeper in form than previously.

Other diseases are clearly the results of disordered immunity and only occur in people who are susceptible. I include here conditions such as streptococcal infections, glandular fever, herpes zoster, myalgic encephalomyelitis (M.E.) and AIDS. The depth at which they occur will reflect the energy of the person, i.e. the state of the immune system. Table 5.2 illustrates the application of these ideas to a list of infectious diseases with superficial, acute disease at the top and deep, internal, chronic disease at the bottom. Be careful with this since conventional disease labels are fixed labels which has more to do with rigid thought patterns than the person who has the symptoms! Consider this as a guide to deciding on the severity of the problem and not as a rigid plan to be applied at all costs. It is worth considering that people with strong energy manifest disease which is associated with clear bacterial illnesses such as scarlet fever (streptococci) or boils (staphylococci) that are relatively 'old-fashioned' now. The newer diseases such as AIDS, legionnaire's disease, non-specific urethritis are associated with strange, unusual organisms.

ACUTE DISEASE, STRONG ENERGY

Childhood illnesses - rubella, measles, chickenpox, mumps: normal
Common cold
Staphylococcal infections, e.g. boils - localised superficial problems
Streptococcal infections, e.g. impetigo, cellulitis - spreading superficial problems
Influenza
Glandular fever - acute attack mainly causing sore throat and enlarged neck glands
Acute bronchitis
Pneumonia
Glandular fever - chronic attack with chronic debility and weakness
Myalgic encephalomyelitis
Tuberculosis
Syphilis
Acquired Immune Deficiency Syndrome

CHRONIC DISEASE, WEAK ENERGY

TABLE 5.2: CLASSIFICATION OF INFECTIOUS DISEASE ACCORDING TO ENERGETIC PRINCIPLES

- NORMAL CHILDHOOD ILLNESSES[9] -

MEASLES

This is an almost universal disease of childhood with epidemics every other year. There is passive immunity obtained from the mother particularly if the child is breastfed. Most cases occur in childhood. The incubation period is 10-14 days. It is the strongest of the childhood illnesses of this type and is responsible for a high mortality in countries where malnourishment is common.

Symptoms

The first sign is a catarrhal stage which is common to most if not all the infectious fevers of childhood. There is little difference from the common cold with runny nose, sneezing, harsh irritant cough. The eyes are invariably affected with swollen eyelids, red and sore eyes (conjunctivitis). There may be photophobia. At this stage it is very difficult to distinguish from the common cold. There are, however, the presence of Koplik's spots which are tiny areas the size and appearance of a grain of salt with surrounding inflammation. They are present in the mouth on the mucosa opposite the upper

---

[9] The skin rashes of childhood appear as macule, papule, vesicle and pustule. These terms are explained in Chapter 11 - Dermatology.

molars. They appear around 3 to 5 days before the rash.

The rash arrives around day 3 to 5, begins behind the ears and rapidly spreads to the sides of the neck, forehead, face and then the trunk and limbs. As the rash appears the fever subsides and the child becomes subjectively improved. It is pink at first and deepens to a dull or purplish red. As it does so the appearance is more papular and areas coalesce into larger patches. There is generalised lymph node enlargement. The process from appearance of the rash takes place over about 24-48 hours and then fades to a brownish colour. By the end of 7-10 days the rash has gone.

Complications:

COMPLICATION	SYMPTOMS TO LOOK FOR
Febrile convulsions	Increasing fever, irritability, stiff neck, photophobia, twitching
Pneumonia	Cough, breathlessness, increasing fever
Otitis media	Earache, fever remains high
Corneal ulceration	Continuing eye symptoms which worsen, pain in the eye

TABLE 5.3: COMPLICATIONS OF MEASLES

Treatment:

There is no specific conventional treatment. Antibiotics will be used in cases of complications. Some practitioners use antibiotics in uncomplicated cases of measles to "prevent" further infection such as otitis media or pneumonia. This practice is dangerous as any infection which does then occur will be by organisms resistant to that antibiotic. That is not to mention the problems usually posed by antibiotics.

Alternative management:

I tend to be a therapeutic nihilist when faced with these diseases of childhood since I consider them to be normal and so do not interfere if progress is also normal. I would treat actively if eruption of the rash was not full or stopped at some stage. This will be accompanied by a continuing fever and feelings of ill-health. In these cases there is a risk that either a complication will appear or problems in later life. If children have a simple, naturopathic approach or are treated with homoeopathy or acupuncture they actually seem to be better after the illness than before. It is as if they have been exposed to an influence and an experience that they have passed with success.

Children who have had antibiotics during the course of measles undoubtedly take longer to recover to full health, to regain energy and appetite. Some may go on to develop syndromes of 'never well since' with a variety of manifestations. These complications, as well as problems in the ears, eyes and lungs, are prevented by prompt treatment by alternative medicine. Similar problems occur in children who are debilitated prior to the illness.

In terms of Chinese medicine, this illness is seen as being due to Wind-Heat invasion. This does not mean that the problem comes from the outside but that the manifestation is on the exterior of the body. It is due to the release of heat toxins which gathered during the time in the uterus.

It is an almost invariable event of childhood and is necessary for the normal development of the immune system. If it does not appear or is only mild (perhaps the rash does not fully appear) then there may be problems later with other, more chronic disease. This is because a healthy immune system will experience this condition at the appropriate time, i.e. childhood.

If the immune system is weakened in some way then the disease may be seen in later life. This is the reason why it is a common observation that childhood diseases in adult life commonly lead to complications. Following this argument a little further, if measles vaccination is used to try and prevent the appearance of the disease then the immune system will consequently be weakened because this avenue of expression has been removed. There is some evidence to suggest this is true with cases of encephalitis, multiple sclerosis and other neurological disorders linked to previous infection with the measles virus.[10] This raises questions about measles vaccination and the deliberate introduction of measles virus deep into the internal structures of the body.

---

[10] Annals of Neurology 1981; 9:17-20.

MUMPS

This is a viral illness which may go unrecognised in some cases because it can be mild in its manifestations. The incubation period is 18-24 days. It affects young children and adults and is very unusual before the age of 2 years. The main areas involved are the salivary glands, central nervous system and endocrine glands such as the pancreas, ovaries and testes.

Symptoms:

The beginning of the illness is non-specific with fever, headache, poor appetite. Pain at the angle of the jaw heralds the development of parotid salivary gland swelling. This is usually bilateral but is occasionally one-sided. There is swelling of the three groups of salivary glands - parotid, submandibular and sublingual although the parotid is the classical site and usually the most noticeable. Dry mouth with a coated tongue is a key feature.

The illness is more severe in adults and there may be a few days of fever, shivering and stiffness in the jaw before the glandular enlargement. In this post-pubertal group the gonads are affected with the male affected much more than the female. One in four such males will develop orchitis and if this is bilateral then infertility is a risk. This is extremely rare. There is pain and swelling of the testis with or without a high fever and there may be mental symptoms of a mild delirium or mental depression.

The central nervous system may be affected with the development of meningitis or encephalitis. This occurs in 5% of people with mumps. It is the commonest viral cause of encephalitis. The symptoms include headache, delirium and hallucinations. The nervous system manifestations may be the only evidence of mumps - 30% with these symptoms have no salivary gland symptoms. There can be paralysis due to affection of the cranial or peripheral nerves and this can be permanent.

Pancreatic involvement is evidenced by pain in the epigastrium, vomiting and anorexia. There may also be endocrine involvement in some with glycosuria which may persist into the convalescent phase.

Rarely the heart, liver, joints and breasts may be involved.

Complications:

COMPLICATION	SYMPTOMS TO LOOK FOR
Orchitis	Pain and swelling in testes - affects 25% of those affected who are post-pubertal. Sterility may occur if both testes are involved. This is very unusual and in any case is virtually always transient.
Pancreatitis	Epigastric pain radiating through to the back. Vomiting
Oophoritis	Iliac fossa pain in females. Only if post-pubertal
Meningitis, encephalitis	Occipital headache, neck stiffness, photophobia

TABLE 5.4: COMPLICATIONS OF MUMPS

Treatment:

There is no specific conventional treatment although corticosteroids may be given for the complications which are usually seen in adults. Care of the mouth is important.

Alternative management:

The general comments I made with regard to measles are relevant here. Care of the mouth is particularly important in cases of mumps because the salivary glands are affected causing dry mouth. It is interesting to note that it is glandular tissue of varying types which is particularly affected in this illness.

In terms of Chinese medicine, this a case of Invasion of Wind-Heat of Shaoyang type leading to Stagnation of Qi (swelling behind the ears). In most cases it is mild with little constitutional upset.

RUBELLA

This is also a viral disease which can be so mild that its effects are unnoticed. About 50% of cases go unrecognised particularly in the under fives. The peak incidence is at 15 years of age. Most cases occur in childhood so that by the age of 18-20 years around 80% of people have had it. The incubation period is 2-3 weeks. The person is infective from 1 week before the rash appears until 4 days after it appears.

Symptoms:

Usually the rash is the first indication of the disease although adults may suffer more systemic symptoms with an initial illness of painful stiff neck, headache and general malaise for 24 hours. Some people may have a mild conjunctivitis, sore throat with slight redness of the soft palate and inside of the mouth. There is generalised enlargement of the lymph glands but especially the suboccipital and post-cervical groups. If there is marked lymph gland enlargement the spleen may be palpable.

The rash is small, discrete, pink and macular. The spots are around 1-3mm in diameter. They are seen first on the face and neck rapidly spreading to the trunk. It rarely lasts more than 24-48 hours.

Complications:

COMPLICATIONS	SYMPTOMS TO LOOK FOR
Arthritis	Pain and swelling of small joints in the hands and feet. It appears in adults by around 7 days, may be severe for a few days but subsides by 3-4 weeks.
Meningo-encephalitis	Headache, neck stiffness, photophobia
Foetal abnormalities	There is a risk of foetal abnormality if a pregnant woman contracts the disease. The risk varies from 70% during the first 4 weeks to virtually zero at 4 months. The results may be low birth weight, microcephaly, cataract, deafness, congenital heart defects and delayed teething. A termination of pregnancy is offered in such cases. There were 362 confirmed such infections in 1987[11] There are 20 cases each year of congenital rubella syndrome.

TABLE 5.5: COMPLICATIONS OF RUBELLA

Treatment:

There is no specific conventional treatment.

Alternative management:

The general comments made under measles are also relevant here. Rubella is not a problem in most cases. The issue is around mass vaccination campaigns aimed at teenage girls although recently a combined vaccination including rubella has been introduced for children aged around 15 months. It seems expensive to routinely vaccinate every female in the country when most of them will contract rubella naturally.

There is usually no attempt made to assess immune status prior to vaccination so most will be unnecessary both from a financial viewpoint and a medical one. Also there is no hard evidence that artificial rubella immunity lasts for a significant period of time. It may in fact only last for a few years and therefore push susceptible people into childbearing years - the very situation to be avoided.. A much better idea is to have rubella "parties" where any cases of rubella in the area invites other children to meet them and so pass it on naturally. Again, rubella is one of the normal childhood diseases necessary for healthy development and prevention of this event is potentially hazardous.

In terms of Chinese medicine, this is similar to measles in that it is seen as an attack of Wind-Heat invasion. It is milder than measles and rarely an issue unless in pregnancy.

---

[11] "Immunisation against Infectious Disease" DHSS leaflet, 1988.

CHICKENPOX

This is a viral illness also known as varicella and is due to the same organism as herpes zoster (shingles). It is possible to contract chickenpox from a case of herpes zoster and vice versa. It usually appears in the 5-15 years age group. The incubation period is 14-21 days.

Symptoms:

In children the first sign is usually the appearance of an itchy rash but in adults there may be a short constitutional upset. They also have a more severe illness. People who receive corticosteroids or immunosuppressants are particularly severely affected. Chickenpox is the feared infectious disease in units treating childhood leukaemia where an infection may kill due to the suppression of the immune system implicit in the treatment of the disease.

All herpes infections have similar appearances of the rash. The first appearance is that of a macule which, over a period of 18-24 hours goes through the stages of papule, vesicle and pustule. The rash is more marked on the trunk and in areas such as the axilla. The mucous membrane of the mouth is also affected. New spots continue to appear throughout the illness so cropping is seen - spots at different stages.

Complications:

COMPLICATIONS	SYMPTOMS TO LOOK FOR
Skin infections	Redness around the pustules and more discharge from them. In very severe cases there is bleeding into the vesicles
Encephalitis	Occipital headache, neck stiffness, photophobia
Pneumonia	High fever, cough, breathlessness, the child is ill. Although rare in children some 20% of adults may develop respiratory symptoms.

TABLE 5.6: COMPLICATIONS OF CHICKENPOX

Treatment:

There is no specific conventional treatment. Symptomatic treatment by bathing and keeping the skin cleanis important for prevention of skin infection. Antibiotics will be given if there is such infection.

Alternative management:

The general comments made about measles are also relevant here. This is a useful illness from an alternative point of view since it usually mild, there is no vaccination currently available and there is no conventional treatment. It is innocuous in most people.

In terms of Chinese medicine, this is caused by an Invasion Damp-Heat. All the herpes virus infections are Damp-Heat in nature as evidenced by the appearance of the vesicles and pustules.

- DISEASES OF DISORDERED IMMUNITY -

WHOOPING COUGH

This is a bacterial disease caused by Bordetella pertussis. There is an epidemic every three to four years with any age affected but especially children. The greatest risk to children is during the first year of life when it may be life-threatening. The incubation period is 8-14 days.

Symptoms:

The initial symptoms are those of a catarrhal nature with runny nose, red, sore and watery eyes and a harsh cough. This is a common picture of many childhood illnesses and is relatively non-specific. The child becomes progressively more "mucussy" and the cough worsens.

After 7-10 days the typical paroxysms of coughing appear. They last for several minutes and the child becomes red in the face (blue in severe attacks). There may be subconjunctival haemorrhages at this time with ruptured blood vessels in the conjunctivae leading to the appearance of bright red areas in the conjunctivae. Nose bleeds may also occur.

An attack usually ends in retching or vomiting. It is here that the characteristic whoop is heard which is a sharp inhalation of breath after a prolonged bout of coughing. The whoop is not common and is more likely to be heard in severe cases or in very young children (under 1 year).

At this time the child is actually less infective although thoroughly miserable with swollen eyelids and a constant sticky nasal discharge. The paroxysms are precipitated by factors such as cold air, smoky atmosphere, stress, sudden noises and posture. They are classically worse at night at around 2-3am. The attacks are maximal around the third week and subside by 6-7 weeks. The cough may return with any subsequent upper respiratory tract infection for up to a year later.

Complications:

COMPLICATIONS	SYMPTOMS TO LOOK FOR
Otitis media	Pain in the ear, fever high or returns, redness of eardrum
Pneumonia	High fever, cough, breathlessness, the child is ill
Cerebral haemorrhage	Headache, central nervous system symptoms such as paralysis, numbness.
Convulsions	Unconsciousness, jerking of limbs

TABLE 5.7: COMPLICATIONS OF WHOOPING COUGH

Treatment:

There is no specific conventional treatment available. Antibiotics are usually given to eradicate the bacterium responsible. Such conventional treatment does *not* affect the symptoms and the only help offered is supportive in the sense of remedies for the cough (of limited benefit) or to treat complications.

Alternative management:

I would always treat whooping cough since it is not a "normal" disease of childhood and is due to a pre-existing lung weakness. It is very amenable to treatment by alternative medicine. I have seen children who have had problems for weeks to find that a single homoeopathic remedy can relieve it almost overnight. It should be noted here that this is much more difficult if the person has received antibiotics. If the illness has been long-term then treatment of any underlying lung condition may have to be undertaken after the acute episode has subsided.

In terms of Chinese medicine, this is known as "hundred day cough" and reflects the duration of many cases. It is considered to be due to Wind-Heat invading the Lung leading to Phlegm-Fire in Lung.

- CHRONIC INFECTIOUS DISEASE -

In this section, I have listed four diseases. They are good examples of chronic disease associated with organisms. They illustrate the point that what is important is the depth of the pathology not the supposed organism which may or may not be present. There are many infectious diseases recognised by conventional medicine and I have listed those which are more common in their relevant Chapter. For example; common cold, influenza and acute bronchitis are discussed in the Chapter dealing with respiratory diseases. I would recommend you to either consult the index or to go to the Chapter which deals with the area affected by a particular disease.

GLANDULAR FEVER

This is a viral illness caused by a herpes-like organism called the Epstein-Barr virus. It affects people mainly in the 15-25 year age group. The incubation period is variable 1-4 months but often 4-20 days. Many people are affected by the virus but only a few develop symptoms.

Symptoms:

The onset may be gradual or sudden. There is a fever of around 104°F (40°C) and a sore throat with sometimes a membrane over the tonsils. The degree of discomfort is more than with the usual tonsillitis and swallowing may be difficult and painful. Lymph gland enlargement is generalised but more marked in the neck. They are usually tender. The spleen is palpable in one third to one half of cases. For this reason anyone with glandular fever must avoid all sports. Ruptured spleen is an unusual complication but leads to 15% of deaths from this illness.

Rashes are seen in around 5% of cases and can take several forms. Macules may appear at the end of week one and resemble rubella whilst some develop petechiae on the hard and soft palates.

The fever is of variable duration. Jaundice occurs in around 5% although liver involvement is present in virtually all cases as determined by liver function tests become abnormal. Chronic tiredness occurs in about 15% of individuals according to the textbooks but in my experience is much more common.

Complications:

COMPLICATIONS	SYMPTOMS TO LOOK FOR
Meningitis, encephalitis	Occipital headache, photophobia, neck stiffness
Peripheral neuritis (rare)	Tingling and numbness in the hands and feet
Mesenteric adenitis	Abdominal pain resembling appendicitis
Haemolytic anaemia	Jaundice, pallor, tiredness and other symptoms of anaemia
Rupture of spleen (very rare)	Severe abdominal pain, shock with low blood pressure, rapid and thready pulse.

TABLE 5.8: COMPLICATIONS OF GLANDULAR FEVER

Investigation:

The white cell count shows atypical monocytes in most cases. 80% of cases show a positive reaction to the Paul-Bunnell test. One fifth of people never become positive.

Treatment:

There is no specific conventional treatment. It is supportive only although antibiotics are usually given. Penicillin causes the appearance of a rash in over 90% of cases with an associated marked debility. In the US this can lead to charges of negligence for which there is no legal defence.

Alternative management:

In terms of Chinese medicine, this is due to an Invasion of Damp-Heat. Most cases occur in students either still at school or at university. It seems to be a result of excessive work and study as well as emotional stress particularly about examinations and career choices. This combination of factors typically depletes Spleen energy and so makes the body susceptible to such an invasion.

Treatment needs to be aimed at these underlying factors as well as the acute manifestations. Typically the acute illness subsides into a chronic period of ill-health lasting anything from a few weeks to many months. The distinction between this and conditions such as M.E. and post-viral syndromes in general is rather blurred.

In such people there needs to be consideration of many aspects of the their life such as diet, relaxation and rest, attitudes to work and study as well as relationship issues which may be present.

In some the diagnosis may not be clear because the "tests" are normal and it may be difficult to distinguish between this and M.E. In fact the label is unimportant since the causes are similar and treatment and diagnosis is primarily taking place on an energetic basis (by homoeopathy, acupuncture and so on).

I have treated people who have tested positive for glandular fever. As their condition fluctuated with treatment and relapses with stressful situations the tests have also fluctuated. They tend to be negative at times of good health and positive at times of poor health. If the pathology is more on the energetic level, the tests will be negative. You will see blood tests become positive when the problem affects the blood. Conventional immunologists cannot understand such changes as, in conventional thought, you either have something or you have not - the idea of change is completely alien.

HERPES INFECTIONS

Herpes viruses are related and lead to a group of diseases which are recognised by the nature of the rash. This goes through the stages of macule, papule, vesicle, pustule and scab. Herpes diseases tend to chronicity so chickenpox may lead to herpes zoster in later life and herpes simplex is recurrent.

HERPES SIMPLEX

There are two types of herpes simplex depending upon the area affected. Type I affects the lips and around the mouth and is the typical "cold sore" with which most of us are familiar. It recurs with debility and upper respiratory tract infections.

Type II affects the genital area and buttocks and is common since a great increase in numbers in the 1970's. It is transmitted via sexual contact. It typically recurs when there is reduced immunity perhaps when overworking or as a result of sexual activity.

Treatment:

An anti-viral agent, acyclovir, is now available for this condition and it does seem to prevent appearance of the rash in some people. It may then "leak" out to appear at the edges of where the drug is applied (it is applied locally). Some people would probably have to apply it all over their bodies to prevent it! Others may find that the rash does not appear but then they develop internal problems perhaps in the bowel, lungs or brain.

Alternative management:

In terms of Chinese medicine, all the herpes viruses cause conditions considered to be Damp-Heat in nature. Type I is an affection of the Stomach where the DampHeat flareups up into the Stomach channel and Type II is DampHeat invading the Liver channel. Suppression by acyclovir may lead to conditions of internal DampHeat. Some cases of herpes simplex correspond to invasion of the Lung and Stomach Channels by Wind.

Treatment needs to be constitutional in nature and results are usually very impressive for such conditions. You would expect this to be so since they manifest on the skin.

HERPES ZOSTER

This is a disease of the skin which is related to chickenpox. The same virus is involved in the two diseases. In this case the virus irritates the posterior root ganglion (sensory) of the spinal cord and so produces symptoms in the distribution of that nerve. The thoracic or lumbar area are usually involved but any area from the head to the lower limb may be affected.

The disease is also known as shingles and is typified by the appearance of a vesicular rash (classical herpes appearance) in the distribution of the posterior nerve root of one or more segments of the spinal cord. It may also be seen in the area of distribution of the V cranial nerve - trigeminal.

It occurs mainly in the middle-aged and elderly and is triggered by stress or other episode which leads to lowered immunity. Some cases occur in people with an underlying malignancy or pneumonia. On occasion it can occur after a shock such as a fall or bereavement.

There is an initial illness of mild constitutional disturbance and fever. Pain develops in the affected areas and at this stage may be mistaken for any number of conditions ranging from musculoskeletal problems to coronary thrombosis. After 4 days the rash appears which passes through the typical stages of a herpes infection - macules, papules, vesicles and pustules. These rupture and so dry, crusting areas are seen. These may separate and leave white anaesthetic areas. The disease is usually unilateral.

As the rash appears the pain worsens and becomes neuralgic in nature. There is a continual burning soreness which is worse for contact or there may be an intermittent stabbing. Itching is seen in some people. Some cases persist and lead to post-herpetic neuralgia. This is a particularly debilitating condition since the pain is virtually continual.

The ophthalmic division of the V cranial nerve may be affected especially in the elderly and so the conjunctiva and cornea are affected. This may lead to keratitis and severe damage affecting sight.

Post-herpetic scars are usually permanently analgesic and in some cases the muscles of the relevant segment may be affected leading to paralysis which is also usually permanent.

Treatment:

In recent years an anti-viral agent has been used to treat herpes infections such as simplex and zoster (see above). Analgesics may also be given. People with herpes zoster require two weeks away from work, partly due to the systemic nature of the illness and because they are infective.

Alternative management:

Early treatment with acupuncture is well-recognised to prevent the complications of post-herpetic neuralgia. Alternative treatment will help the sometimes severe symptoms.

Attention may have to paid to the underlying condition since shingles occurs in people who already have some imbalance due to shock, an injury, emotional stress and so on.

MYALGIC ENCEPHALOMYELITIS (M.E.)

This is also known as postviral fatigue syndrome, postviral syndrome and Royal Free disease. It is a relatively new disease although it was first described in 1934. It seems to be commoner as the years pass and affecting younger people. Many conventional practitioners deny its existence but with increasing awareness and the presence of support groups such as M.E. Action[12] it is being taken more seriously.

It may occur in epidemics. It is a vague, ill-defined disease in many people with great disagreement over its origin, course and in some quarters even its existence. Many conventional textbooks still do not even mention it.

Women seem to be prone to its development three times more likely than men. It chiefly affects the 30-40 years age group. It typically begins after an upper respiratory or gastrointestinal tract infection from which the person does not make a full recovery.

Symptoms:

These can be vague and ill-defined which reflects the degree of depletion present in this condition. Virtually any symptom can be present which is why this diagnosis may be a "catch-all" for people who are difficult to categorise conventionally.

Muscle fatigue and pain are common with general malaise. The tiredness may, on occasions, be severe. Some people remain in bed all day and literally can do nothing. Others have to use wheel-chairs because they are too weak to walk.

Headache, dizziness and fainting attacks may occur. The extremities are cold. Gastrointestinal symptoms include nausea, flatulence and diarrhoea. Mentally, there are problems with memory and concentration. The emotions are unstable with outbursts of anger or weeping. Sleep disturbance is common - either difficulty getting off to sleep or continual waking during the night. A rather unusual symptom is hyperacusis (sensitivity to sound) which, interestingly is commonly seen with withdrawal syndromes from tranquillisers. The key, as always, is the individual and the symptom picture will vary from person to person.

---

12 M.E. Action, PO Box 1302, Wells, Somerset BA5 2WE

People with ME can be broadly divided into three groups depending upon their progress. This is common with most chronic diseases. These three categories are:

1. Recovery after a variable length of time.
2. Relapses/remissions for years with relapses at times of undue physical or mental stress.
3. Chronic progressive disability.

These groups reveal the state of energy of each person with those in the first being the strongest and those in the last being the weakest.

Diagnosis:

Conventional physical examination is normal as are laboratory tests and so the diagnosis is one of exclusion. In some people there may be evidence of a recent infection, usually viral. The commonest ones seen as Coxsackie A and B, echo and Epstein-Barr viruses. The latter is associated with glandular fever.

Treatment:

There may be several approaches depending upon the doctor who sees the person and their personal preferences or speciality. People may be given antibiotics if there is evidence of any continuing infection although this is more likely to be the precursor to the illness. Antidepressants are probably the most common medication offered, with or without tranquillisers. I have met some people recently who have been given antidepressants and told by their practitioner that they are pain killers. It may be that there is a move to prescribe these drugs more frequently for such people. Counselling and psychological approaches are used by more enlightened practitioners.

Alternative management:

This illness is a mixed bag of conditions in which each individual will have factors of varying importance. It is clearly an attempt by the body to switch off and gain some rest. It often affects people who work hard and find it difficult to let go and relax. This may be why it is seen more commonly in women who are taught by our society to look after the needs of others even to the point of ill health. Men on the other hand may find it easier to stop and rest. These are only tendencies, of course, since ME is seen in men. The other factor which may be in operation here is that diseases which have a psychological component are usually under diagnosed in men since the male orientated profession is reluctant to label men as having psychological difficulties.

In terms of Chinese medicine, the condition may be, at least at its outset, one of External Pathogenic Factor Invading as a consequence of underlying depletion of Qi or Blood. The origin may lie in such factors as overwork, emotional stress, not wanting to say "no". There is invariably overuse and abuse of antibiotic prescriptions. These can only make the problem worse since they deplete the Qi. So you see syndromes such as External Pathogenic Factor Remaining, Qi or Yang deficiency, Blood or Yin deficiency. Damp in the muscles and channels is common in those with marked degrees of aching and muscle weakness.

A woman I treated with this condition had 2 years of upheaval due to a change of husband's job and his working away. She had to sell the house on her own and look after the children. After that period of time the family moved house (some 400 miles) to be with the husband. She moved to a new job, the children started a new school and then she developed toxoplasmosis which is an unusual infection caught from cats. She was told she had the problem because she cleaned the cat-tray out each day! After 4 months of treatment with antibiotics she was so weak that she could only get out of bed for 4 hours each day. Her energy was depleted to the point that her life was merely sleeping, eating and resting. The issue here is that the infection comes after - *it is the result not the cause.*

Treatment should be aimed at removing any Pathogenic Influence Remaining together with attempting to remedy the underlying condition. The use of drugs will only serve to worsen the already weakened state. Since Qi deficiency and Damp accumulation are common, it is clear why antidepressants are often prescribed and produce short term relief in some. Antidepressants are hot energetically and so stimulate the Qi and dry up the dampness. They primarily affect the Heart and Liver. In the short-term, there may be less aching and depression as the Damp is dried and the Heart and Liver Qi are heated and moved. Long-term of course, they can only disperse and weaken the Qi and further deplete the Yin and Blood.

ACQUIRED IMMUNE DEFICIENCY SYNDROME (AIDS)

I have spent quite some time and space discussing this disease because it raises several important issues about the conventional view of infectious disease. It is still quite uncommon but diseases of this severity reveal the fundamental, philosophical differences in conventional and alternative medicine.

AIDS was recently recognised as having been a cause of death in the UK in a seaman in 1959[13]. It is a new disease and was first recognised around 1979 in the USA. Its name indicates that it is an acquired weakness of the immune system. In conventional medicine this as seen as being due to the effects of HIV (Human Immunovirus). The person becomes vulnerable to certain infections and various rare malignant tumours develop.

T lymphocytes, which are involved particularly with resistance to viral and fungal infections, are affected. B cells which are involved primarily with resistance to bacterial infection are left intact. The reduction in lymphocytes is associated with the development of viral and fungal infections, parasitic infestations and certain tumours. This collapse of the immune system indicates the severity of the condition. It is conventionally considered to have a 100% mortality. In reality, around 85% of people with AIDS seem to die of the disease although any such figures have to viewed extreme caution because of the short period of time since the disease appeared.

It was recognised fairly early that there are similarities between this disease and serum hepatitis in that a virus is involved, that antibodies are present which are an indicator of infection and that transmission may take place some time after initial infection. Transmission is similar in terms of contact with blood and body fluids. Increasingly, people with syndromes diagnosed as AIDS have no evidence of HIV infection. The simplistic suggestion that all people with AIDS have HIV infection and that all HIV infection leads to AIDS is not correct. As practitioners, if you give people this information, it can help relieve the sense of inevitability which many people are given in their dealings with conventional medicine.

There is much discussion about the origins of AIDS. There are several theories but the ones which seem most reliable are those which relate the disease to susceptibility. How can someone's immune system be so weakened that it lets in such a virus and, subsequently, opportunistic viral, fungal and parasitic infections? In Africa, the disease is most prevalent in the very countries where smallpox vaccination was pursued the most vigorously in the push to eradicate smallpox.

In the 1920's, trials of a polio vaccine were held which involved the injection of monkey serum into humans. There were already simian immune deficiency syndromes and one could argue that transmissible agents crossed from one species to another. This was always considered to be impossible but recent events in animals with regard to bovine spongiform encephalopathy ('mad cow' disease) has shown that such transmission can and does take place.

The origin of the disease continues to be a source of discussion in conventional circles. In terms of susceptibilities which I have already discussed, the cause is the weakening of the general immunity of the population. AIDS is seen in those with severely weakened immune systems. This may be in babies where the immune system is immature or where it has been weakened by such things as drug abuse, suppressed disease, poor diet, irregular life-style and so forth. In Edinburgh in 1989 it was stated that 60% of HIV positive people had used intravenous drugs. Consequently, HIV is a weak pathogen and only affects those with severely depleted immune systems.

The most dangerous situation for any immune system, healthy or not, is a bypassing of the normal layers of the immune system by the injection of contaminated blood or body fluids. The first groups to be affected were drug addicts who injected (13%) and male homosexuals (71%). This situation mirrors serum hepatitis which has the same methods of transmission. The other similarity is that whilst most people with HIV disease suffer little or no illness as a result, although they may still be infectious to others, a minority develop AIDS. The commonest practice involving injection of disease material into the bloodstream is vaccination (see below).

No-one knows how many people who are HIV positive go on to develop full blown AIDS. It presumably depends upon many factors such as constitution, life-style, drug use/abuse[14], work

---

[13] Lancet, July 7th 1990: 51.
[14] I would include the use of prescribed drugs here as well as 'recreational' drugs.

practices, sexual practices[15]. Conventionally, the incubation period for the disease is seen as being very variable and on average is 28 months with a range between 9 months to 11 years. This latter figure is movable as time passes by and we move further and further away from the date of original discovery. HIV infection is viewed in conventional circles as merely a stage on the way to developing AIDS. This is not true and is one of the fallacies which needs to be challenged as it serves to undermine and disempower people. Any appearance of disease is dependent upon the state of the immune system and this is a reflection of the factors mentioned above.

The first stage in this process is that contact is made with the virus. This is by means of sexual intercourse or passage of blood or body fluids into the body. There is no other recorded case of transmission. If the person is susceptible then "infection" occurs. It is not possible to be affected by the virus by kissing, embracing or non-sexual forms of contact.

After a latent period which is not accurately known since it varies so much, antibodies are produced against the virus. This is the state of HIV positive. It is important to realise here that HIV positive only indicates that antibodies are present. Lack of antibodies, i.e. HIV negative may still mean that the virus is present. This is shown in Table 5.9. Thus, HIV negative people may still be infectious.

It is not very clear from the literature how long it takes for a person to become HIV positive after contact but it can certainly take three months and occasionally longer. Some people never develop antibodies. During this period, a person would be negative but infectious. In a study of HIV negative homosexual men engaged in high risk sexual behaviour (see below), almost one quarter (23%) were found to have the virus. Most of these remained HIV negative for up to 36 months. The value of one test is nothing and the value of two tests even if separated by some months is limited.[16]

HIV positive, i.e. showing antibodies to HIV, is *not* the same as AIDS. The syndrome may, or may not, follow at some later date. This is misunderstood in general when people talk about an AIDS test. There is no such thing. AIDS is a clinical diagnosis based on a particular symptom picture. The test is for antibodies to HIV. There is a great controversy raging at the moment about the exact role of the virus in the development of the syndrome because there are some people who develop clinically a state of AIDS and yet have never had any sign of HIV. Peter Duisberg, professor of molecular biology at Berkeley, a well-known proponent of the theory that HIV has a minor role to play in AIDS, states that it is the immune system which is the main problem. The body does a good job, in most cases, of dealing with the virus. It is when other factors which I have already mentioned come into operation that the syndrome of AIDS develops.

As with general public health measures to prevent infection of any kind, there are certain practices which can minimise the amount of contact with HIV. According to the Terence Higgins Trust, a group specifically set up to deal with issues around HIV and AIDS, there are several categories of risk. High risk categories are anal intercourse and vaginal intercourse without condoms, any act which draws blood, any sexual practice which involves contact with urine or faeces, sharing sex toys, and sex during the menstrual period if the partner has open cuts or grazes or sores on their hands or body.

Medium risk is oral sex by woman to man, even if he withdraws before ejaculation, oral sex by woman to woman if active partner has bleeding gums, mouth ulcers etc., oral sex by man to woman if he has mouth problems as above, vaginal intercourse with condom.

No risk is regarded as stimulation using hands either mutually or solo, general body contact, stroking or body kissing, ejaculation of semen onto body, sex toys (providing they are not shared). The health education message of "safe sex" can be seen as something of a misnomer. "Safe sex" is not possible, only "safer sex".

Added to the uncertainties about the testing for antibodies, is the certainty that if a person's HIV status becomes generally known there is a social stigma. People lose their jobs, children are banned from school, there may be general social ostracism. Insurance or mortgages are almost impossible. It may be very difficult even if it is discovered that the test is negative since some may take the view that if there is no risk why have the test in the first place? If the test is positive then there is pressure to take conventional medication.

---

[15] There is a recognition in Chinese medicine that excessive sexual activity particularly when emotionally disturbed, under the influence of drugs or when tired is more depleting to the body's energies.

[16] New England Journal of Medicine June 1st 1989: 1458-62.

If people are thinking of checking their HIV status then I would consider the following to be useful pieces of advice:

- Have counselling before the test to discuss the issues which are important to you. It may be preferable to use a counsellor who is not involved in the unit doing the testing since vested interests are better avoided.
- A normal test does not *prove* there is no problem.
- A positive test only tells you if you have antibodies. It gives you no information about your general level of health.
- Medical confidentiality is not absolute so have the test under an assumed name and certainly never through medical practitioners you know unless you are absolutely certain of their reaction. Specialist clinics for sexually transmitted disease tend to be more helpful.
- Be very careful about who you tell since the consequences of this becoming generally known can be severe.
- The main issues are around health and general life-style and these can be addressed whether you know your HIV status or not.

The ideas above can be summarised as in Table 5.9.

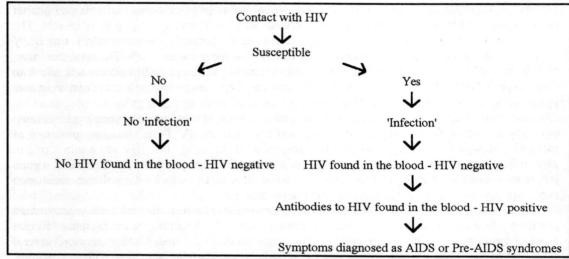

TABLE 5.9: FLOWCHART OF SEQUELAE OF CONTACT WITH HIV

Symptoms:

The initial symptoms of HIV infection are acute fever with lymphatic gland enlargement. This can be similar to influenza or glandular fever. It lasts for a few days and is followed a symptom free period. Whether there is progression to further clinical conditions clearly depends upon the general state of health of the person. If the lifestyle is one of depletion then this tends to lead to deterioration in the immune system. If the lifestyle is more moderate and strengthening then there is every reason to suppose that a long and healthy life will result. The view that AIDS is inevitable in all persons with HIV infection is more a reflection of conventional medical states of mind rather than the actual realities of the situation.

As mentioned above, some cases of AIDS are not associated with HIV at all and are somewhat of a puzzle for conventional medicine. This would support the belief that it is other factors (co-factors as they are called) which are important. If enough co-factors are present then AIDS may result irrespective of the presence of HIV.

Symptoms which may indicate the development of AIDS or a pre-AIDS syndrome are:

- Generalised lymphatic gland enlargement.
- Profound fatigue, persisting for weeks with no obvious cause.
- Unexplained weight loss (more than 10lbs in 2 months).
- Severe night sweats that may occur on and off for several weeks.

- Fever lasting more than 10 days.
- Diarrhoea lasting more than 1 month.
- Cough lasting more than two weeks and not due to smoking. This may be associated with shortness of breath, persistent sore throat and difficulty in swallowing. The white spots of "thrush" may be visible in the mouth.
- Signs of individual cancers such as purplish or pink blotches in the skin (Kaposi's sarcoma).

The three main problems for people with AIDS are infections, cancers and other immune disorders.

Infections are due to viruses, fungi or parasites. Pneumonia due to the unusual parasite Pneumocystis carinii is the commonest disorder. The commonest fungal infection is Candida albicans ("thrush"). The commonest viral infection is herpes simplex ("cold sores"). Other infections found with AIDS are unusually severe attacks of herpes zoster ("shingles"), toxoplasmosis and tuberculosis.

Two types of cancer are seen with AIDS. Kaposi's sarcoma (KS) which is a rare cancer of skin presenting as purplish blotches and lymphoma.

Other immune disorders include haemolytic anaemia and idiopathic thrombocytopenic purpura.

Treatment:

The main conventional treatment is to treat infections as they arise by means of antibiotics, antifungal and antiviral agents.

There is a drug available to treat the supposed cause, the HIV infection. In common with many treatments directed at viruses, it is toxic since the cell has to be killed in order to get at the virus. Zidovudine (also known as AZT) is increasingly used to treat both people with AIDS and people with asymptomatic HIV infection. Originally developed as a chemotherapy treatment for cancer, it was 'rediscovered' to be used in this situation.

You may find that AZT is used as treatment merely because of a low CD4 lymphocyte count. This is a notoriously unreliable test to assess immune function since it can change according to several factors including exercise, stress levels and diet.

The drug has many side-effects including nausea, insomnia, myalgia, severe headache, rashes, vomiting and fever. A severe polymyositis syndrome of muscles aches and pains can occur with prolonged therapy The most harmful effects are on the blood which are serious and frequent. About one third of people develop anaemia usually after six weeks of treatment. Most of these need repeated blood transfusions every three or four weeks on full drug dosage. Even before the anaemia becomes apparent the red blood cells change in size and start to swell up. Neutropenia may develop before 6 weeks. Thrombocytopenia may also be seen.

Alternative management:

Many of the approaches described in Chapter 6 and the treatment of cancer are also valid here. A multiple approach must be taken for serious, chronic degenerative conditions. The complication here is with conventional treatment which is heavily suppressive and strongly advocated by conventional practitioners. Energetically, you should consider AZT to be similar in action to the chemotherapy agents used in cancer. This is discussed in Chapter 6.

The key is the immune system, as in so many cases, and it is important to pay attention to diet, mental/emotional factors as well as perhaps a specific therapy. The people who do the best in terms of quality of life and length of life are those who pursue an alternative approach.

If you look again at Table 5.9, you can see how if the person improves their state of health will move up to the top. The proof for this is that some people become asymptomatic and then become HIV negative as the blood clears and the antibodies disappear.[17]

---

[17] There are many practitioners of alternative medicine who are working with HIV positive people and people with AIDS. As with the alternative treatments of cancer, they are undersupported although there are some well organised support groups in the UK and particularly the US who are more involved in such treatment. Recently the work of Chinese medical practitioners in Africa has proved that Chinese medicine has much to offer for patients.
An unpublished trial by Professor BoPing Wu of the Academy of Traditional Chinese Medicine in Beijing working in Tanzania summarised the treatment of 158 HIV positive patients between 1988

People with HIV infection and AIDS will require a lot of support since there is much misunderstanding, both inside and outside the medical profession. I would rate this to be as much as a problem as treating people with cancer. The issues around cancer are discussed fully in Chapter 6. In the end, the person chooses the treatment they wish. If we can offer support, practical help and measures which can increase the strength of the immune system then definitely beneficial results will be obtained.

- HISTORICAL DISEASES -

I have named the following historical diseases since they are rarely seen in the UK. However, their importance lies in the widespread use of vaccination in the belief that such practices will prevent their re-emergence. I discuss vaccination in detail on Page 70.

TETANUS

This is a bacterial infection caused by Clostridium tetani. It is found in ground which is contaminated with the faeces of many animals such as the horse and cow. Spores develop which resist heat and dryness and so can survive for long periods. There has never been a recorded instance of tetanus resulting from the bite of a domestic animal.

The bacterium grows in conditions where there is no oxygen and so in deep penetrating wounds particularly where there is much tissue damage. Crushing injuries in agricultural workers are a special risk as are neglected wounds, e.g. battlefield injuries.

The bacterium produces toxins which affect the central nervous system. Symptoms develop after a quiescent period of variable time depending upon the site of the wound and its proximity to the central nervous system.

The first signs are those of restlessness with muscle twitching then stiffness of the neck. Soon the jaw muscles are affected (hence its popular name of "lockjaw"). Later there is more generalised stiffness and convulsions. These are precipitated by stimuli such as noise or light. Death, if it occurs, is due to exhaustion, cardiac insufficiency or pulmonary collapse.

Some cases are very mild and certainly not all lead to such severe problems.

Treatment:

Injections of antitoxin are given as soon as there are suspected problems and antibiotics to remove any remaining organisms. Convulsions are treated with anticonvulsants. Treatment is mainly supportive to deal with any manifestations in a particular case.

The key is wound hygiene and so tetanus is rare now in the developed world where wounds tend not to be neglected. Vaccination is still routinely given to all children and many people are given boosters in casualty departments around the country in response to minor wounds and the bites of dogs and cats. I would estimate that many are given unnecessarily even from a conventional viewpoint.

Antibiotics are usually injected at the same time to "prevent" wound infection. As mentioned later, the use of antibiotics for prophylaxis is usually pointless. Either no infection would have occurred anyway or if it does it will then be resistant to the antibiotic given.

DIPTHERIA

This is a bacterial disease caused by Corynebacterium diptheriae. The main feature of the disease is that the organism produces a toxin which affects the heart and the central nervous system. This is not true in every case and some people may only have a very mild attack.

and 1991. The T4 cell count increased in 31% and 7% became HIV negative.

Symptoms:

The incubation period is very short in the order of 2-4 days. The nose and tonsils are the usual sites of affliction. The person is clearly ill with malaise, pallor, mild fever. There is sore throat with a characteristic greyish-white membrane on one or both tonsils which is firmly attached. There will be enlargement of the relevant lymph node groups. In severe cases toxins are released which affect the cardiovascular and/or central nervous systems.

This disease is rarely seen in the West now and is a problem due to poor housing, poor nutrition and inadequate public health measures. Therefore, there has been a great reduction in the numbers seen in the last 50 years or so with the result that most people have never seen a case. In 1984 there were 2 cases in the UK.

Treatment:

Injections of antitoxin are given to neutralise the toxins released by the organism. Supportive treatment may be required if circulatory failure intervenes.

COMPLICATIONS	SYMPTOMS TO LOOK FOR
Circulatory collapse	Low blood pressure, rapid and thready pulse, grey and pale complexion, reduced urine output, proteinuria
Nerve involvement	Altered speech, regurgitation of fluids into the nose when swallowing, blurred vision, double vision, difficulty swallowing, numbness and tingling in the limbs (legs more than arms)

TABLE 5.10: COMPLICATIONS OF DIPTHERIA

Alternative management:

The importance of this disease for alternative medicine lies merely in the public health application of its vaccination. No practitioner in the West is likely to see this condition.

POLIO

This is a viral disease which is transmitted by the faecal-oral route. The large epidemics of the 1940's and 1950's were almost certainly associated with the fad of tonsillectomy. Removal of such an important lymphatic gland at the entrance of the lung and stomach has potentially serious consequences. Since that time, the number of cases has gradually declined and now the only cases are either caused by the vaccine or are due to ingesting contaminated food or drink. This does not happen in the West because sewage and drinking water are separated. Epidemics tended to occur in the late summer and early autumn.

Symptoms:

Many people in an epidemic will be infected with virus but only a minority develop symptoms and not all of these develop severe symptoms. The virus affects the motor nerve cells in the spinal cord leading to paralysis.

The incubation period of 7-12 days. There is mild fever, generalised aches and pains which in some leads on to weakness and paralysis. The site of the paralysis depends upon the part of the spinal cord and brain which is involved. In some instances the muscles of respiration are affected requiring mechanical assistance to prevent death due to asphyxiation.

Treatment:

There is no definitive treatment available. Prevention is important and public health measures to protect water and food supplies are essential. If a person develops symptoms then complete rest will minimise the severity of the attack. Massage and physiotherapy play an important part in aiding recovery.

Alternative management:

The importance of this disease for alternative medicine lies merely in the public health application of its vaccination. No practitioner in the West is likely to see this condition. There are treatments available such as massage, Chinese herbal formulae, Ayurvedic treatment and the like and such natural approaches are used in those areas where polio is still found.

- ANTIBIOTIC USE -

Antibiotics, strictly speaking, are drugs which kill bacteria or prevent their growth. For the purposes of discussion in this section, I want to include all the drugs which are used against infecting organisms. These are antifungal, antiviral, antiprotozoal and antiparasitic drugs.

Such chemicals can be used either when an infection occurs or as prophylaxis (to prevent the occurrence of infection)[18]. Prophylactic use tends not to prevent infection but to lead to the appearance of resistant organisms when infection does actually happen.

There is a general view in some conventional circles that antibiotic use is harmless or at least only leads to minor problems. This is nonsense and is particularly dangerous in the case of children who are often more susceptible to the harmful effects. There are the well-known problems of diarrhoea and vaginal thrush due to eradication of the usual bacteria resident in those sites as well as disturbance to Vitamin B utilisation. Also the use of antibiotics leads to a general weakening of the immune system. This is well recognised amongst mothers of young children who may have received recurrent doses of antibiotics. The child then becomes susceptible to every apparent passing infection.

Energetically the antibiotics affect the digestion particularly leading to low energy and the development of mucus and mucus-related disorders such as middle ear disease, adenoid and tonsil enlargement, diarrhoea, poor weight gain and development and so on.

Different antibiotics tend to be used for different types of infecting organism but this is not particularly important for the practitioner of alternative medicine. What is necessary is to know the usual dosages and how to withdraw them when appropriate.[19]

The situations to be cautious about are those people who take antibiotics for serious or life-threatening disease and those who take them for chronic conditions. If it is a case of serious or life-threatening disease then conventional advice is necessary. In the situation of chronic infection, it depends upon the individual situation and I would refer you to the relevant disease category in this book.

In all other cases, the course of action is relatively straightforward. If the person's energy is strong and the condition is mild with no or little suppression then stop the antibiotic as you treat. In this way there will be no interference with your treatment.

If the person is weak and/or there is marked suppression then treat as the antibiotics are taken and continue to treat constitutionally after the acute phase has subsided. In this way there will not be the release of unmanageable symptoms in a weak person.

In all cases, I would refer you to the information about recognising serious symptoms in Table 5.15 on Page 79.

In terms of Chinese medicine, most antibiotics are cold and damp in nature leading to depletion of Spleen Qi deficiency, Damp accumulation in the Middle and Upper Jiaos and perhaps Qi depletion of other organs as a consequence especially the Lung and Kidney. There is often Heat in the Lung after such treatment particularly in the case of children. If the original diagnosis is one of External Pathogenic Factor then the consequence may be External Pathogenic Factor Remaining.

The sulphonamide group of antibiotics seem to be of a different type and lead to superficial heat reactions and I would say they are warm and dispersing in nature. They are especially a problem, therefore, in people with Blood or Yin deficiency conditions.

Antifungal and antiprotozoal agents seem to have the same effects as most antibiotics except

---

[18] In good conventional practice, prophylaxis is restricted to specific situations where risk is known and not merely suspected. In routine clinical practice, a different pattern of behaviour is often evident. "Failure to establish and adhere to such guidelines has made unnecessary chemoprophylaxis the commonest form of antibiotic misuse in hospitals". "Antimicrobial Chemotherapy", Edited by D.Greenwood (Bailliere and Tindall, 1983). I would only say here that I would add 'and general practice' to this extract.

[19] "Prescribed Drugs and the Alternative Practitioner", Dr S Gascoigne (Ashgrove Press, 1992).

they are stronger in their action. Antifungal drugs particularly affect the Liver and Spleen leading to nausea, vomiting, hypochondriac pain and in some cases, jaundice.

The so-called antiviral drug, AZT, used in the treatment of HIV infection and AIDS, was developed as a cancer chemotherapy drug. Its effects are similar to other agents which are described in Chapter 6.

- VACCINATION[20] -

Vaccination is the practice of introducing 'foreign' matter into the body to prevent disease. The term originally derived from using cowpox to protect against smallpox. The process intends to render people immune from toxin or infection. It is widespread now and mass vaccination campaigns are carried out particularly on children. The practice developed from a procedure carried out by a Dr Jenner in 1792 when he used cowpox to try and prevent the development of the more serious smallpox. The historical facts are that Edward Jenner, a country doctor, noted that dairymaids who had contracted cowpox were protected against smallpox. He inoculated a healthy boy, James Phipps, with pus from the arm of Sarah Nelmes, a dairymaid who was suffering from cowpox. Some weeks later he inoculated Phipps' arm with material from a case of smallpox. The boy remained healthy. Jenner published these results and the medical profession immediately took on the idea. On the basis of this evidence the Western medical world has undertaken to vaccinate everyone of us against several diseases. Large scale vaccinations of the population were not used however until earlier this century and were compulsory until the 1950's and are still so in the USA.

The idea that you actually eradicate disease is, at the least, philosophically contentious. If it is possible, where do the underlying imbalances go to? There is no such thing as perfect human health. If people are prevented from having relatively mild infectious diseases what are we creating for the future? People who are already ill are the ones who have difficulties with childhood diseases. Of 132 deaths from measles discussed in the Lancet, half were in children with serious chronic disease or disability and had at best a short expectation of life. That is, they were due to die soon anyway.[21] As the same article stated, "The effect of measles vaccination on mortality has proved difficult to assess. This is surprising ......"

To understand vaccination, it is important to have some understanding of conventional ideas on immunology. It has been noted that when a person is infected by a particular organism, they produce antibodies against that organism. The deliberate introduction into the body of disease products or modified micro-organisms is designed to stimulate the production of antibodies. If in the future the person comes into contact with such substances, they will produce defence reactions much quicker and more efficiently than would otherwise be the case.

This sounds very reasonable and is the information we have been given since childhood. A great industry has built around this practice. However, the immune system is much more than the presence or absence of antibodies. These exist in the blood and so, hierarchically, are at a deep level of the person. The immune system as a whole is made up of many different layers from the superficial tissues such as skin, secretions such as sweat and tears, defence mechanisms within each organ such as mucus production in the lungs. Once disease has descended into the deeper levels then, and only then, are antibodies produced. You could say that antibodies are only produced when the disease is at a deep level. That is, when it is already a relatively severe problem for the body. This is only a physical list of defences of course and there is no mention of energy which is an added protective layer outside the skin.[22]

Vaccination is the deliberate introduction of toxic material into the bloodstream, bypassing all these subtle levels of the immune system, and so would seem to be, potentially, very dangerous. In addition, it is clearly not the best way to remove a person's susceptibility since other levels need to be addressed at the same time. We only develop an infectious disease, and indeed any disease, if we are susceptible. The question to ask is does vaccination change that susceptibility and if so, is it in the direction of health or of disease?

The opinion of the conventional profession is that vaccination 'is a good thing' and is responsible for the disappearance of some infectious diseases or the fall in death rate of others. This is

---

[20] Although the terms vaccination, immunisation and inoculation have slightly different definitions, I shall use the word vaccination to embrace them all.
[21] Lancet, August 1st 1981.
[22] I discuss levels in Chapter 2 and how the blood is one of the deepest organs of the body.

not true. There are many reasons why disease undergoes change over the years. Some like scarlet fever, for which incidentally there is no vaccination, become very much milder whilst others become more severe. Complex sociological, economic, political factors are usually in operation. The only factor with which there is *no* correlation is medical practice. [23]

The death rate from infectious diseases *has* dramatically fallen in the last 100 years[24][25]. This is used to support past, present and future vaccination schemes. If we consider the true cause of infectious disease,susceptibility, and that organisms are the effect not the cause, perhaps things are not as they seem.

If one looks at the available data it becomes clear that the death rates from infectious diseases began to decline long before mass vaccination came along.

Table 5.10 reveals that a great reduction in the death rate from tuberculosis took place before the common use of antibiotics in the 1940's or mass vaccination in the 1950's. The first sanatorium was not opened in New York until 1910 so it is clear that improvements in living standards which began in the latter part of the 19th century are responsible for changes in death rates.

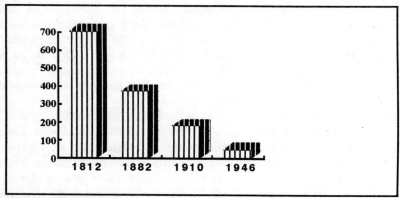

TABLE 5.10: DEATH RATE IN NEW YORK FROM TUBERCULOSIS (/10000) [26]

Considering combined death rates from scarlet fever, diptheria, whooping cough and measles amongst children, it is clear that nearly 90% of the total decline in mortality between 1860 and 1965 occurred before the introduction of antibiotics and mass immunisation. (seeTable 5.11).

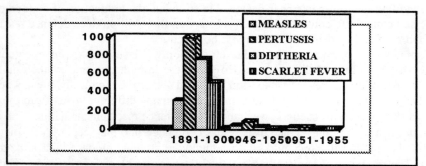

TABLE 5.11: DEATHS PER MILLION CHILDREN UNDER 15 YEARS OF AGE [27]

---

[23] "Medical Nemesis" by Ivan Illich (Bantam, 1976).

[24] It is often stated that modern medicine, including the use of vaccines and drugs such as antibiotics has been responsible for the improvement in life expectancy. In fact this is not as large a change as assumed. In 1841 in Britain, a man of 50 years had a life expectancy of 20.0 years. In 1976 it was 22.7 years. This is a remarkably small improvement. The overall increase in life expectancy from birth has been due to decreases in infant mortality. This has declined due to changes in living conditions and not to medical treatments.

[25] More recent advances may be put into perspective by the following. "There have been considerable advances in some rare conditions but with perhaps two exceptions, peptic ulcer and renal failure, there is no major common disease in which it is possible to demonstrate convincingly that those receiving the best treatment in 1985 are much better off than those who received the best treatment in 1960." Oxford Textbook of Medicine, Volume 1: Page 2.1 (Oxford University Press, 1987).

[26] "Medical Nemesis" by Ivan Illich (Bantam, 1976).

[27] Epoch, Volume 4, M. Nightingale 1982-3.

It is certainly true that vaccination has an effect on the body, I am not claiming otherwise. However, the perceived result may not be the real result. If you apply the principles of energetic medicine to vaccination we can postulate the following:

There are two possibilities following vaccination. It can either have an effect or it cannot. The vaccination can only affect the person if they were already susceptible to that particular disease. If there is no susceptibility then neither the disease nor the vaccination can affect the person.

If the person is susceptible then three basic reactions are possible:

i) Mild, with local irritation - this infers that there is a connection energetically with the vaccine but the person's energy is not strong enough to entirely throw off the injected material. It therefore remains in the system manifesting later as a chronic condition. In terms of Chinese medicine this may be analogous to a case of pathogenic factor remaining in the body.

ii) Stronger reaction such as fever where the body's energy is strong and may throw off the vaccine completely.

iii) Very strong reaction such as encephalitis, brain damage, meningitis, paralysis. There is susceptibility but the person's energy is so weak that the vaccine enters deep into the body and damages vital organs or in some cases causes death.

So, if a person has a vaccination and later does not develop the disease, there are several possibilities:

* not susceptible - vaccination has no effect, would not have developed disease anyway
* no contact
* unrecognised - this is common since medical practitioners are reluctant to diagnose, e.g. whooping cough in those who have been vaccinated as this would lead to doubts being cast upon the effectiveness of the vaccine
* immune system damaged - the energy of the person has been impaired to the extent that manifestations of acute disease are not possible. At some time in the future there may be the appearance of a chronic disease.

At this point I want to mention the effects of smallpox vaccination which in the latter years of use caused far more deaths than the actual disease.

Between 1953 and 1961 in a population of 47 million there were 11 deaths from smallpox. In the same time there were 37 deaths from the vaccination but in only 1/2 million people vaccinated. This gives an excess of deaths in the case of smallpox vaccination 316 times that of the disease itself.[28]

In the 25 years ended December 1962, nearly 2/3 of the children born in England and Wales remained unvaccinated for smallpox yet only 4 children under 5 died from smallpox. In the 1/3 who were vaccinated, no less than 86 children under 5 were killed by vaccination and many more were seriously injured by it. [29]

In a military hospital in 1944, 100 consecutive cases of smallpox were studied and 96% of those were vaccinated. 70% had been vaccinated within the last two years. 14 cases died and of these only 1 had not been vaccinated. It can be concluded that vaccination failed to prevent smallpox and death from smallpox.

However smallpox is no longer a problem since there have been no recorded cases since the late 1970's. It has always been attributed to the practice of vaccination but I would suggest that contact tracing and isolation were at least as important if the effectiveness of the vaccine is as indicated above.

What is more important for people today is the use of vaccination for diseases of children. These may either be the 'normal' diseases of measles, mumps, rubella or for those illnesses which are now very rare in the West such as polio, diptheria and tetanus.

---

[28] Reports of the Registrar General.
[29] Parliamentary reply, February 12th 1964.

MEASLES VACCINATION[30]

Mass vaccination began in 1968 with an uptake rate of 71% in 1986 (in some areas 29%, in others 89%). In the case of measles the death rate showed a similar marked fall before the introduction of mass vaccination and before the introduction of antibiotics in any great quantity. The argument for the introduction of measles vaccination is that it kills some children. Whilst this is true we have to consider whether it protects *at all*. The graph in Table 5.12 illustrates the changes in deaths from measles over the past century. It is clear from this the effect on death rate of mass vaccination.

An epidemic of measles in the US in 1990[31] has cast doubts on whether vaccination is so effective for this disease as formerly thought[32]. There were the highest number of cases for the previous 10 years. It seemed from comments by scientists at the Centre for Disease Control in Atlanta that up to 40% of cases had been vaccinated. Since only half of children had been vaccinated the conclusion is self-evident - vaccination is of no use. As a result, the Centre of Disease Control has recommended that everyone have a *second* vaccination. Some states have introduced legislation to make this legally enforceable. Presumably in ten years we shall see pressure for a third vaccination ..... and a fourth .... and a fifth.

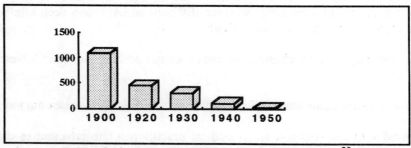

TABLE 5.12: DEATHS PER MILLION FROM MEASLES[33]

There are several possible known sequelae of measles vaccination. These include:

- Fever in up to 15% - begins 5-6 after vaccination and lasts for 2 days
- Febrile convulsion will occur in some with fever
- Rash in 5% - begins 7-10 days after vaccination and lasts for 2-4 days
- Encephalitis
- Encephalopathy
- Syndrome of muscle weakness, wasting, tingling and numbness (Guillain-Barre syndrome)
- Reye's syndrome
- Squint
- Blurred vision and other visual disturbances
- Hearing loss
- Lack of co-ordination and balance
- Arthralgia
- Arthritis
- Allergy
- Bruising or other bleeding abnormalities
- Weight fluctuations in the weeks or months after vaccination[34]
- Decreased lymphocyte number and activity[35]

---

[30] In developing countries, there is the use of high strength vaccine in children under 1 year of age which causes *increased* mortality - Lancet, October 12th, 1991: 903-906
[31] General Practitioner, August 24th 1990.
[32] In 1978, an announcement was made in the USA of the goal of eliminating measles by 1982. History has revealed the worth of this rather grandiose scheme.
[33] Epoch, Volume 4, M. Nightingale 1982-3.
[34] American Journal of Clinical Nutrition 1977; 30: 592-98.
[35] Clinical Immunopathology 1981; 21: 341-50.

RUBELLA VACCINATION

In the case of rubella, German measles, the problem is not with the person with the disease but the foetus in cases of pregnancy. Therefore, vaccination of pre-pregnant females is advocated as the answer to this problem. It was introduced in 1970. However over 2% of susceptible pregnant women still develop rubella and so rubella is now given to children of both sexes between the ages of 12 and 24 months. In spite of high vaccination rates there was no detectable reduction in the numbers of babies born with congenital defects.[36]

As vaccination was offered only to females before 1988 it provided a good opportunity to study the differences in the occurrence of the disease in males and females. A Glasgow practice investigated people's immunity to rubella after a vaccination take-up level of 86-87%. There was no significant difference in the incidence of German measles between males and females.

Certainly, any vaccination offered should only be done after the immune status of the child has been ascertained. Since many cases of rubella are sub-clinical, children may in fact have had the disease without knowing. Any immunity gained from the vaccination lasts for a variable length of time and there is little information concerning long-term immune states. Reinfection does occur in vaccinated individual individuals with figures quoted of around 50% and if in pregnancy can lead to foetal abnormalities.[37]

Complications after the vaccine are common especially the joint pains which are seen in adults with more severe cases of the natural type of rubella. 26%-40% of those receiving vaccination in mass campaigns develop arthralgia.[38]

The most effective way of attaining immunity seems to be "rubella parties" where children are actively put into contact with someone with rubella in order to develop the disease and gain natural immunity.

There are several possible known sequelae of rubella vaccination. These include:

- 40 days after vaccination a typical reaction is pins and needles, pains in the arms or pain in knee with desire for crouching
- multiple nerve problems with weakness and tingling
- tingling and weakness of the hands (carpal tunnel syndrome)
- Syndrome of muscle weakness, wasting, tingling and numbness (Guillain-Barre syndrome)
- reduced platelet count
- suppression of cellular immunity
- blurred vision (optic neuritis)
- pins and needles, numbness in the face

MUMPS VACCINATION

This is a relatively new vaccination in the UK and was introduced in 1988. At the same time mumps was made a notifiable disease. This will make the subsequent analysis of the effects of mumps vaccine impossible since the figures before and after that date cannot be directly compared. It is given as part of the measles, mumps, rubella vaccine (MMR) at the age of 12-18 months.

---

[36] Sir Henry Yellowlees, UK Chief Medical Officer, February 26th 1976.
[37] "Vaccines" by Plotkin and Mortimer (Saunders, 1988).
[38] Science, March 1977.

There are several possible known sequelae of mumps vaccination. These include:

- low grade fever
- inflammation of the parotid gland
- pain and swelling of the testes (orchitis)
- weakness, numbness and tingling (neuritis)
- encephalopathy
- nerve deafness
- allergic reactions
- a post-vaccination syndrome of glandular swelling, tiredness and malaise

WHOOPING COUGH VACCINATION

Mass campaigns for this vaccine began in 1956 with a 67% uptake rate in 1986. The changes in the death rate from this disease during this century are shown in Table 5.13 - date of mass vaccination marked with an arrow. The case of whooping cough vaccination is very much of topical interest as we are constantly being exhorted to vaccinate against this illness even to the point of mass marketing techniques being used on television showing the distressing picture of a child suffering from whooping cough. This is not a technique which is employed to enable people to make a rational decision. The problems surrounding whooping cough vaccination have been known for years and several authorities warn of the dangers of neurological damage following such procedures. In fact, several European countries have now stopped such vaccinations.

A great problem with determining whether vaccination leads to specific conditions is that there is no gathering of data. An important issue with regard to mass vaccination is that is a world-wide experiment with human immune systems and no-one is gathering information in an organised way. In an attempt to remedy this, Harris Coulter, the well-known author and medical researcher, questioned many people about the health of their children following vaccination. His books "The Pertussin Vaccine: A strong contra view" and "DPT - A Shot in the Dark" detail the results of his work in the US. It seems that side-effects from the vaccines and especially whooping cough vaccination are far more common than previously known. In his first book he says 'Our estimate of the prevalence of these disorders is based upon a study done in 1979 at UCLA under FDA sponsorship. Its findings (confirmed by two other studies) suggest that at least 1000 babies die as a result of DPT vaccine every year, with these deaths being classified as SIDS (Sudden Infant Death Syndrome)...... The UCLA/FDA study also suggests that at least 11-12000 cases of permanent damage (mostly neurological) are caused by the vaccine every year.'

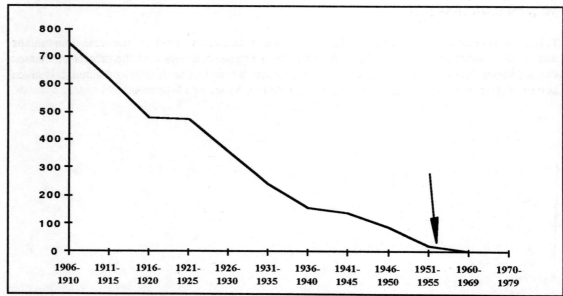

TABLE 5.13: DEATHS FROM WHOOPING COUGH PER MILLION CHILDREN AGED UNDER 15 YEARS [39]

---

[39] Epoch Volume 4, M. Nightingale 1982-3.

Trials in Sweden of an acellular whooping cough vaccine (the type usually used in the UK is whole cell vaccine) were stopped after a report of three deaths from the vaccine. The Swedes are very cautious about such trials and stated that they thought it "unethical to test a dubiously needed vaccine on their population." [40]

There are several possible known sequelae of whooping cough vaccination. These include:

- local swelling and pain
- fever
- anorexia
- irritability
- vomiting
- sleepiness
- crying - cannot console
- episodes of decreased responsiveness and flaccidity
- convulsion
- acute encephalopathy leading to death or permanent brain damage

MENINGITIS VACCINATION

This is a relatively recent introduction. There are areas of the UK where meningitis is more common than usual. In view of this, vaccination has been introduced. A similar scheme has been in operation in New Zealand for several years where babies under a week old are given vaccines. In 1987, in New Zealand, the Health Department began a trial of vaccinating children against meningitis. There was a high incidence of adverse effects leading to abandonment of the trial after public outcry. The campaign was eventually restarted with booster injections for everyone except those who had a reaction to the first thereby rendering useless any analysis of results.[41]

Meningitis is clearly a serious disease but the best way to attempt to avoid these disorders or to minimise their effects is to strengthen the immune system. Alternative medicine is very good at this because it has the philosophical base with which to help. More information on this and the raising of healthy children can be found in Chapter 19 - Children's Health.

There are several possible known sequelae of meningitis vaccination. These include:

- fever
- local pain and redness

TETANUS VACCINATION

Routine vaccination for tetanus began in 1961. It is routinely given to everyone in this country. The disease is a rare infection gained from infected penetrating injuries. Wound hygiene is of paramount importance in these situations and there is doubt as to the efficacy of the vaccine. Certainly, there are homoeopathic remedies available that can specifically prevent problems after perforating injuries. Immunoglobulin is given to those with a high likelihood of developing the disease such as neglected perforating wounds.

There are several possible known sequelae of tetanus vaccination. These include:

- local reaction in up to 95% - the likelihood of this increases with each dose
- oedema
- redness in 25-30%
- enlarged lymphatic glands
- fever
- numbness, pins and needles (peripheral neuropathy)
- convulsions
- allergic reactions

---

[40] New Scientist 1989, 1689,24.
[41] Leaflet "Immunisation - Introduction to a New Perspective" by Marcus Williams.

DIPTHERIA VACCINATION

Diptheria, the third component of the triple vaccine (DPT), is extremely rare in this country and yet the vast majority of the population is still vaccinated. The rationale behind this seems dubious to say the least. What is the point of vaccination against a non-existent disease?

The late Dr Robert Mendelsohn, a US paediatrician, was well known for his opposition to many conventional treatments of little or no use. He stated that there is as much likelihood of contracting diptheria in the US as being bitten by a cobra.[42]

There are several possible known sequelae of diptheria vaccination. These include:

- local reactions
- encephalopathy - this has been reported in 1 study and showed an increase in central nervous system damage[43]

POLIO VACCINATION

Polio is another disease which rarely occurs in the Western world. When polio does occur it usually does so only in vaccinated cases rather than in unvaccinated. Vaccination, using a live vaccine (see Table 5.14) is the deliberate introduction of live polio virus into the environment. There are repeated instances of parents developing the disease after catching it from their recently vaccinated children.

The factor in the development of polio is living conditions and so in societies where sewage has been separated from drinking water it is extremely rare.

The immune status of the person is important as seen with the epidemics of polio in the 1940's and 1950's in people who had their tonsils removed. Polio virus is found in those who do not contract the clinical disease with the ratio of infection with no symptoms to disease being 1000:1 in children and 75:1 in adults. Certainly, of all the vaccinations polio is the most "natural" in terms of how it is administered. The worst thing to do to the body is to inject infective material directly into the blood stream as occurs with the rarely used Salk vaccine. Therefore, of the two types of polio vaccine - the live oral or the killed injection you have a dilemma - introduce live polio virus into the community or risk damage to the immune system with injected morbid material.

However neither may be particularly effective in terms of protection. Despite the introduction of vaccination into Africa, Asia and South America the disease has actually *increased* considerably.[44] The decline in polio cases in Europe occurred at exactly the same time as the decline in the USA although there was no mass vaccination in Europe at the time.

COMMENTS

The foregoing discussion of vaccination may present information which is new to you. Certainly, during my training at medical school and beyond, I was completely unaware that these ideas existed. There is clearly a subconscious, if not deliberate, attempt to hide the truth. I would only ask you to consider this information and decide for yourself. Many people have serious misgivings about vaccination and seek help from alternative practitioners. I would hope that the information I have quoted here and other sources will be more widely available in the future.[45]

---

[42] "Confessions of a Medical Heretic" by Robert Mendelsohn (1984)
[43] British Medical Journal 1981, 282: 1595-99
[44] World Health Organisation Bulletin, 1980.
[45] A clear and concise description of vaccination and its problems is contained in "Mass Immunisation - A Point in Question" by Trevor Gunn (Cutting Edge Publications, 1992). This is published in booklet form and is useful to have in the waiting room or to be given to patients.

VACCINATION	AGE
Diptheria, tetanus, whooping cough (pertussis) -DTP or triple vaccine	May vary according to the preferences of your region but when I qualified it was 5, 7 and 13 months. Now it is more likely to be 2, 3 and 4 months.
Polio (oral)	With the DTP vaccine
Meningitis (haemophilus influenzae - HIB)	With DTP and MMR vaccines
Measles, mumps and rubella (MMR)	12-18 months [46]
Diptheria, tetanus and polio (oral) booster	5 years
Tetanus booster	every 5 years
Rubella	Females aged 10-14 years
Bacille Calmette Guerin (tuberculosis) BCG	As a baby in inner city areas where tuberculosis is increasing. At about 12-14 years otherwise
Polio (oral) booster	18 years

TABLE 5.14: CURRENT VACCINATION SCHEDULE IN UK

VACCINE	PRESENTATION	CONVENTIONAL CONTRAINDICATIONS
CHOLERA	Killed organisms injected	Acute illness, fever, hypersensitivity (may result from repeated vaccinations).
DIPTHERIA	Toxin injected (alone or as part of DPT or as part of DT)	Acute illness, fever.
HEPATITIS B	Killed organisms injected - two types, one from human plasma and the other from yeast cells	Severe infection
HEPATITIS B - for contacts	Human immunoglobulin	Lasts a few weeks only. Not to be given within 3 weeks of a live virus vaccination. Live virus vaccinations must be given over 3 weeks before or 3 months after.
HEPATITIS A	Human immunoglobulin	For contacts. Lasts a few weeks only. Live virus vaccinations must be given over 3 weeks before or 3 months after.
INFLUENZA	Killed organisms injected	Hypersensitivity to egg, acute illness, fever, pregnancy. Children under four years.
MEASLES	Live organisms injected- contains neomycin and polymyxin (alone or as part of MMR).	Acute illness, fever, lymphatic system malignancy, pregnancy, people receiving immunosuppressants, corticosteroids or radiotherapy, allergy [47] to neomycin or polymycin, hypersensitivity to egg.
MEASLES, MUMPS, RUBELLA (MMR)	Live organisms injected	See individual entries under measles and rubella
POLIO	Live organisms (oral) - usual in UK - contains small amounts of penicillin, streptomycin, polymyxin, neomycin.. Killed organisms (injection) - contains small amounts of penicillin, streptomycin, neomycin.	Acute illness, fever, vomiting, diarrhoea, malignancy of the lymphatic system, in the first four months of pregnancy, hypersensitivity to the antibiotics contained in the vaccine.

[46] This vaccine (MMR) is given even with a history of these diseases or previous vaccination of measles.
[47] Allergy here indicates any allergic reaction to a substance of mild nature. Hypersensitivity refers to severe allergic phenomenona which would include wheezing, cyanosis, breathing difficulties, low blood pressure, fainting, shock, urticaria.

RUBELLA	Live organisms injected (alone or as part of MMR)	Acute illness, fever, malignancy of the lymphatic system, pregnancy, people receiving immunosuppressants, corticosteroids or radiotherapy, hypersensitivity to neomycin or polymycin. Avoid pregnancy for one month after vaccination.
TETANUS	Toxin injected (alone or as part of DPT or as part of DT)	Acute illness, fever.
TUBERCULOSIS (BCG)	Live organisms injected - unless newly born everyone must have skin test first to check for hypersensitivity to the vaccine	Acute illness, fever, positive sensitivity to the vaccine, generalised septic skin conditions (if eczema is present than may be vaccinated on normal skin area), people receiving immunosuppressant drugs, corticosteroids, radiotherapy, malignancy of the lymphatic system
TYPHOID	Killed organism injected	Under 1 year of age, acute illness, fever, typhoid outbreak, hypersensitivity (may result from repeated administration)
WHOOPING COUGH	Killed organism injected (alone or as part of DPT)	Acute illness, fever, history of severe reaction to a previous dose. Special care in those with cerebral damage, history of convulsions in child or immediate family.

TABLE 5.15: COMMONLY ADMINISTERED VACCINATIONS - METHODS AND EFFECTS

The conventional contraindications are reasonable as far as they go but I would add some of my own. These are not the accepted medical view

Avoid vaccination in any chronic disease but particularly neurological conditions of any type, allergic conditions or conditions where allergy is a factor, current treatment with any drug which depletes the immune system including antibiotics, pregnancy, breast feeding, anyone with an immature immune system - this is certainly everyone under the age of six months of age but strictly speaking means anyone under about 18 years of age.

VACCINATION AND FOREIGN TRAVEL

Some people say to me that they accept the arguments about vaccination in this country but what about travel to other countries? If the statements about vaccination in this country are true then they must also hold true for diseases such as hepatitis, typhoid, cholera and so on.

In terms of compulsory vaccinations, these are restricted to yellow fever in some African and South American countries. In addition, specific vaccinations such as cholera or typhoid may be compulsory from time to time in areas where there is currently an outbreak. All other vaccinations and treatments are recommended only.

It would seem sensible to avoid contact as much as possible with contaminated food and water, biting insects and so forth. Travel does entail a certain degree of risk. It is clear from the information above that vaccination does not remove such risk. We all have to make decisions for ourselves based upon knowledge and what we would like to do.

- HOW TO RECOGNISE SERIOUS CONDITIONS IN ACUTE INFECTIOUS DISEASE -

A common question that is asked by alternative practitioners is how to recognise when people may have disease which is life-threatening or dangerous. In such cases hospital treatment may be required or the help of a conventionally trained practitioner. The table below is a guide to problems to look for. In children you obviously have to be more circumspect because their symptoms change more quickly. If you treat a person with such symptoms then more frequent monitoring will be necessary. In terms of acupuncture you would treat the person every day or so and in the case of herbs perhaps give enough for two or three days. In these situations it is important to be available by telephone.

SYMPTOMS	COMMENTS
FEVER VERY HIGH	104°F (40°C) and above. This indicates potentially severe disease. There is strong vital energy but the process may damage the person.
FEVER MILD	Perhaps 99-100°F (37.2-37.8°C) - may indicate mild disease but could be the beginning of severe disease in a weak person, i.e. vital energy too weak to generate fever.
FEVER PROLONGED	Most fevers last a day or so. If several days have elapsed then this is of concern that the person is not strong enough to throw off the problem.
DEHYDRATION	This may result from loss of fluids, e.g. diarrhoea and vomiting or lack of intake. In babies look for dry skin/lips, decreased skin elasticity, strong urine, scanty urine or even dry nappy, sleepy, lack of responsiveness. In older people there will be reported thirst also.
SYMPTOM SEVERITY	The stronger the symptoms, e.g. lots of diarrhoea, lots of vomiting then this is potentially serious. However be careful since weak people have weak symptoms, e.g. pneumonia in the elderly or people with A.I.D.S. may present only with breathlessness - no cough and no fever. It is important to assess each case carefully.
SITE OF SYMPTOMS	Are these in the superficial levels of the body or involving internal organs? If symptoms occur indicating pathology in the lung, kidney, liver, heart or central nervous system then these are clearly more worrying. In terms of Chinese medicine, worry more if the symptoms are at deeper levels of the Taiyin, Shaoyin and Jueyin.
PROGRESSION	Assess the direction of the pathology. By this I mean is it moving to internal organs or more superficially? It is of concern if symptoms start to appear indicating pathology at a deeper level, e.g. in the case of the respiratory system this would be illustrated by sore throat with fever progressing to cough then breathlessness and finally confusion - an effect on the deepest level (mental).
PULSE DIAGNOSIS (CHINESE MEDICINE)	If you treat a person with an External Pathogenic Factor and the pulse is superficial, floating and even overflowing then after treatment you would expect the pulse to moderate. If this does not occur it indicates that the External Pathogenic Factor may be stronger than the upright Qi. Careful assessment of the case is then necessary as treatment is likely to be difficult. The next thing to happen may be collapse of the person.

TABLE 5.15: HOW TO RECOGNISE SERIOUS CONDITIONS IN ACUTE 'INFECTIOUS' DISEASE

- SUMMARY -

The presence of organisms does not necessarily indicate disease since they are invariably found in 'normal' people.

Any pathogenic influence of organisms must be the *result* of an imbalance and not the cause.

Symptoms are the key to treating these diseases.

Ignore the organism and take the case.

Make a judgement as to the severity of the case based on the symptom picture.

Antibiotics are safe to stop *unless* the condition is severe or it is a case of long-term prescription.

Antibiotics are usually used inappropriately.

6 CANCER

OBJECTIVES.
At the end of this Chapter you will be able to:
State the philosophical differences of alternative and conventional medicine regarding cancer.
Describe the features of a benign and malignant tumour.
State the conventional management of a malignant tumour.
Compare this with the alternative medical approach.

- INTRODUCTION -

Cancer is a very powerful symbol in our society and leads to great consequences for the affected person and their family. In some respects the fear and loathing of this disease has been overtaken by the issues around AIDS. Cancer is very common in our society with, on average, one person in three developing the disease and one in four dying of it. Very few families are untouched by such a common condition.

Cancer has always been with us and was described by the ancient Greeks but in recent years there has been a genuine increase in incidence. This is in line with the increasing incidence of chronic disease. Contrary to popular belief this is not due to more efficient means of diagnosis (the vast majority of people are still diagnosed by the tried and trusted methods of old) or due to increased life-expectancy. Changes in life-expectancy have not occurred significantly over the past 50 years and yet more and more cancer has appeared in recent years.[1] [2]

It is often quoted that there is a war against cancer and terms such as these reveal much about conventional views of cancer. The idea that disease comes from the outside and has little or nothing to do with the person with the disease are, of course, seen here also. The cancer is seen as something which is alien and has to be attacked.

Cancer does not come from elsewhere, our bodies manufacture it and manifest the energetic imbalance in this way. This is no different, in principle, from other diseases. The only difference is that cancer may be severe and life-threatening. My feeling is that the emotion which is generated around cancer is not so much related to this but to older ideas associated with diseases such as leprosy, syphilis, tuberculosis and plague. The person is often shunned and stigmatised by the diagnosis of cancer, they are seen as being victim, yes, but also tainted with a deeply disturbing influence. People are treated in ghetto-like institutions, they are subjected to treatments which seem,

---

[1] "Chronic Disease and Public Health", Edited by Lilienfeld and Gifford (John Hopkins Press, 1966). This reveals that there has been a real increase in the incidence of chronic disease including cancer. This is when other changes such as the age of the population has been taken into account.
[2] There has been an increase in cancer of 11% in the last 40 years in real terms, i.e. taking account of population changes. National Cancer Institute (USA). See "Politics of Cancer" by Epstein (Sierra, 1978).

and indeed often are, worse than the original disease.

I am reminded here of the description of the death of Charles II and the similarities with the treatment of some people with cancer . The King fell ill with a kidney complaint and a series of physicians proceeded to bleed him, use cupping glasses with scarification, administer purgatives, blister the skin of his shaven head ending with red-hot cautery. For four days and four nights he was 'treated' by fourteen physicians. At the end of this time he apologised for 'an unconscionable time a-dying'.[3]

I see many similarities with the treatment of cancer today. Some people are given treatment which is severely depleting ending in complete collapse of the immune system. Some people are given treatment when they are clearly in a terminal or pre-terminal state.[4] This is a big problem for individuals and their families since they may feel hope and relief that 'something is being done' whereas the conventional view is that death is inevitable. In such cases there is only increased suffering at the time of death because they have been weakened unnecessarily. Not only do people worry about dying but also about *how* they may die.

It is this disquiet with the conventional treatment of cancer that has driven practitioners to seek out alternatives. When I trained in medicine and subsequently in practice, I had no idea that such alternatives even existed, let alone their claimed success rates. It is important in any discussion of cancer to include these so that people can make up their own minds about treatment. Alec Forbes, who helped found the Bristol Cancer Help Centre, said that he chose cancer as the disease to treat by means of alternative medicine because it is the condition which is treated particularly badly by conventional medicine and particularly well by unorthodox means.[5]

- TUMOURS -

The generic term for lumps of any description is tumour and it means nothing more. Confusingly, the word tumour is often used as a euphemism by the conventional profession to indicate cancer. The idea of a lump, and the possibility that it may be cancer, strikes terror into the hearts of most people. However, not every lump is cancerous, although in most circumstances, conventional medicine will try to exclude this from the diagnosis.

Tumours are differentiated into benign and malignant and this distinction can only be definitively discovered by examination of the cell type after removal from the body. The issues around this I shall discuss later. The two words are very different in their associations.. Benign conjures up feelings of friendliness, harmlessness, quiescence and this is revealed by the common root with benevolent. The term malignant is quite different. Sharing a root with malevolent, you can see how a completely feeling arises. Now thoughts appear of evil, invading, despair, pain and death.

These ideas can be interpreted in visual form. When people are asked to visualise lumps you will find that two appearances are commonly seen as indicated in Figure 6.1. This can be helpful in clinical practice by asking people to visualise their tumour and to provide images of it being transformed into healthy tissue. In this way people can gain insights into their disease as well as how they feel about it. If improvement occurs then the images will change to become less diseased and more positive. There are several excellent books on this subject which outline the methods used and the responses that are possible.[6]

---

[3] "The Last Days of Charles II" by Raymond Crawford.

[4] I have seen many occasions where a diagnosis of cancer has been made with a prognosis of several months only and yet patients are still treated with chemotherapy. It is difficult, if not impossible, to see the therapeutic rationale of this. If patients are not going to recover then why give them treatments which make them feel so ill? The answer lies partly in the doctor's desire to 'do something'.

[5] Lecture given by Dr A Forbes at Bristol Cancer Help Centre, 1984.

[6] "Getting Well Again" by Carl Simonton, Stephanie Simonton and James Creighton (Bantam, 1981).
"Mind As Healer, Mind As Slayer" by Kenneth Pelletier (Allen and Unwin, 1977), Pages 251-262 refer specifically to the management of cancer by visualisation methods.
"Love, Medicine and Miracles" by Bernie Siegl (Rider, 1986).

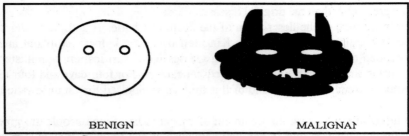

FIGURE 6.1: COMMON IMAGES OF BENIGN AND MALIGNANT TUMOURS

The duality of benign and malignant pervades the whole issue of tumours and cancer. If people have a benign tumour then there is a tremendous feeling of relief. If people have a malignant tumour then great fear ensues leading to a desire to attack the cancer. There are many military metaphors in medical practise and none more so than in the field of cancer treatment. It is no accident that wars are fought against cancer and against foreign armies. Terms are used such as surgical strike, magic bullet, aiming and targeting. Always the emphasis is on aggressive treatment. Only the lump is considered as if the person were merely an extraneous attachment.

- CANCER -

Cancer is the generic term which is applied to malignant tumours. The name is derived from the Latin for crab and this indicates its nature of grabbing at neighbouring tissue and invading. It is the second commonest cause of death in the Western World. The commonest cancers are in the lung, large bowel and breast.

Since the conventional philosophical view is that disease comes from the outside, the causes of cancer are perceived as being external in origin. This is the basis of health education schemes to change behaviour, follow a more 'healthy' lifestyle and avoid known causes of cancer. This is shown below in Table 6.1.

EVENT	TISSUE AFFECTED
Ultraviolet light	Skin
Tar based substances	Skin
Aniline dyes	Bladder
Asbestos	Pleura
Benzene	Blood (leukaemia)
Vinyl chloride (PVC manufacture)	Liver
Radiation	Blood (leukaemia)
Tobacco smoking	Lung, lip, tongue
Drugs - female sex hormones	Breast, uterine cervix
Alcohol	Liver
Diet	Large intestine, oesophagus, stomach
Viruses	Uterine cervix - not proven

TABLE 6.1: KNOWN OR SUSPECTED CAUSES OF CANCER

The alternative view is that of susceptibility as discussed in relation to infectious disease in Chapter 5. Hence the 'causes of cancer' become merely triggers that lead to cancer in susceptible people. The real cause becomes a disordered vital force that manifests as a depleted immune system.

The immune system is the part of the body which guards against external invasion and checks internally to detect abnormalities. Cancer is arising all the time in our bodies.[7] When the immune system is healthy, these areas are detected and dealt with before the problem becomes noticeable. If the immune system is depleted in some way then the cancer can grow and become clinically identifiable.. The alternative approach is to help the immune system become strong again to deal with the cancer itself. Malignant lumps are manufactured by the body and do not arrive from outside the body. The most appropriate method of management is to encourage the body to transform that tissue

---

[7] "Treatment of Inoperable Cancer" by W. Herberger (John Wright and Son, 1965)

- matter and energy - into healthy cells. In this way there is no waste. Surgery, where parts of the body are lost forever, means that this is not possible.

Prevention of cancer lies in maintaining a healthy immune system in all senses of the word. The tonsils, which are groups of lymphatic glands in the throat, serve to act as one of the first lines of defence. If they are removed our immune systems are weakened. It has been noted that children who have their tonsils removed are three times more likely to develop Hodgkin's disease, a malignant disease of the lymphatic system.[8]

Psychological traumas are the most powerful suppressors of the immune system. It has been known for many years that cancer follows a psychological shock such as a bereavement, separation or other major life change.[9] Galen in the Second century AD stated, "Melancholic women are more subject to tumours than sanguine women." Burrows in 1723 said, "Cancer is caused by the uneasy patterns and passions of the mind with which the patient is strongly affected for a long time." Sir James Paget in 1870 wrote, "The cases are so frequent in which deep anxiety, deferred hope and disappointment are quickly followed by the growth and increase of cancer that we can hardly doubt that mental depression is a weighty addition to the other influences favouring the cancerous constitution."

We see two diametrically opposed systems - conventional medicine sees the cancerous lump as the problem which must be attacked at all costs to remove it . "Cure" is only seen in terms of the size of the lump without any mention of the person. Ironically, or not depending on your point of view, all the conventional treatments damage the immune system.

Alternative medicine sees the person and their immune system as the issue to be dealt with and so treatments are aimed at strengthening not depleting. The so-called non-toxic cancer therapies, of which there are many, have been called the Gentle Method.[10] The person's energy is gently strengthened to the point where they, themselves, transform the cancer. Our bodies have made it and our bodies can remove it. The lump takes second place and may not change in size for a long time. It may even increase in size in the short term. A conventional doctor would see this as failure of the treatment.

The conventional definitions of response depend entirely on the behaviour of the cancer itself with no mention of the person.

Complete response	Complete disappearance of all detectable disease
Partial response	More than 50% reduction in the size of the tumour
No response	No change or less than 50% reduction
Progressive disease	Increase in size of tumour at any site

TABLE 6.2: CONVENTIONAL CRITERIA FOR RESPONSE OF CANCER TO TREATMENT. [11]

You can see there is no mention of the person, quality of life or subjective changes in health. The condition of the person, conventionally, is not viewed in any depth. Any increase in general well-being, appetite etc are considered as being of overwhelming importance in alternative medicine. Although welcomed by conventional practitioners, there are seen as of less importance than the overriding issue of tumour size. The general condition of the person is mainly seen as important in withstanding conventional treatments such as radiotherapy or chemotherapy.

I describe some cases later and it will be clear then that, in common with the response of any disease to treatment by alternative medicine, the actual lumps can become larger for a short time. The person will feel better in themselves with more energy and reduced systemic symptoms.. In terms of conventional medicine this would be termed treatment failure. It is one of the difficulties of treating people with cancer that opposite criteria may be used to indicate success.

---

[8] Lancet 1971, Vol 1: 431, Lancet August 16th, 1980: 338-9, Journal of Paediatrics 1958; 52: 339-61.

[9] In "Mind As Healer, Mind As Slayer" by Kenneth Pelletier (Allen and Unwin, 1977) there is an excellent account of the commonly found personality traits found in people with cancer. See Pages 134-149.

[10] "The Gentle Method" by Brenda Kidman

[11] "Clinical Medicine" by Kumar and Clark (Bailliere and Tindall, Second Edition 1990): 351

SYMPTOMS

In this section, I will discuss the general principles of symptoms seen in malignant disease. I have listed the details of each specific cancer in the relevant section of that organ.

Conventionally, these are seen as a result of the presence of the cancerous lump itself. Any complaints before this was evident are ill-understood by conventional practitioners. If you talk to people with cancer they may at first say that the lump was the first problem they noticed. On further questioning, they will admit to perhaps feeling tired, run-down or other more specific problems for some months or years before the diagnosis was made.

Some specific symptoms can be related to the lump itself. They may be understood as resulting from a progressive enlargement which tends to invade surrounding tissue. The swelling itself is more or less obvious, depending upon its location. There may be enlargement of associated lymph glands. This is commonly due to inflammation and is a defence reaction. In some cases the cancer may have spread to these lymph glands. The lump is usually felt as being hard, irregular and immobile due to its invasion of surrounding tissue. This is in contradistinction to benign tumours which are usually soft, smooth and mobile as they are surrounded by a capsule of tissue.

If the cancer is in an enclosed space such as the skull then symptoms of pressure will be evident sooner and more severely. In this case, therefore, you see symptoms such as headache, vomiting, visual disturbances and eventually tiredness leading to confusion, sleepiness and coma.

A cancer in a hollow tube such as the gastrointestinal tract or adjacent to structures such as the common bile duct will lead to obstruction of that tube. In the case of the large intestine this leads to symptoms such as abdominal distension, constipation, colicky pain and eventually vomiting. In the case of the biliary system, there is the development of jaundice.

Since cancer may be an invasive process, bleeding will occur if the cancer breaks through onto a body surface such as the skin, mucous membrane, cervical canal and so on. This is why bleeding is always taken seriously. Symptoms such as haematemesis, haemoptysis, abnormal vaginal bleeding, bleeding in the stools may indicate cancer. This clearly depends on other factors such as age and lifestyle since there are many causes of each of these symptoms.

Pain and weight loss are usually thought of as common, early symptoms. In fact these symptoms occur late in the development of the disease and not in every case. Pain may be due to involvement of nerves, organ distension or general pressure. This is why the pain is often dull and constant. Pain of this nature nearly always indicates a serious condition since energetically it reveals severe depletion of the person's energy. Pain which is sharp and changes from time to time is often indicative of a less severe condition. Weight loss occurs particularly with cancer of the lung and gastrointestinal tract. It is not seen in people with cancer of the breast or brain.

People will also have symptoms and modalities according to their own individual condition which is of much more importance to practitioners of alternative medicine.

In rare situations, cancers produce hormones and syndromes of over production of hormones may present. They are usually antidiuretic hormone (ADH) or adrenocorticotrophic hormone (ACTH). I would refer you to the section on the endocrine system for details of the clinical picture seen.

The key clinical picture which may indicate cancer includes:

* short history - weeks or months rather than months or years
* progressive - symptoms which develop over a short time with new ones developing indicating a progression, e.g. cough for 8 weeks with occasional haemoptysis over the past 3 weeks and the recent development of breathlessness
* lump
* bleeding

If you see any of these, particularly the first two, you must always think of cancer as a possible diagnosis.

CONVENTIONAL DIAGNOSIS

Conventional medicine always seeks to establish whether a lump is benign or malignant and the precise nature of the tissue before any treatment or decisions about management are made. This is because the tumour is considered to be the primary target for treatment.

Cells are examined microscopically to determine their appearance. The cells are obtained by means of a biopsy. This can be performed by surgery with local or general anaesthesia or by methods such as cervical smear, sputum sample, aspiration by syringe and needle (usually for breast lumps).

When cells are examined under the microscope, there is a remarkable resemblance to the diagrams on Page 82 of visualised lumps. A benign tumour is an accumulation of cells which reproduce in abnormal numbers but remain within the tissue of origin. They are relatively well behaved and do not stray outside a surrounding capsule. They are regular in size and shape, do not divide quickly and resemble their tissue of origin. A benign tumour may occasionally grow so large that it becomes a cosmetic problem or press on neighbouring structures. This is particularly true in the brain because the rigid skull does not allow expansion and so pressure symptoms are common.

Malignant tumours contain cells which are capable of invading adjacent tissues and disseminating to form deposits in distant sites (metastasis). They are delinquent in their nature and do not behave as normal cells. They do not seem to realise who they are or where they are. This loss of identity is clearly a serious problem and reflects the deep pathology which must precede diagnosis. The cells are irregular in shape and size, divide rapidly, do not resemble so much their tissue of origin and may outgrow their confining capsule.

I would repeat here that this is an imbalance of control rather than a problem with a few individual cells. The body has an overall control system to enable cells to know what they are, where they are and how much they should divide, develop and grow.

Although the distinction between benign and malignant is often clear-cut, this is by no means always the situation. Some cancers are designated latent (carcinoma-in-situ). That is, they have the microscopic appearance of cancer but do not break out of their capsule and remain in their tissue of origin. This serves to illustrate that there are different degrees of malignancy and carcinoma-in-situ will be present in someone whose immune system is relatively strong. In this case the cancer is being held in check, not receding and not advancing.

CONVENTIONAL CLASSIFICATION OF MALIGNANT TUMOURS

The classification of tumours follows their cellular appearances. Names are given to indicate their tissue of origin. Some cases are difficult to decide histologically and reflect a very malignant process. Of course, the more malignant the disease then the more depleted the person.

1. Carcinoma: tissue of endodermal or ectodermal origin e.g. skin, bowel mucus membranes.
2. Sarcoma: tissue of mesodermal origin e.g. muscle, bone.
3. Leukaemia/lymphoma : white blood cells/tissue from the lymphatic system.

Within each class there may be a subdivision depending on the precise cell type. For example, lung cancer may be squamous cell carcinoma, adenocarcinoma, small cell undifferentiated or large cell undifferentiated.

The differences only matter to a conventional practitioner as some are affected more by radiotherapy or chemotherapy.

STAGING

After a diagnosis of malignant disease has been made, investigations are performed to determine if the cancer has spread to distant sites. This is termed staging. Primary cancer is present only in its original site and the cells, although abnormal, are going to bear the closest relationship to those of the organ in which they are found. Secondary cancer is where cells appear in sites a distance away from the primary. Conventionally, these cells travel round the body either by the blood, lymphatic system or across body cavities and settle in distant sites. This process is known as metastasis.

The staging may be done in several ways. At the time of the original biopsy, lymph glands which drain the affected area may have also been removed. Scans are performed of bone and liver. A search is carried out in likely areas for evidence of further disease.

An assessment is made of the size of the primary tumour, the extent of local spread, lymph gland involvement and whether spread to distant parts has occurred. Staging is an indication of the degree of malignancy of the tumour and of the state of the tumour-patient relationship. Many tumours are classified according to a TNM classification, T=tumour, N=nodes, M=metatasis. T0 or T1 is an indication of the size of the tumour, M0 or M1 is an indication of whether there are metastases or not.

In some cases the cancer which has been diagnosed may be a secondary itself. For example, if a cancer becomes evident in the liver and is in several sites at once, it is likely that it has spread from somewhere in the gastrointestinal tract. In this case, a search will be made for the primary since treatment cannot begin until this is found and analysed. The fact that a primary is so small as to be undetectable means that the energy of the person must be very weak.

In alternative medicine, what is important is the energy of the person. People who are relatively well localise a problem in one area of the body - whatever that problem may be. If their energy is depleted, the disease tends to spread and perhaps affect more internal levels or more important organs. Secondary cancer arises in those who are more depleted. Whether these cells travel round the body like being on the M25 motorway waiting to exit at various sites is, I think, irrelevant. The body is just as capable of making secondary cancer cells as it is of making 'primary' cancer cells.

Whether a cancer spreads or not is a function of the state of the person's energy. Conventional practitioners see it as a function of time and treat cancer as a surgical emergency. This haste and pressure can only serve to produce more anxiety and worry which in turns leads to further strain on the immune system. A large primary tumour indicates a healthier situation than a small primary tumour which may have spread early.

These views of alternative medicine and the health of people with cancer can be summarised as in Table 6.3.

The position on this chart of any individual is a function of their vital force, of the strength of their immune system, of their upright Qi. It is *not* a question of time. If a person is very weak then they will move from the top to the bottom very quickly. This occurs when someone has a normal investigation one year and invasive cancer, perhaps with secondaries, the next. If someone has a relatively strong immune system then they will tend to remain at the top of the chart. Treatment here by *any* method will tend to be successful. Conventionally, surgery is used for primary tumours and this is relatively successful. This is what is to be expected. Treatment for people at the bottom of the chart by methods which serve to further deplete the immune system would be expected to make more people die. This is in fact what happens in many cases. [12] [13]

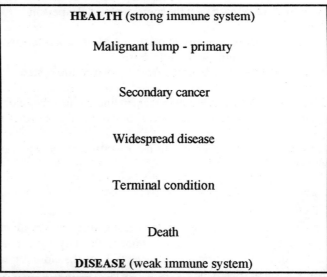

HEALTH (strong immune system)

Malignant lump - primary

Secondary cancer

Widespread disease

Terminal condition

Death

DISEASE (weak immune system)

TABLE 6.3: RELATIONSHIP BETWEEN STAGE OF CANCER AND STRENGTH OF THE IMMUNE SYSTEM

Alternative practitioners may be, and often are, accused of delaying the diagnosis so preventing the "correct" treatment can be applied. It can be seen from the discussion above that time is not the

---

[12] "Cancer, The Alternative Method of Treatment of Cancer" by Isaac Bryant (Roberts Publications). There are several references here to increased death rates in patients subjected to radiotherapy or chemotherapy.
Lancet March 15th, 1980; 580-2. This is an account of the *decreased* survival time of those with breast cancer treated with surgery and chemotherapy compared with those who only have surgery.
[13] It is one of the paradoxes of conventional medicine that the treatments with powerful effects on the immune system are reserved for those patients who are weakest.

issue - it is the strength of the person.

Cancer spreads to different situations depending upon its original site. The first spread is locally and to the relevant lymphatic glands (see below). Subsequent spread to distant sites in some cancers is indicated in Table 6.4. Details of each are to be found in the relevant Chapter.

PRIMARY SITE	SECONDARY CANCER FOUND IN:
Lung	Liver, bone, brain, adrenal glands
Stomach	Liver, bone, brain, lung
Colon	Liver, lung
Breast	Liver, bone
Kidney	Liver, bone, lung
Prostate	Bone

TABLE 6.4: SITE OF SECONDARY CANCER

It is important to know the lymphatic drainage of the body since if you detect lymphatic gland enlargement you will be able to know where to look for possible problems. These can be summarised as in Table 6.5.

LYMPHATIC GLAND GROUP	AREA DRAINED
Axillary	Front of chest, breast, upper back and shoulder, upper part of front and side of abdomen, upper limb
Supraclavicular	Skin of face and neck, external ear, lung, stomach (left side)
Inguinal	Penis, scrotum, vulva, perineum, abdominal wall below umbilicus, gluteal area, lower limb

TABLE 6.5: MAIN GROUPS OF LYMPHATIC GLANDS AND THE AREAS THEY DRAIN[14]

TREATMENT

Here I am considering the conventional treatment of malignant disease. The main aspect is to consider whether the cancer is primary or secondary. There are a few general principles which can be applied to all tumours:

- In the case of primary tumours only then the treatment is usually local by either surgery or radiotherapy or a combination of both.
- If secondaries are present then systemic treatment with chemotherapy and/or hormone therapy will be given.
- There is an evaluation of the response to treatment as illustrated by Table 6.2 on Page 84.

These basic principles of treatment may change according the preferences of the surgeon or physician in charge. Some people are given chemotherapy very early, others are given radiotherapy. There are many differences seen in clinical practice. You should view the information above as merely a guide since in reality any combination can be seen.

SURGERY

This is the conventional treatment of choice for most primary cancers. It may be used alone or with other treatments depending upon the cancer type and the preferences of the consultant in charge. After the development of anaesthesia and antisepsis in the latter part of the nineteenth century, surgery became very popular within the medical profession with ever more drastic operations being developed. Today, it is the first line in people with cancer.

There are risks involved with any surgery or anaesthesia. These are detailed in Chapter 4 - Investigations.

---

[14] "Gray's Anatomy" Edited by Williams, Warwick, Dyson, Bannister (Churchill Livingstone, 1987 - 37th Edition).

RADIOTHERAPY

The tumour is localised by the radiologist and multiple daily doses of radiation are given for a specified period of time. The practice in the UK is to give the maximum permitted dose of radiation over one course and so people rarely have second courses. In the rest of Europe there seems to be lower doses given and so the courses can be repeated.

Radiation damages normal and malignant cells and so the radiation dose is aimed as accurately as possible. Despite this, there are marked symptoms with many people. Treatment is usually continued for 3 to 6 weeks and causes what is basically a radiation-sickness syndrome of malaise, fatigue, nausea, anorexia and vomiting. This usually lasts for several months starting either during treatment or just after. It typically recurs with relatively normal periods in between.

The overlying skin becomes reddened and can break down. There are oral and pharyngeal reactions and thrush can be a problem. The bone marrow is affected if a large area is irradiated. The status of the blood is checked regularly. Hair loss is not a feature unless treatment is directed at the head. Hair loss in this case is permanent.

Radiotherapy to the gastrointestinal tract can cause dysphagia, dyspepsia, diarrhoea, tenesmus and mucus per rectum.

Such treatment can be used in the case of secondary cancer to reduce the size of the cancer. In this case, it is only ever temporary in its effect and is aimed to give symptomatic relief only.

CHEMOTHERAPY

Chemotherapeutic agents are toxic, cumulative in their effect and the use of several at the same time magnifies the effect. In other words, they all cause toxic side-effects, these are worse the longer the treatment or the more agents are used. They frighten people because they are very concerned about the extreme effects. They are used routinely in about 50% of people with cancer although it has been found that they are only of use in about 5% of cases.[15] [16]

The early agents were derived from nitrogen mustard, a chemical warfare agent. There are many different types now and they have effects in different parts of the cell metabolism. All cells have similar metabolism and so treatment will affect all cells especially those which are rapidly dividing such as those in the gastrointestinal tract, bone marrow and skin (therefore, hair loss).

The drugs are very potent and the difference between the ineffective and toxic dose is small. The maximum dose given is governed by the toxicity to the normal cells. They are usually given repeatedly over periods of several months to several years. The toxic effect is monitored by noting symptoms and by regular blood checks. It is the state of the blood which is the controlling factor in the size of the dose given and the length of treatment. There may be intermittent administration to allow normal tissue to recover such as once every 3 or 4 weeks. There may be combination chemotherapy in which several agents are given together such as in the treatment of leukaemia.

There are many side-effects because the agents are not selective and so some damage to normal cells is inevitable. In the gastrointestinal tract there are mouth ulcers, nausea, vomiting, and diarrhoea. There is hair loss which is usually reversible after the therapy ends.

The blood is quickly affected and after 3-6 treatments most people have problems with tiredness, weakness, hair loss and signs of anaemia. Blood checks are done regularly and treatment may be stopped in those whose blood is affected severely.

There are often psychological problems involved in the illness and these may be magnified during treatment. Childhood growth may be stunted if treatment is given for a prolonged period of time.

Intellectual impairment can occur, particularly in the treatment of children. Fertility is reduced in the case of postpubertal people, males being more affected than women.

Chemotherapy agents are also carcinogenic and so cancer may develop after their use.

---

[15] Scientific American November 1983, Volume 253. Article by John Cairns of Harvard University.
[16] It is useful to think about the following observation. Chemotherapy cannot possibly kill *all* cancer cells since it kills normal cells at the same time. To kill all tumour cells by such a method would require the death of all cells. Consequently, either chemotherapy is symptomatic, i.e. merely reduces the size of a cancer or the immune system will remove any remaining cells. The immune system is the area which is particularly damaged by chemotherapy and so less likely to be of help. This is a paradox which conventional medicine does not attempt to address.

HORMONAL THERAPY

Some malignant tumours develop in organs subject to hormonal control. Such cancers may also be hormone dependent and so manipulation of their hormone environment may affect their growth. Examples of such organs are the ovary, testis, uterus, and breast.

Several methods may be used to apply this principles of treatment. The source of the hormone can be withdrawn either chemically or surgically, a drug which blocks the hormone may be prescribed or its opposite hormone can be administered. These options are summarised in Table 6.6.

SITE OF PRIMARY CANCER	TREATMENT METHOD
Breast	Administration of tamoxifen (oestrogen blocker) Removal of ovaries Administration of aminoglutethimide (adrenal blocker) Removal of adrenals Administration of androgens
Testis	Administration of oestrogen
Prostate	Administration of oestrogen Removal of testes
Ovary	Administration of progesterone
Uterus	Administration of progesterone

TABLE 6.6: SUMMARY OF HORMONAL TREATMENTS

ALTERNATIVE TREATMENTS OF CANCER

The essence of treatment by alternative medicine is to support and strengthen the immune system. At the same time methods may be applied to the cancer itself but this is a secondary issue. The prime concern is the state of the immune system. When this has been dealt with the body will remove the cancer itself. All the non-toxic cancer therapies have these aims in common.

Since all disease is manifest on all levels of the person it is helpful to consider treatment at all of these levels to attain the best results. I tend to take multiple approaches with people to achieve this. Visualisation, dietary treatment and a specific form of alternative therapy are the minimum treatments I recommend.

The Hoxsey treatment is now situated at a clinic in Mexico after the US Government drove it out of the USA in the 1970's. The three strands of their treatment are healing through a positive attitude, diet and a herbal tonic. It is successful in having an 80% cure rate[17] and these are usually people who have been through conventional medicine and are now categorised as untreatable. In conventional terms, they have a life-expectancy in months rather than years.

Relaxation techniques can be taught quite easily and are extremely helpful. There is no doubt that visualisation adds power to the practice. Visualisation is an integral part of Buddhism and Hinduism and is a powerful tool for changing states of mind. Work has been done by physicians around the world to show that such treatments have proven, quantifiable results.[18]

Dietary treatment can be applied in many ways depending upon the system of medicine practised by the practitioner. My own methods, which reflect the principles of Chinese medicine, are at variance with some of those used by other alternative cancer treatments. Diets consisting of large quantities of raw, cold food perhaps with the use of juice fasts, enemas and such like are detoxifying in nature. They aim to rid the body of the harmful substances which accumulate with time and lead eventually to disease such as cancer. From the Chinese medical perspective however, they also remove valuable substances from the body and in cases of depletion, this may make some people worse. Detoxification treatments cause energy and fluid to be flushed out of the body. I have seen people with cancer and other serious degenerative diseases start such treatments and deteriorate

---

[17] Mildred Nelson, "Hoxsey - A treatment for cancer", US Film 1982. 'Cure rare' or survival rate are the terms used to mean that the patient has survived for a certain period of time - usually 5 years. Conventionally, these are used to indicate whether a treatment is successful or not. I quote survival times as used by conventional medicine for each cancer in their relevant Chapters.

[18] "Getting Well Again" by Carl Simonton, Stephanie Simonton and James Creighton (Bantam, 1981). This book was a great revelation to me. I read it when I was in general practice and prior to this I had great doubts about whether patients could recover from serious chronic disease. An invaluable account of the power of visualisation.

because their problem was not so much too many toxins as too little energy or fluid.

The precise details of diet depend upon the energetic diagnosis but there are several basic principles. The digestion, energetically, can be likened to a cooking pot on the stove. If cold and raw food is put into it then more energy has to be applied to the pot. Similarly, if people eat such food then more energy is required to digest the food. If there is already a digestive weakness or generally depleted energy this will be made worse. This is the reason why some people with cancer who eat only raw and cold food in large quantities can get rapidly worse. I have definitely seen people die due to following such diets.

Dietary advice needs to be matched to the needs of the individual. General comments that are valid for most people are the need for cooked, warm food, no salt, no chemicals, the use of unbleached grains, no alcohol, tea or coffee. The emphasis needs to be on vegetables, fruit (cooked) and grains. The principles of such treatment can be studied in several books on the subject of Chinese dietary therapy.[19]

Death is in the minds of everyone who has any contact with cancer and it is important that this is at least acknowledged. People may, through a mistaken sense of protection, not be told their diagnosis. This is preventing the person having access to information with which they may change their lives. I am not happy with people being told conventional prognoses which are notorious in their inaccuracy. However, everyone has a right to knowledge about their body so that they can choose a course of action appropriate to them. The management of people with cancer is difficult but issues need to be faced and explored so that emotions may be worked with and ultimately released. Suppression, particularly around the time of death, can only lead to more suffering and pain. There are several excellent texts which explore this.[20] Certainly some people do not want to know and it is important to respect this, but I believe that we should expect to tell people and to discuss the issues with them. The sense of relief that many people experience when they are shown that honesty and trust goes a long way to removing some of their problems. The hospice movement has, in the past few years, become a major benefit to people who are seriously ill and dying. Although they may depend upon drugs particularly for pain-relief, they are certainly aware of the issues which face people at death and are a great source of help. If people cannot be at home for their final days or weeks, a hospice can offer an appropriate alternative to hospital.

Everyone has a basic human right of access to medical information so that informed decisions can be made. Practitioners who withhold such information invariably do so because they, themselves, cannot deal with the emotions generated. It is the abdication of a practitioner's responsibility not to inform people.

There needs to be the application of a specific method of treatment in addition to visualisation and diet. People with cancer are suffering from severe, degenerative disease and require help to deal with this. The main treatments which I advocate are herbalism with or without acupuncture and homoeopathy. In this way, the immune system of the person may be strengthened and internal blockages or deficiencies can be remedied. In my experience, the people who do best are those who reject conventional treatment and follow the methods outlined here. In this way, everything is designed to strengthen them and nothing depletes them.

In terms of Chinese medicine, many different syndromes can be diagnosed as cancer. The common occurrences are of Stagnation of Blood or Phlegm with underlying Yin or Yang deficiency. Such Stagnation is evident by the lump of the cancer but there is always an underlying chronic condition which is the predisposing factor in its development. The person's condition must be individualised for the most appropriate treatment to be applied.

The conventional treatments of radiotherapy and chemotherapy are part of an ancient method of treating tumours by means of escharotics. An escharotic is something which burns and has been used for centuries by herbal healers to 'burn' the tumour. Of course, the modern methods are much stronger and there is no way of using balancing treatments as with a complete herbal formula. Tamoxifen is an

---

[19] "Chinese System of Food Cures" by Henry Lu (Sterling, 1986).
"Prince Wen Hui's Cook" by Bob Flaws and Honora Wolfe (Paradigm 1983). This is particularly useful for a description of the underlying principles of Chinese medicine and their application to diet.
[20] "On Death and Dying" by Elisabeth Kubler-Ross (Tavistock Publications, 1986). An excellent account of the states of mind encountered during terminal illness and methods to ease the progression to acceptance.
"The Tibetan Book of Living and Dying" by Sogyal Rinpoche (Rider, 1992). This uses the insights of Tibetan Buddhism to help all of us gain an increased awareness of life and death. I cannot speak too highly of this book which is written by one of the foremost spiritual teachers in the West.

oestrogen blocker which is used after the primary treatment of breast cancer and is designed to prevent an recurrence. In energetic terms it should be considered the same as radiotherapy and chemotherapy. All these treatments are hot in nature, they damage the Spleen Qi and heat and dry the Blood particularly of the Liver and Kidney. If the person is already deficient in Blood then Yin deficiency may result.

The aim of conventional treatment is to melt the Stagnant lump of Phlegm or Blood with heat and this may have some results if the person is Yang deficient to begin with. If the person is Yin or Blood deficient, then the hot nature of the treatment may cause further Phlegm production as the Yin becomes more deficient. This would be evidenced clinically by the appearance of secondaries. In some people of course, the only way to remove a Phlegm lump is to dry all the body fluids and these are the people who die whilst having conventional treatment.

CASES

Describing case histories is the best way to summarise the approach I have described and to discuss issues around the treatment of cancer. I have outlined two cases here of radically different outcomes.

CASE 1

A woman of 40 years presented for treatment after a lump was removed from her right breast some 2 years previously and diagnosed as cancer. There was no other treatment given and 6 months before attending the clinic, she developed lumps in the scar of the operation and in the skin in several sites. These were diagnosed as secondary cancer in the skin. Bone and liver scans were normal She was given a course of chemotherapy for 6 months. There was no change in her condition except now she had developed breathlessness to the extent she could not walk upstairs without stopping.

She was told at this stage there was nothing more that could be done for her. She began a course of herbal treatment together with acupuncture, visualisation practice and sessions with a healer. The first reaction to treatment was that she felt better in herself with increased energy. Later the breathlessness began to subside. Within 3 months her skin lumps had disappeared. She was no longer breathless and could now walk with no problems.

After another 4 weeks she then noticed a lump begin to appear in her left breast. This gradually enlarged over a period of a week to become as large as a goose egg. This can now be classified as a primary cancer and if you study the Table 6.3 on Page 87 you will see that she has actually become more healthy. She came originally with a secondary cancer and now had a primary. You would then expect this to reduce with treatment and eventually disappear. The conventional view, of course, sees this as another cancer which has to be treated in the same way as the first lump.

I informed her of my view of her progress but she decided to opt for a course of radiotherapy - 5 doses each week for 4 weeks. The breast lump quickly disappeared but within 1 week of the treatment she developed pain in the vertebrae and ribs. This was due to secondaries in the bone - worse than a secondary in the skin. Over the course of the next few weeks, many secondaries in bone appeared and were treated each time by radiotherapy locally. All the time her health was deteriorating and unfortunately she died some 4 weeks later.

There are several things to bring out here for discussion. People can improve even when apparently at an advanced stage of disease despite treatment by powerful suppressors of the immune system. Internal levels such as increased energy and well-being are the first changes seen. Treatment, if curative, may lead to the reappearance of old symptoms which in this case was primary cancer. People have strong faith in conventional medicine even if it has proved ineffective or caused a worse disease.

My personal view is that, in the end, every person chooses their own treatment plan and management. I do offer an alternative path for people and am, increasingly, keen that they have full knowledge of options. I have no problem offering people hope with my method of treatment since I know that this, in itself, can be therapeutic. I discuss conventional treatments and their effects with people so that they can decide which course of action is most appropriate for them.

CASE 2

A woman aged 44 years came for treatment. She was diagnosed as suffering from bone cancer some 10 years previously. The original site was the left mastoid area which was treated with radiotherapy. Over the years, different areas of bone would be affected by cancer and each time radiotherapy was given. Each time the problem would disappear from that area only to reappear somewhere else.

Some 4 weeks before she sought alternative treatment, she developed generalised lymphatic gland enlargement, cough and breathlessness with multiple bony secondaries. Her other symptoms at that time were marked tiredness with very chilly feelings at 4am causing her to wake up. These are an indication that the energy is severely depleted.

The conventional treatment recommended was chemotherapy despite a poor prognosis and the likelihood of severe side-effects. She chose to decline this and decided to have treatment by means of Chinese herbs and acupuncture. She was also given dietary advice and recommended visualisation.

Again, the first changes were in general energy with increased well being, disappearance of the cold feelings in the morning and easing of cough and breathlessness. After 3 months of treatment virtually all the lymphatic glands had reduced in size and disappeared. She then began to develop pain behind the left ear with a feeling of 'drawing down' in the external auditory canal. On examination with an auroscope, there was a large, greyish cystic swelling obstructing the whole canal. This was the cancer affecting the mastoid area and surrounding tissues. Her hospital consultant wished to treat with radiotherapy. As in Case 1, this is reappearance of the original primary cancer and is a curative event. Interference at this stage is dangerous and may lead to irrecoverable suppression. In this case, the decision was made to stay with alternative medicine only. Her view was that this was the only treatment which had ever really helped.

Over the course of the next 6 months, the cystic swelling reduced in size and eventually disappeared. She still gets some pain in the left mastoid area some 2 years later but she remains well, is back at work and has few problems. I have no doubt that if she had received chemotherapy when it was recommended that she would not be alive.

The major difference between the two cases is that the second person had more faith in alternative treatment and managed to stay with the process. People are very fearful during their treatment, particularly if there is the appearance of unpleasant or worrying symptoms. They need a lot of support from us as practitioners, from their family, as well as information so that they can make informed decisions about treatment.

Cancer, and its treatment, draws a clear distinction between the opposing views of alternative medicine and conventional medicine. I believe that the more we can provide of an alternative path will be greatly appreciated as well as being of great benefit to people's health. Ultimately, we can only offer what we believe to be true and so the priority is to have competence and confidence in our practice. This, together with diet, visualisation, healing and specific treatments, will definitely provide a vital service to people with serious health problems.

- SUMMARY -

The conventional view of cancer is that it is caused by external events.

The alternative view is that cancer is the result of a depleted immune system - susceptibility.

Conventional treatment focusses on the lump - surgery, radiotherapy, chemotherapy, hormones.

The alternative approach focusses on the state of the immune system by means of diet, visualisation and specific methods such as herbs or homoeopathy.

Cancer tends to spread to surrounding lymph glands and then distant sites.

The most effective results are obtained through multiple approaches. Mental and emotional issues are factors which need to be dealt with - visualisation, counselling, issues around death and dying.

The conventional diagnosis may be cancer if you see any symptoms which have a short history and are of a progressive nature.

7 CARDIOVASCULAR SYSTEM

OBJECTIVES:

At the end of this Chapter you will be able to:
Describe the differences between the alternative and conventional views of the heart and circulation.
List the symptoms attributable to disturbances of the cardiovascular system.
State when a symptom(s) would indicate a serious underlying condition.
Describe the main symptoms of diseases covered in this Chapter.
Explain the relevant management by an alternative practitioner of each disorder.
Explain how to differentiate lymphatic gland enlargement according to its clinical appearance.
State the symptoms attributable to disease of the blood.
State how to recognise a serious situation.
Explain the relevant management by an alternative practitioner of each disorder.

- INTRODUCTION -

The cardiovascular system consists of the heart and blood vessels. It is seen in conventional medicine as a physical object with the heart pumping blood through the vessels to complete a circuit. This view can be likened to a domestic central heating system in that there is a pump and tubes carrying fluid. Thus, there is a separation from its non-physical aspect.

ASSOCIATION	COMMENTS
Propels Blood[1]	This is the familiar view of the heart as a pump
Governs Blood vessels	This association is familiar to the Western view.
Houses the Mind	Sometimes the word spirit is used. This is the site of consciousness and many disorders which are psychological in manifestation are classified, energetically, as Heart disorders.
Paired organ is Small Intestine	This connection explains why anxiety due to a Heart disturbance may lead to problems in the lower part of the body. The heat of the anxiety may be conducted through into the Small Intestine or Urinary Bladder leading to cystitis, colitis and so on.
Opens into the Tongue	Heart disturbances can be manifest by speech problems such as stuttering. Blueness of the tongue is seen in conventional medicine as being caused by heart disease in some cases.
Complexion	This is very much affected by the function of the heart.
Arteries and arterioles	This is also understood from a conventional viewpoint
Colour - red	The Heart is said to 'stamp the Blood red'. It is interesting to note that many prescribed drugs for the heart are red in colour - despite the 'scientific' base of conventional pharmacology.
Taste - bitter	Each major organ has an associated taste. In this case excess bitter food can damage the Fire element.
Season - summer	The energy of summer is of luxurious growth and blossoming. This can be compared to the energy of the Heart which is the major organ circulating blood around the body as well as housing the mind - our innermost spirit.
Element - Fire	The Element correspondence reveals the connection of Chinese medical theory to nature. Each Element is connected to the others to provide, in health, a harmonious balance.
Time - 11am to 1pm	The 'time' of an organ is when its energy it at its maximum. This explains why heart attack is commonly seen at around midday as it is an excess of energy in the heart. Cardiac insufficiency, which is a deficiency of heart energy, is commonly seen around midnight.
Emotions - joy and happiness	This association explains why loneliness and separation have such an effect on the heart.
Mental aspect	Responsibility, gratitude, appreciation, politeness, humility.

TABLE 7.1: HOLISTIC ENERGETIC VIEW OF THE HEART[2]

Vitalistic principles[3], as listed in Table 7.1, reveal that the heart houses the mind and so has

---

[1] All organs which are capitalised, e.g. Blood, Heart, Kidney indicate that I mean the energetic view of that organ and not the narrowly defined physical structure of Western science.

[2] An excellent source for information about the energetic organ systems of Chinese medicine is, "Between Heaven and Earth" by Beinfield and Korngold (Ballantine, 1991). I mention the main points here to perhaps shed some light on a wider view of the organs. Homoeopaths may recognise remedy pictures in these descriptions as these are merely another way of describing the same energetic entity.

[3] It is interesting to note the similarities between the ideas of Chinese medicine and those of homoeopathy. The homoeopathic remedy Aurum metallicum (gold), for example, reveals symptoms of depression, hopelessness, negativity on the mental level and retrosternal oppression with breathlessness on the physical. Gold is the most precious metal and the Heart is the precious organ which houses our mind, our consciousness.

an important function in mental and emotional aspects. The comments on the right of the Table are to explain the associations which are made by energetic medicine. The information in this Table is derived from Chinese medicine and will be most familiar to practitioners of this. However, the underlying energetic principles are common to all methods of alternative medicine and so there will be glimpses of recognition for other practitioners - see footnote 3 as an example.

The emotion which Chinese medicine associates with the heart is joy although it may be more helpful to think of emotions such as love and compassion. In the West, this is seen on days such as February 14th - St Valentine's Day - when a heart is pictured in conjunction with ideas about love. This reveals again the basic split in Western life where the doctor is a 'fixer' of the machine and energetic aspects are reserved for special occasions.

The major factor to affect the heart, therefore, would be separation - separation from the love of others and separation from our own love. Heart disease is more common in isolated social groups such as some immigrant communities[4] and people who are socially more isolated or deprived.[5][6][7][8] The heart is the core - *coeur* - the innermost part and terms exist in common language such as heartache, broken heart, heartfelt and open-hearted.

There is no understanding in conventional medicine of the mind. Disturbances of the heart on an energetic level causing symptoms such as anxiety, depression and so on are categorised as psychiatric disorders. I have listed psychological disorders together in Chapter 16 for ease of study. In reality, it is common to see groups of symptoms such as palpitations, breathlessness and anxiety indicating that the heart as a complete entity is involved. This denial of anything other than the physical is seen in other organs of course. In clinical practice a psychological disturbance may be due to any organ imbalance. The differentiations are discussed in detail in Chapter 16 - Psychological Disorders.

- BASIC ANATOMY AND PHYSIOLOGY -

As I mentioned above, the conventional view of the cardiovascular system can be likened to a domestic central heating system. Although this may seem a simplistic view, in reality this is the underlying idea behind many conventional treatments. The anatomy of the cardiovascular system can be diagrammatically represented as in Figure 7.1. which I shall refer to as I discuss particular diseases such as cardiac insufficiency. This will help explain the conventional theories which underpin many diagnoses and treatment.

There are several basic facts of anatomy and physiology which it is useful to know. I consider that most courses in these subjects are over detailed and reflect orthodox thinking rather than the particular needs of the alternative practitioner. I have listed the objectives which I consider useful to achieve as a preliminary to study of cardiovascular disease. These are detailed in Table 7.2.

---

[4] The mortality from ischaemic heart disease in the UK was studied for the years 1979-83. It was highest in those born in the Indian subcontinent and especially young Indian men. In others cases there was increased mortality amongst Irish, Scottish and Polish-born immigrants. BMJ 1991 Mar 9; 302(6776): 560-4.
Such differences can be due to complex reasons. It is certainly true that most immigrant groups tend to be isolated within the wider community. Racist attitudes serve to further isolate and alienate them. These factors may partially explain why heart attack rates in Northern Ireland and Scotland are amongst the highest in the world and certainly far in excess of those in England.
[5] The presence of ischaemic heart disease in middle age is related to poor socio-economic conditions in childhood rather than any so-called risk factors at the time. BMJ 1990; 301: 1121-3.
[6] Deaths from cardiovascular disease in general is related to infant mortality rates rather than current factors. British Journal of Preventative and Social Medicine 1977; 31: 91-5.
[7] People with heart attacks have been found to have an above average death rates in their siblings, tend to come from larger families and are more likely to have had fathers who were unemployed. These factors in childhood have long-term effects on the heart. Lancet 1986; i: 1077-81.
[8] A study of people who were born in Hertfordshire, UK in 1911 revealed a lower death rate in those who weighed more at birth and were being breastfed at 1 year. The differences in death rate were very large. Lancet 1989; ii: 577-80.

As a preliminary to study of disease of the cardiovascular system you are able to:
Identify the surface anatomy of the heart and great vessels
State the location and names of the peripheral pulses
Describe the main structure of the heart, arteries, veins and describe how the whole is divided into the systemic and pulmonary circulations
Describe the events, including electrical activity, during the cardiac cycle
Discuss the movement of fluids between the capillaries and the intercellular spaces

TABLE 7.2: OBJECTIVES FOR ANATOMY AND PHYSIOLOGY AS PREREQUISITE FOR STUDY OF DISEASE OF THE CARDIOVASCULAR SYSTEM

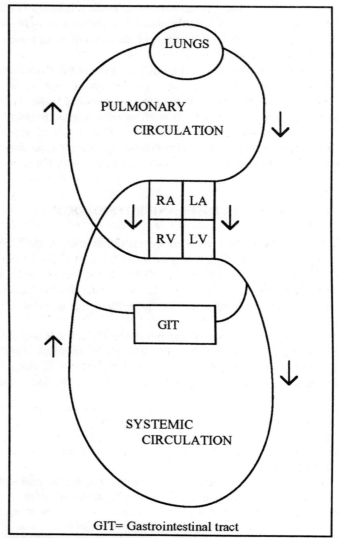

GIT= Gastrointestinal tract

FIGURE 7.1: DIAGRAMMATIC REPRESENTATION OF THE CARDIOVASCULAR SYSTEM[9]

- PATHOLOGICAL PROCESSES OF THE CARDIOVASCULAR SYSTEM -

As I discussed in Chapter 3 - Basic Pathological Processes, the major pathological process of conventional medicine is inflammation. This is considered to be the root of many disease processes. However, in the case of the cardiovascular system there are several processes which are specific to this system although they may have an effect on other organs due to an effect on blood supply.

[9] RA = right atrium, RV= right ventricle, LA = left atrium, LV = left ventricle.

ATHEROMA

The main process to consider is the development of atheroma which builds up in layers on the interior of arteries - atherosclerosis. This is a fat-based substance which gradually obstructs the flow of blood. The main constituent of atheroma is cholesterol and so theories have been developed attempting to connect the intake of cholesterol with an increase of atherosclerosis.

The development of such deposits in arteries is clinically related, at least conventionally, with ischaemic heart disease. Atheroma in the coronary arteries is considered to be responsible for the obstruction to blood flow in the disorders of angina pectoris and heart attack. In reality, there is a poor relationship between the development of atheroma and symptoms. Some people have arteries which are so blocked it would seem a miracle if any blood reached the heart yet have few or no symptoms. Others who have little obstruction by atheroma may have a severe heart attack. The key is the function of the heart and this is related to its energy rather than its structure. Alternative medicine, therefore, may produce improvements in symptoms despite apparently severe obstructive disease.

The factors which lead to the development of atheroma are low physical activity, smoking, excessive intake of fatty food and emotional stress. Many advertising schemes have been devised to try and encourage people to change their habits. They only succeed if they are locally based and the enthusiasm for their application is generated in everyone. I would suggest that the success of these are due as much to their reduction of separation and loneliness as to any physical changes which are focussed upon by conventional medicine.

The conventional response to raised cholesterol levels is to restrict fat in the diet and to prescribe drugs which lower these levels. There is no evidence that such a strategy changes the incidence of heart disease[10] [11] unless they produce an effect on the level of emotions as described above. It is to be remembered that chole*sterol* is a vital precursor of many steroid hormones such a cortico*steroid*s, oe*strogen*, proge*sterone*, testo*sterone* and so on. The connection is revealed by the similarity in names. Fat is also essential for the absorption of Vitamins A, D, E and K.

Cholesterol is manufactured in the liver and it is this organ which is responsible for high cholesterol levels. There is a relationship between heart disease and the intake of refined carbohydrates[12]. Merely to restrict fat intake is insufficient yet this is the target of the medical profession and pharmaceutical industry. The root cause is, in any case, a liver and digestive system imbalance and this is related to diet but also to emotional states.[13] The best way of reducing cholesterol levels is to deal with reactions to stress and to strengthen the function of the liver and digestion. If the amount of fat in the diet is reduced and cholesterol lowering drugs[14] given, there is a reduction in serum cholesterol for about 6-9 months and then it starts to rise again. After about 12 months or so the level is the same or higher than before. This is a common observation with many drugs. AZT[15], for example, which is given to people with AIDS or who are HIV positive, may lead

---

[10] There has only ever been one trial which has been acceptable in terms of design to show that reduction in cholesterol levels leads to a fall in clinical events due to atherosclerosis. It did however lead to an *increase* in deaths from other causes. Other trials have revealed no difference in outcome between experimental and control groups. "Oxford Textbook of Medicine, Second Edition", Edited by DJ Weatherall (Oxford University Press, 1987).
[11] There have been many surveys which connect low cholesterol levels with an increased incidence of cancer. We may be exchanging one problem for another. Lancet 1989; Jun 24th.
[12] "The Saccharine Disease" by Cleave (Wright, 1974).
[13] A study researching cholesterol levels showed that these were increased in people threatened with unemployment. These were much higher if there was sleep disturbances. BMJ 1990; Sept.8: 461.
[14] It has been known for many years that the use of cholesterol-lowering drugs leads to serious problems. A trial of clofibrate in 1978 revealed an increase in suicide, aggressive behaviour and accidental death. A US trial in 1980 showed that low cholesterol levels are linked to an increased risk of cancer Journal of Chronic Disease, Vol. 33, 1980, 311-312. It would seem to only reason to prescribe such drugs is if the cholesterol level is very high, that is, at least in excess of 12 mmol/l (Normal 1.2-7.0 mmol/l).
[15] A recent trial of AZT has revealed what many of us suspected. That is, there is no benefit from taking this drug. The result is that it has relieved a lot of pressure which people experienced at the hands of the medical profession. This was the famous Concorde trial which was presented at international conference in June 1993. A subsequent trial, to lead to further confusion, has suggested that AZT *does* prevent the onset of AIDS . The truth of course, is that a drug originally developed as cancer chemotherapy which is seriously damaging to blood has *no* possibility to prevent the onset of disease and must hasten it.

to an increase in lymphocytes for about 6 months and then the levels fall at around 12 months so that the person is usually worse off. This is an amelioration followed by a worsening and is suppressive in nature.

In terms of Chinese medicine, raised cholesterol levels usually correspond to Phlegm in the Blood. It is important to consider particularly the function of the Spleen and the Blood and its related organs - Heart, Liver and Kidney.

CASE OF RAISED CHOLESTEROL LEVELS

A man aged 52 years came for treatment. He had a past history of a heart attack some 2 years earlier followed by heart bypass surgery. He subsequently had a deep venous thrombosis in his left leg from which the vein for the bypass had been removed. His main complaints were persistent pain and swelling in the left leg. At times the swelling was so severe that water would leak out. He worked in a stressful job with a lot of pressure and worry. His cholesterol level had originally been 9.7 mmol/l (normal 1.2-7.0 mmol/l) which had been reduced to 7.9 mmol/l with drug treatment. He had stopped drug treatment because he was not happy with the side-effects and his cholesterol had increased to 9.4 mmol/l.

I treated him with acupuncture and herbs which resulted in an improvement in his general mental and emotional state. He felt happier and calmer. His leg improved and the swelling reduced in size. He had little in the way of pain and started to practice Tai Chi exercises. His cholesterol level over a period of 4 months reduced to 4.7 mmol/l. His Chinese medical diagnosis was Kidney and Spleen Yang deficiency with Phlegm and Damp accumulation.

This case shows that one problem is stacked on top of another by conventional medicine until people have several conditions at the same time. If the root is not addressed there can be no hope of general improvement. The main issue here is his reaction to stressful and worrying work and there is no point treating the surface - the high cholesterol level - without paying attention to deeper issues.

Atheroma is a generalised disease and some people present with heart problems, others may have cerebral symptoms whilst others develop renal disease. Several manifestations may be seen in the same person. Once the arterial wall has been damaged by the deposition of atheroma, there may be consequences other than obstruction. These include thrombosis, embolism and haemorrhage. The main distinction between these processes is that the manifestations of atheroma/ischaemia are gradual whilst the others are sudden. Ischaemia, a gradual process, leads to syndromes such as angina pectoris, dementia, transient ischaemic attacks, renal damage and so forth. The sudden processes of thrombosis, haemorrhage and embolism lead to syndromes such as heart attack, 'stroke', pulmonary embolism, deep venous thrombosis and so forth.

HAEMORRHAGE

Haemorrhage is bleeding and may occur in different sites and due to different underlying conditions. It must always be taken seriously although by no means every situation is severe. There are 5 situations to consider:

- trauma (injury)
- inflammatory disease
- tumours
- degenerative processes
- disorders of clotting

Injury is self-evident either from the appearance or the history. The treatment required will depend upon the severity of the injury. The more serious situations will have to be dealt with in hospital although there are alternative treatments available which can help to minimise further damage and aid recovery. In an ideal situation these can be employed along with conventional reparative techniques.

Inflammatory disease is the commonest situation in outpatient practice. Disorders such as acute bronchitis, ulcerative colitis, peptic ulceration and so forth may all be associated with bleeding. In these situations, the severity of the situation will be reflected by the amount of bleeding. If it is recurrent, persistent or severe then this would indicate a greater seriousness. It is important in every situation to assess the symptom of bleeding together with the complete symptom picture. I describe cases, particularly in Chapter 13 - Gastrointestinal system and Chapter 18 - Gynaecology where bleeding is a feature and how it can be managed.

Tumours may cause bleeding and are the thing which most people worry about. It is important to take the symptom in context with the rest of the clinical picture. If, for example, coughing of blood occurs on one occasion in a person of 20 years with an acute chest problem - cough, sputum of yellow colour and malaise - perhaps there is no need for worry. If however there is coughing of blood over several weeks in a 55 year old man who smokes, this is a completely different situation and may require further investigation and consideration.

Degenerative processes which lead to haemorrhage are primarily to do with atherosclerosis. Arteries become weakened as the fat deposits build up in their walls. They may rupture and cause haemorrhage, the symptom picture depending upon the organ affected. Stroke occurs if there is haemorrhage into the brain and this is a relatively common situation in the Western world.

Disorders of clotting are unusual and certainly so in clinics of alternative medicine. The two main causes of these are conventionally are:

- capillary damage
- thrombocytopenia

Capillary damage is the commonest situation and may be due to old age, Vitamin C deficiency[16] and treatment with corticosteroids, penicillin and sulphonamide antibiotics.

Thrombocytopenia, a low platelet count, is uncommon but as there is little treatment available conventionally, you may see people with this condition in the alternative clinic. Some cases of thrombocytopenia remain a mystery conventionally - idiopathic thrombocytopenic purpura. Other may be due to drugs of many kinds such as quinine, cancer chemotherapy, sulphonamide antibiotics, thiazide diuretics, corticosteroids and others. Bone marrow disease can interfere with the manufacture of platelets. Some people have antibodies to platelets and this is an example of autoimmune disease.

The conventional treatment of haemorrhage depends upon the cause and the original disease will be dealt with in its usual way. Thrombocytopenia is treated either with corticosteroids or by means of removal of the spleen - splenectomy. The spleen has various functions but one is to remove old platelets and red blood cells from the circulation. If the spleen is removed then the platelets present will survive for longer. There is no attempt to remedy the underlying cause. The other function of the spleen is in the manufacture and maturation of lymphocytes and so splenectomy has a profound effect on the condition of the immune system. People are more likely to develop severe infections and may be given long-term antibiotic therapy. As I pointed out in Chapter 5, such antibiotic use does not prevent the existence of infection but ensures that any infection which does occur is resistant to the antibiotic taken.

In terms of Chinese medicine, bleeding may be due to Spleen Deficiency not Holding Blood, Heat leading to Reckless Blood or Stagnation of Blood.

CASE OF THROMBOCYTOPENIA

A man aged 24 years came for treatment with a platelet count of 22000/mm^3 (Normal 150000-350000/mm$^{3)}$ At the time of diagnosis his count had been 3000. He had antibodies to platelets showing that this was an example of an autoimmune thrombocytopenia. The treatment conventionally was with prednisolone - a corticosteroid - and the advice to have a splenectomy. His past history was interesting in that he had lived in the Third World for 2 years and had suffered an attack of giardiasis. The treatment for this is metronidazole which can cause low white blood cell counts although there is no mention of an effect on platelets. Also, corticosteroids which he was currently taking can cause low platelet counts!

His other symptoms were bowel problems of diarrhoea several times each day, urgent bowel motions after meals, pain in the epigastrium and excessive rumbling in the abdomen. In terms of

---

[16] Overt scurvy, Vitamin C deficiency, may be unusual in the UK but there are many people who eat inadequate diets either in terms of quantity or quality. This is particularly true in the elderly and those who live alone. It is always worth checking what people eat on a daily basis. You only have to see the average trolley of goods in your local supermarket to know what many people's diets consist of.

Chinese medicine his diagnosis was Spleen Yang deficiency. The Spleen has a function in holding Blood and in cases of deficiency may lead to bruising and bleeding. This would be consistent with a conventional diagnosis of thrombocytopenia. The cause of this in his case was a history of bowel disturbances perhaps with inadequate diet and antibiotics use (metronidazole) as an added factor.

He was committed to alternative medical treatment and declined the offer of a splenectomy. This would not cure his condition but just lead to less platelet destruction. It would also severely limit his ability to travel as his immune system would be damaged. He was treated mainly with herbs to strengthen his digestive (Spleen) function and as his symptoms improved then his platelet count recovered. After several months it became more normal at $100000/mm^3$ and his treatment continues. An important part of his treatment was dietary changes and he practised visualisation daily.

THROMBOSIS

This is clotting and there are complex mechanisms in health to ensure there is balance so that neither extreme of haemorrhage or thrombosis can occur. Various situations may lead to thrombosis in the blood vessels and some of these are discussed in relation to deep venous thrombosis. In the context of degenerative disease and atheroma, as the arteries become progressively more blocked clotting becomes more likely. This is due to several factors including reduced flow of blood, roughened arterial surface providing places for a clot to adhere and alterations in the thickness of blood. This situation can lead to thrombosis in an artery and the clinical picture will reflect the site of the clot. If it occurs in the brain there will be stroke whilst in the heart there will be heart attack.

EMBOLISM

An embolus is, usually[17], part of a clot which detaches and circulates around the blood system. It becomes lodged in a small blood vessel and produces symptoms as it then obstructs blood flow. The main clinical situations are stroke where an embolus breaks off from perhaps an atheromatous carotid artery or pulmonary embolism which occurs secondary to a deep venous thrombosis. If I can remind you of the diagram on Page 97, emboli from the systemic veins will become lodged in the lungs, emboli from the systemic arteries become lodged in the organs, e.g. brain, kidneys etc or the extremities.

OEDEMA

Oedema is excess fluid in the tissues and arises because fluid leaks out of the circulation. There are several mechanisms of oedema production in conventional thought.

Fluid is normally present in the intercellular spaces to provide nutrients to cells and remove waste products. When this is increased, oedema becomes evident. There are factors which allow fluid into these spaces and which drain it away. In health these are in balance.

The factors which allow fluid to escape the circulation and enter the intercellular spaces are:

• arterial pressure greater than osmotic[18] pressure
• capillary permeability
• balance of sodium (extra cellular) and potassium (intracellular)
• volume of water in the body

The factors which drain fluid away from the intercellular spaces are:

• osmotic pressure greater than venous pressure
• capillary permeability
• patency of veins and lymphatics

---

[17] Other items which may form an embolus are atheroma, injected air, tumour cells and fat (from a broken bone).
[18] Osmosis is a process where water passes from a less concentrated area to a more concentrated through a semi-permeable membrane. Osmotic pressure, therefore, is the pressure exerted, in this case by blood, that draws water into the more concentrated area.

These factors are summarised in Figure 7.2. Any changes of the relative balances in the above may lead to the collection of fluid around the cells.

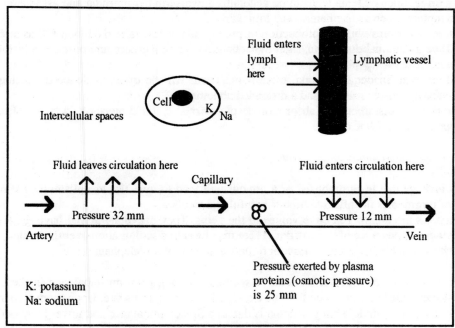

FIGURE 7.2: FORMATION OF INTERCELLULAR FLUID

CAUSES OF OEDEMA

Increased capillary permeability

- Allergy - may be general or localised. If general then it tends to be in the upper part of body. There may be other symptoms of allergic reaction such as runny nose, sneezing, wheezing, diarrhoea, and urticaria.
- Inflammatory processes of any type.

Increased sodium levels in the extra cellular spaces.

- Dietary sodium in food or prescribed drugs, e.g. commonly available formulations of paracetamol and Vitamin C contain large amounts of sodium.
- Disturbed sodium-potassium balance in some kidney disorders.

Increased fluid volume.

- Clinically, this usually occurs secondary to increased sodium levels.
- Retention of water due to kidney disease perhaps with scanty urination or no urine, e.g. nephritic syndrome causing oedema in the face.
- Hormonal imbalances leading to oedema related to changes in the menstrual cycle - this is the mechanism of fluid retention when taking oral contraception or hormone replacement therapy.

Decreased plasma osmotic pressure due to reduced protein in the blood.

- Kidney disease such as nephrotic syndrome or chronic glomerulonephritis lead to the loss of protein in urine. Such oedema tends to be generalised, worse in the morning and associated with urinary symptoms such as haematuria and loin pain.
- Liver disease interferes with the production of protein and so levels in the blood fall as a result. There will be abdominal distension, right hypochondriac pain, jaundice and possibly a history of drug or alcohol abuse.
- Malnutrition is an inadequate intake of protein. There will be other evidence of inadequate nutrition such as muscle wasting and a distended abdomen.
- Malabsorption is a disturbance of absorption despite normal diet and metabolic activity. Diseases of this type include coeliac disease.

Reduced flow in lymphatic and venous systems.

- Venous blockage due to thrombosis or a tumour will tend to give rise to unilateral oedema. In the case of thrombosis the affected limb is painful and swollen.
- Varicose veins are due to defective valves in the veins. They are bilateral and have the typical blue, distended appearance of varicosities. There may be skin discolouration over the ankles.
- Lymphatic system blockage due to tumour or parasitic infestation (elephantiasis).

In terms of Chinese medicine, oedema is seen as resulting from an imbalance in the Lung, Spleen[19] or Kidney. Oedema can, therefore, be classified according to its site. Upper body oedema is due to a Lung imbalance, middle body oedema is due to a Spleen imbalance and lower body oedema is due to a Kidney imbalance. It is possible to compare the allergic oedema described above as being a Lung disorder in Chinese medicine, malabsorption diseases would be a Spleen disorder and the nephrotic syndrome would be a Kidney disorder. It can be seen that the Chinese view of a cause of the oedema may or may not agree with conventional ideas.

It does serve to explain conditions when conventional medicine cannot do so. There is a condition called idiopathic oedema of women. This rather grandiose terminology means that oedema occurs in some women due to an unknown cause. It tends to appear or become worse either at the end of the day or before a period. There may be associated symptoms such as those which occur in pre-menstrual tension, abdominal bloating and sudden weight changes. There is no explanation in conventional medicine other than an assumption of "hormonal imbalance". Such women are given diuretics as a symptomatic measure. They come to rely on this medication until such time as it ceases to work and the oedema, which is never completely controlled, starts to worsen.

In Chinese medicine, it is often due to Spleen imbalance and explains why there is an association with craving for sweet food as well as being worse pre-menstrually. It is a problem on the energetic level and so cannot be diagnosed by the gross physical methods of conventional medicine. Alternative medical treatment is very effective. It is not enough, however, just to try to cleanse fluid out of the system. The energy of the digestion needs to be strengthened and then the fluid is controlled. Many women enter a vicious cycle of dieting, excessive exercise and measures such as slimming aids or diuretics. These will serve only to further deplete the digestive energy and lead to more oedema.

- CLASSIFICATION OF CARDIOVASCULAR DISEASE -

Disease of the cardiovascular system is very common in the West causing 50% of all deaths. The conventional classification of disease is according to its perceived cause - infection, degenerative processes such as atherosclerosis, thrombosis and so on. It is of more importance to an alternative practitioner to relate the disease labels to symptom pictures and underlying energetic states. The classification in Table 7.3 is determined by alternative views of disease.

Hypertension is missing from this list although it is invariably found in conventional textbooks in the section on cardiovascular disease. I describe hypertension in Chapter 9 - Urinary

---

[19] The Spleen, as understood by Chinese medicine, is responsible for many digestive processes. Such action is described as transformation and transportation and is described more fully in Chapter 13 - Gastrointestinal system.

system, since I feel it is primarily a disorder of the kidney. It may well have effects in other areas but it is a misapprehension to state it is a cardiovascular disease.

```
┌─────────────────────────────────────────────────┐
│          SUPERFICIAL, ACUTE DISEASE             │
│                                                 │
│ Pericarditis                                    │
│ Peripheral vascular disease                     │
│ •    Veins                                      │
│ •    Arteries                                   │
│ Angina pectoris                                 │
│ Myocardial infarction (heart attack)            │
│ Cardiac failure                                 │
│                                                 │
│          INTERNAL, CHRONIC DISEASE              │
└─────────────────────────────────────────────────┘
```

TABLE 7.3: CLASSIFICATION OF CARDIOVASCULAR DISEASE

- PERICARDITIS -

This is an unusual condition which, as its name implies, is an inflammation of the pericardium. The pericardium is the protective lining around the heart and so disease here is milder than disease situated in the heart itself.

The pericardium may be involved with other disease such as heart attack, autoimmune conditions, tuberculosis and malignancy. In these cases there will be the symptoms of the original condition as well as the clinical appearance of pericarditis. However, viral pericarditis as described below is the commonest type.

Symptoms:

Viral pericarditis is commonest in young adults. There may be a preceding fever but the main feature is a sharp pain in the centre of the chest which may radiate to the neck and shoulders. It is better for sitting forward and worse for lying down, movement and breathing. The symptoms are similar to pleurisy but the presence of palpitations confirm that the disturbance is in the heart. The condition lasts for several weeks.

This illness occurs in people who are overworked and have a pre-existing heart imbalance. This is essentially energetic rather than structural. There are often relapses at times of stress or overwork.

Investigations:

Diagnosis is made clinically with the help of ECG changes seen in the first week of ST segment elevation which changes to T wave inversion. After recovery the ECG is normal.

Treatment:

This is by means of aspirin or non-steroidal anti-inflammatory agents. Corticosteroids are given in severe cases.

Alternative management:

The main issue here is to treat the underlying Heart imbalance after the acute attack has subsided. People are often sensitive to external events in many senses and a combination of stress, worry and overwork has usually precipitated the attack. Some cases of pericarditis are secondary to more severe disease such as heart attack. These will be clear from the associated symptoms.

- PALPITATIONS -

At this stage, I want to discuss palpitations as they are a common symptom of heart disease. This category of disease in conventional medicine is denoted as 'disorders of rhythm and rate'. In conventional medicine, they are classified according to the particular appearance of the ECG. In this way, a precise pattern of disorder can be observed related to the passage of the electrical impulse across the heart muscle. It may originate from the sino-atrial node, atrium, atrio-ventricular node or ventricle.

For an alternative practitioner, this is not practicable since you do not have access to an ECG, interpretation is difficult and such findings are more related to conventional drug use. It is more helpful to relate to symptoms. The cardinal symptom is palpitations. This is an awareness of the heart beating and occurs normally after exercise and in association with certain emotions. Even then if they are excessive or prolonged it would be considered an abnormality.

Conventional medical pulse taking is limited to its rate (normal 72/minute), rhythm (regularity), strength of beat and information about the state of the arterial wall. It does not seek to obtain the subtle energetic qualities looked for in Chinese or Tibetan medicine.

The important thing to determine with palpitations is whether there is underlying structural heart disease. Palpitations may result from emotional/energetic causes or be associated with more structural heart disease disrupting the flow of electrical conduction through the heart. The latter is clearly potentially serious and this is particularly true of those associated with ventricular disease.

Simply stated, a rapid pulse is more than 90 beats per minute and a slow pulse is less than 60 beats per minute. The serious conditions are related to extremes of these or to symptoms arising from the ventricle of the heart. These situations would lead to severe disruption of cardiac function. This would be indicated by chest pain, oedema or loss of consciousness. Similarly, a serious condition may be present if the pulse is very slow (< 50/minute) or very rapid (> 120/minute).

Treatment:

Palpitations with no associated structural heart disease are treated by reassurance with or without drugs such as tranquillisers or betablockers. Increasingly, betablockers are used early in the treatment of such symptoms and even in children. This can only lead to a weakening of heart function with consequences in later life. The treatments of palpitations are summarised in Table 7.4.

MILD CASE	
TREATMENT	TREATMENT LEVEL
Stimulate vagus nerve (vagotonic measures[20]) • Valsalva manoeuvre[21] • Immerse face in water • Carotid sinus massage • Eyeball pressure	1
Betablockers, calcium antagonists	2
The drugs below are almost always used solely for severe cases: Amiodarone, bretylium, disopyramide, flecainide[22], lignocaine, mexiletine, procainamide, propafenone, quinidine, tocainamide	3
Intravenous by means of adenosine, atropine or verapamil	4
Electric shock - DC cardioversion	5
Pacemaker	6
Surgery - destruction of conductive pathway in the heart	7
SEVERE CASE	

TABLE 7.4: CONVENTIONAL TREATMENT OF PALPITATIONS

---

[20] This is to increase the activity of the parasympathetic part of the autonomic nervous system, i.e. relaxatory mechanisms. This is the aspect which balances the sympathetic part, i.e. stimulatory or adrenaline effect.

[21] This is forced expiration against a closed glottis.

[22] A trial of flecainide and eucainide had to be discontinued in March 1989 because there was a higher death rate from arrhythmias in the treated group. Lancet 1991; Apl 20, 337: 969.

Alternative management:

The separation into emotional and structural is very conventional. You cannot separate the function/structure of the heart as a pump of blood from its function/structure in housing the mind. It is vital to treat the person as a whole and particularly think of emotional factors, long-term emotional suppression, separation, shock and bereavement. If a serious condition is suspected then can you deal with it? As a guide, any situation requiring treatment from number 3 downwards in Table 7.4 would be a potentially serious situation.

In terms of Chinese medicine, palpitations indicate a Heart-specific symptom. Therefore, any of the Heart syndromes may manifest palpitations amongst their symptoms.

If the case is complicated by drugs think about whether reduction is possible when you treat. Never reduce rapidly and in the case of ventricular arrhythmias you may need ECG monitoring as slow gradual withdrawal is performed. Remember, MOST cases of palpitations are NOT due to structural heart disease and so can be managed safely.

CASE OF PALPITATIONS

A woman of 45 years came for treatment with symptoms of hot flushes, sweating, anxiety, aggressive feelings and tiredness. She had suffered with palpitations some 8 years before and had a surgical ablation of an area of the heart transmitting electrical impulses. She also suffered with symptoms of abdominal bloating, pains in the abdomen and alternating constipation and diarrhoea particularly in stressful situations. She had symptoms of pre-menstrual tension each month with a lot of breast tenderness.

In terms of Chinese medicine, her diagnosis was Heart and Liver Blood deficiency with Liver Qi stagnation. She would present with palpitations except the operation some years before had prevented these appearing. After treatment involving tonifying Blood and relieving Liver Qi stagnation, she felt much calmer with reduced emotional flareups. During the course of treatment it became clear that problems in her childhood, particularly a violent father, had led to this situation. As she became stronger, she was able to remember more and become more aware of her feelings. Interestingly, her palpitations returned some months after beginning treatment which I viewed as a return of old symptoms. Her consultant considered this to be impossible. These types of cases are difficult to treat as they involve deep emotional states, worrying current symptoms and long-term imbalances. There is much which can be done to help with care and the correct treatment. It is useful to consider additional help with perhaps relaxation, counselling or psychotherapy.

- FAINTING -

This is a temporary loss of consciousness (a few minutes) due to a fall in blood pressure. Less blood reaches the brain and as a protective mechanism, fainting ensues which produces a horizontal position. Thereby blood supply to the brain is increased. There may be several causes of this common condition. The occurrence which may indicate a serious underlying condition is when fainting happens during exercise. This suggests an obstruction to blood flow leaving the heart and must always be taken seriously.

Clearly, any loss of consciousness has to be carefully considered. It is important to determine the associated symptoms, any precipitating factors and sequelae. The common types of loss of consciousness are listed in Table 7.5.

DESCRIPTION	COMMENTS
Classical faint - characterised by sweating, light-headedness, pallor, rapid pulse and then loss of consciousness - blood collects in the lower extremities. More likely in hot conditions and if hungry.	Prolonged standing After illness, loss of fluid as with diarrhoea or vomiting On the sight of blood, unpleasant events Low blood pressure due to loss of fluids or blood Hypotensive drugs Vasodilators
Raised intrathoracic pressure prevents venous return to the heart and so less blood for supply to brain	Excessive coughing, straining to urinate or defaecate
Poisoning	Toxic fumes, drugs
Epilepsy	This can superficially have the appearance of a faint but it lasts for longer, there is jerking of the limbs, there may be biting of the tongue and urinary incontinence
Central nervous system disorders	Head injury, 'stroke', brain tumour. The latter two are discussed in Chapter 14 - Central Nervous System
Severe internal disease	These include failure of major organs such as heart, liver or lungs, diabetes mellitus[23], obstruction to blood flow within the heart

TABLE 7.5: LOSS OF CONSCIOUSNESS AND ITS CAUSES

- PERIPHERAL VASCULAR DISEASE -

DISEASES OF VEINS

VARICOSE VEINS

Veins contain valves which aid the return of blood to the heart. When their function becomes defective, blood circulation is impaired and blood collects in the veins. In this condition, it is the legs which are affected. Any vein can be affected by varicosities, e.g. the anal veins leading to haemorrhoids, the veins at the lower end of the oesophagus in cases of liver cirrhosis.

Varicose veins are particularly common in people who have jobs involving a lot of standing such as office workers although there is a large familial component. It is more frequently seen in women than men. Some cases of varicose veins occur secondary to damage to the veins as in deep venous thrombosis.

Symptoms:

There may be no symptoms other than the appearance of large, dilated veins. It is often the appearance which leads to requests for surgical treatment. Feelings of heaviness or tiredness in the legs are common which are relieved by rest or by elevation of the limbs. Oedema and pigmentation occur in severe cases due to fluid leaving the venous circulation and entering the extracellular spaces. Pigmentation is due to the deposition of blood pigments in the tissues. Eczematous changes with itching and even ulceration can occur and is often associated with infection.

Treatment:

This is aimed towards aiding return of venous blood upwards and so weight loss, gentle exercises, support tights and adequate rest especially with the legs raised are all important. Surgery is a common

---

[23] Diabetes mellitus produces unconsciousness by means of raised blood sugar levels - hyperglycaemia. Hypoglycaemia which may also produce unconsciousness is a consequence of the *treatment* of diabetes mellitus by insulin or oral medication. This distinction is explored fully in Chapter 15 - Endocrine system.

procedure which consists of stripping of the veins (removal of the veins) or by injecting phenol compounds into the vein to cause it to close down permanently. These are performed either for cosmetic reasons or because of severe symptoms. The problem is that the varicose veins return after a variable period of time and it is unusual to see complete removal of all affected veins..

Complications:

COMPLICATIONS	SYMPTOMS TO LOOK FOR
Varicose eczema	Itching, dryness and discolouration of the legs
Varicose ulcers	Ulceration of the leg above the ankle
Thrombophlebitis	Pain, redness, swelling of the superficial veins

TABLE 7.6: COMPLICATIONS OF VARICOSE VEINS

Alternative management:

The treatment of varicose veins can be difficult particularly as this condition has cosmetic considerations. It is certainly possible to relieve many of the symptoms of aching, heaviness and swelling but it is more difficult to deal with the appearance of the veins. Conventional treatment is not the marvellous cure many think it is since not all veins can be removed and they invariably return after some years. The removal of superficial veins can lead to reduced venous return in the legs and so symptoms of swelling and heaviness. There may be a consequent danger of deep venous thrombosis. Other measures include increased exercise, support stockings and losing excess weight.

In terms of Chinese medicine, the syndrome which usually corresponds to varicose veins is Sinking of Spleen Qi due to Deficiency.

SUPERFICIAL THROMBOPHLEBITIS

This is an inflammatory disorder of the superficial veins which is self-limiting in nature and never hazardous to life. It may be associated with trauma, injection of irritant chemicals or, the commonest situation, varicose veins.

Symptoms:

This condition is characterised by pain, swelling, redness and heat of the affected veins. The veins are tender and hardened.

Treatment:

This is symptomatic by means of aspirin or non-steroidal anti-inflammatory agents. The significance of this condition lies in its distinction from the more serious deep venous thrombosis.

DEEP VENOUS THROMBOSIS (DVT)

This is a potentially serious condition and is occasionally encountered in alternative clinical practice particularly with regard to its treatment by anticoagulant drugs. It is a much more serious condition than the previous one and you should know how to distinguish them as the possible outcomes are so different. In this condition it is the deep veins of the calf which are affected.

In health, the blood is maintained in a fluid state and clotting only occurs as a reaction to a specific event. There are several predisposing factors which may lead to clotting in an abnormal situation. These include:

- Reduced blood flow
- post-operative
- elderly
- bed rest
- Direct injury to the calf
- Increased clotting tendency, e.g. post-operative, oral contraception/HRT, cancer, pregnancy

Any risk is increased by smoking.

Symptoms:

There is pain, tenderness and swelling of the affected leg. It is usually in the calf but may extend up into the thigh. There is marked pain on dorsiflexion of the ankle on the affected side. You should enquire about the previous history which may indicate one of the causes above.

Complications:

COMPLICATIONS	SYMPTOMS TO LOOK FOR
Pulmonary embolism	Pleuritic chest pain, haemoptysis, breathlessness

TABLE 7.7: COMPLICATIONS OF DEEP VENOUS THROMBOSIS

Diagnosis:

Ultrasound may be used although the definitive test is by venograms. Dye is injected into the veins of the foot and X-rays taken to look at the deep venous system of the calf and thigh. A thrombosis will be seen as a shadow although the test is not infallible. Radioactive dyes may also sometimes be used.

Treatment:

Anti-coagulant agents are given to prevent any extension of the thrombosis. These do nothing to get rid of that already formed. The danger is considered to be with fresh clot as this breaks off fairly easily and may lead to the pulmonary complications. Anti-coagulation is continued for at least 6 months with regular check-ups at the hospital to ensure that the correct level of anti-coagulation is maintained. Warfarin is the common drug used. Some people may be given such treatment on the assumption of a DVT with no radiological evidence.

Alternative treatment:

In every case you should assess the severity of the condition and the underlying health of the person. It is always a tricky question about whether to come off anticoagulants before the "allotted time" is up - usually 6 months. I would suggest it mainly depends on the person's motivation as well as your assessment of the condition. Withdrawal should be gradual to prevent the rebound effect of increased clotting. I would be less worried if the original situation were due to a specific event such as post-operatively or in response to the oral contraceptive. If there is a long-standing blood disorder it would be wise to be more circumspect.

- DISEASES OF ARTERIES -

RAYNAUD'S DISEASE

This is an intermittent, symmetrical attack of pallor affecting the fingers (occasionally toes also) with no evidence of obstructive arterial disease. It is precipitated by cold and is commoner in women. It is due to spasm in the arteries supplying the ends of the limbs and is almost always a disease of the upper limb.

In some cases it may be associated with an underlying autoimmune disorder such as systemic lupus erythematosus and scleroderma when it is termed Raynaud's phenomenon. Some cases are due to pressure on the subclavian artery by a cervical rib - a rib arising from the 7th cervical vertebra. In other cases it is associated with the use of vibrating tools such as pneumatic drills or chain saws where it is known colloquially as "white finger".

Symptoms:

There is a classic sequence of whiteness, blueness and finally redness which reflect changes in the arterial blood supply to the affected part. The last stage is often quite painful. It can happen in response to very small falls in temperature. The ends of the fingers are the usual site but in severe cases the hands and forearms may be affected. The hands may be cold in most situations but this worsens in cold weather.

Treatment:

This is disappointing conventionally and most people are told to live with the condition. Smoking can make it worse and the avoidance of cold is helpful in stopping the worst attacks. Some people develop symptoms with minimal precipitating factors. Drugs are of no value and cervical sympathectomy is sometimes performed. It is of limited and only temporary help although there are spectacular side-effects such as lack of sweating and flushes in the upper limbs.

Alternative management:

In energetic terms, this is a condition involving a constitutional lack of heat in the interior and so treatment should be directed at this. It is a chronic illness with debility and lack of energy generally and so efforts should be made at strengthening the person as much as possible. It is important for people to keep warm and protect themselves from the effects of external cold as much as possible.

In terms of Chinese medicine, this usually corresponds to a deficiency of the Yang particularly of the Kidney and this explains why the symptoms appear in cold conditions. Tonification of the Yang will lead to relief. This can be by means of acupuncture and moxibustion but herbs and diet are important methods to warm the interior. If there is associated autoimmune disease then the problem is clearly more severe and treatment will be prolonged.

OBLITERATIVE DISEASE

This is a condition of narrowing of the arteries of the legs due to the development of atheroma. It is the same process as occurs with most cases of ischaemic heart disease. 90% of people in this group are male and over 50 years of age. There is a definite association with smoking as there is with all the diseases of an atheromatous nature in the cardiovascular system.

Symptoms:

Intermittent claudication is the term applied to the typical cramp-like pain which occurs in the calves on exercise and which is relieved by rest. The person with this condition states that there is a fairly regular limit to the amount of exercise which can be undertaken (compare angina pectoris). There are decreased or absent pulses in the feet and lower legs. The muscles may be wasted due to the lack of blood supply. The skin shows cyanosis and pallor or it can have a reddish dusky appearance. If you press on the toe, for example, it will take a long time for the blood to return to the area when you remove your finger. This is indicative of the sluggish circulation. Hair loss is common in the lower limbs. Oedema will develop if the problem worsens and ulcers may eventually appear or gangrene in extreme cases.

The prognosis is dependent on the severity of the generalised disease and what changes the person make to their life-style. The problems in the legs are only the local manifestation. 80% of people with this condition die from cerebrovascular disease, namely cerebral haemorrhage, thrombosis or embolism manifesting as stroke.

Investigations:

The diagnosis is obvious from the history but investigations may be performed to delineate the extent of obstruction and as a preliminary to surgery. Angiography, involving the injection of dye, will reveal the site and degree of arterial obstruction.

Treatment:

A graduated series of exercises can lead to some improvement in the tolerance level. It is vitally important to stop smoking since high levels of carbon monoxide in the blood after smoking will only lead to less oxygen reaching the already compromised tissues. Loss of excess weight is helpful. Conventionally, any high blood pressure and raised cholesterol levels are treated. Drugs may be used to attempt to increase the circulation in the legs but they are of dubious value.

Vasodilators are the commonest agent used but clearly have problems in trying to open up an artery which is like a rigid pipe! Alcohol is often the most effective. Foot hygiene is essential as any infection in the feet can lead to dire consequences.

Surgical procedures are sometimes undertaken if all of the above are not sufficient to achieve control of the symptoms. If there is a single block in a fairly large artery then it may be possible to remove that. However, most people have diffuse disease and so the only surgical operation is that of lumbar sympathectomy. This is cutting the sympathetic nervous supply in the lumbar region so that the arteries in the legs may dilate more. It is of variable effectiveness.

Alternative treatment:

In terms of Chinese medicine this is Stagnation of Qi and Blood in the channels of the legs. There are several underlying causes of this including Cold and Damp invading the channels, internal Fire due to smoking, alcohol intake and emotional suppression or external injury. Treatment can definitely alleviate the symptoms but the success is also dependent on the changes initiated by the person. Gentle exercise and stopping smoking are essential. It is important to view this as part of a generalised problem and there will be organ disease as well. General warming is helpful and people should be advised to wrap up warmly in cold weather. Appropriate advice is needed about the level of cold food in the diet and the taking of warming soups and stews especially in the colder months.

BUERGER'S DISEASE

This is not as common as the obliterative disease discussed above. It seems to be a particularly severe form of obstructive arterial disease which mainly affects young men who smoke excessively. There are similar symptoms as described above but they are more severe. The pathological process is unclear in conventional medicine. There is evidence of inflammation in the arteries and spasm because of undue sensitivity to nicotine may also be a factor.

- ISCHAEMIC HEART DISEASE -

This is a category of disease which is characterised by chest pain. In conventional medicine, the cause is seen as a reduction of blood flow through the coronary arteries. The heart muscle receives an inadequate supply of blood for its needs and a cramping pain is felt in the chest. The common association is with atherosclerosis. This scenario is a result of the physical approach of conventional medicine. In clinical practice, some people have severe symptoms with little obstruction by atheroma and others, whose arteries are severely affected, have no symptoms. The important factor is function and this is related more to energy than structure. The predisposing factors involved in the development of heart disease are emotional states such as loneliness and separation. This is why heart disease is more common in men. Women find it easier to be connected to others and share experiences. Men tend to be more isolated and out of touch with their feelings. Interestingly, as women strive to emulate men in business, the incidence of heart attacks in women is increasing[24].

The numbers of cases of ischaemic heart disease double for each decade of increase in age. The general tendency is for it to affect younger people but there are also associations with diabetes mellitus, myxoedema, familial hypercholesterolaemia, smoking and high blood pressure. In the case of these conditions, people are affected at a younger age and more severely.

Under the age of 45 years the ratio of men to women is 6:1. Although the passage of women through the menopause is often quoted as leading to an increase in incidence, the increase in frequency

---

[24] The incidence of ischaemic heart disease is highest in the 'developed' world and commonest amongst the poor in those countries rather than the rich.

reflects increasing age alone. Menopause has no effect on this rate. It makes no sense to give female hormone replacement treatment to women in an attempt to prevent heart attacks. Oestrogen and progesterone actually *increase* the likelihood of thrombosis and so obstruction to coronary artery blood flow.

There are two clinical syndromes associated with ischaemia. These are angina pectoris and heart attack (myocardial infarction).

ANGINA PECTORIS

This is the result of an inadequate blood supply to the muscle of the heart. The common cause is due to ischaemia as outlined above but it may also occur in some people who are severely anaemic and the where the blood is weak. The situation which arises is similar to the cramp felt in the legs with undue exercise.

Symptoms:

The main symptom is pain in the chest which comes on with effort and emotional stress particularly in the cold or after a meal. Rest relieves the pain.

There is a remarkably constant limit to the exercise managed before symptoms appear and people typically state that they can only walk 100 yards, 250 yards or whatever before they feel the pain. The pain is variously described as pressing, heavy, gripping, like a tight band around the chest, raw or burning. It is not usually described as sharp, stabbing or like a knife. It is felt retrosternally in the centre of the chest and often radiates to the neck, back, lower jaw, epigastrium or inner aspect of the arms. The left arm is more often affected than the right.

There is varying intensity from mild to severe. There is associated sweating and pallor. Increasing severity of pain, recurrent pain with decreasing periods of relief or pain occurring at night suggests that heart attack may be imminent (so-called crescendo angina). Certainly pain lasting more than 30 minutes is almost certainly a heart attack. The pain will be relieved by nitrates - a vasodilator. Palpitations are a common association with the attacks of pain. Other symptoms include tiredness, shortness of breath on exertion and flatulence.

Clinical examination is often normal and diagnosis can be made on the basis of the symptoms. The presence of such symptoms does indicate fairly advanced disease of the heart and 30% of people with this condition survive 10 years.

Investigations:

Most routine investigations including the resting ECG are normal. An exercise ECG[25] reveals ST depression and is positive in 75% of *severe* cases. It is more often normal in women. Coronary angiography[26] may be performed to determine the presence and degree of arterial blockage prior to surgery.

Treatment:

The symptoms are the main indication as to the progress of the disease. In cases where they are increasing in severity, exercise tolerance is reducing or where there is an acute onset a heart attack may be imminent. In others, where there is a stable exercise limit then this danger is much less.

---

[25] There have been found to be a high number of false positive results with exercise ECGs. That is, an ECG which is abnormal but with no disease. Only about 5-10% of those with heart disease have a positive test and so some centres resort to coronary angiograms in asymptomatic people to determine who has heart disease and who does not. BMJ 1987; 295: 620

[26] There have been estimates of the "appropriateness" of investigations and treatments in conventional medicine. These are done because there are many such investigations and treatments which have not been assessed by means of double-blind clinical trials despite the assertion of the medical profession that these are necessary before procedures are used widely with patients. Such estimates revealed that coronary angiography is deemed appropriate in 49% of cases and coronary artery bypass in 55%. Lancet Vol. 335; June 2 1990: 1317.

Conventionally, drugs are the mainstay of treatment along with advice about losing excess weight and stopping smoking. The removal of cigarettes can lead to improvement in any condition due to ischaemia because of the level of carbon monoxide in the blood of smokers. This obviously reduces the quality of any blood which does reach the organ involved.

The conventional treatment of angina pectoris is listed in Table 7.8. Such a list is helpful to the alternative practitioner since it gives hints as to the severity of the condition in a presenting person. For example, if a person comes for treatment who is taking nitrates, symptomatic and prophylactic, together with betablockers then this is a relatively severe case. If, in addition, the person is waiting for investigation with a view to surgery then this would indicate a further stage of severity.

Nitrates are vasodilators and consequently decrease the pressure in the circulation so that the heart has to work less. They also relax the coronary arteries and so may increase blood flow to the heart.

Betablockers block the effect of adrenaline and so reduce heart rate and the amount of work done by the heart. There is no effect on the amount of adrenaline produced and so betablockers are essentially 'anaesthetic' in their action. That is, they prevent people having awareness of how they feel. There are many types and all share similar names, e.g. propanolol, atenolol, sotalol. They have common effects which include tiredness, cold extremities, slow pulse, cardiac insufficiency, wheezing, impotence and depression. Sudden withdrawal can lead to a heart attack as the heart is now exposed, unprotected, to the full force of circulating adrenaline.

Since they block the effect of adrenaline, they have an effect in relieving anxiety. After the recent awareness in the medical profession with the problems of tranquillisers there have been many more prescriptions of betablockers for the treatment of anxiety. I have even seen them given to children for school phobia. These practices are potentially very dangerous as these drugs effect the heart. Long-term they can only be weakening and you would expect to see later syndromes of fatigue or heart disease. They are also used to treat tremor, migraine and hypertension.

Calcium antagonists are a relatively new group of drugs which have similar effects to betablockers and may be considered to be of a similar severity of action. They reduce muscle contractions by interfering with calcium exchange. Other effects include slow heart rate, peripheral oedema, nausea, rash, headache, jaundice.

TREATMENT	TREATMENT LEVEL
Nitrates • symptomatic • prophylactic	1
Betablockers, calcium antagonists	2
Surgery • Angioplasty • Coronary artery bypass	3

TABLE 7.8: TREATMENT OF ANGINA PECTORIS

Surgery is offered to those whose symptoms are not relieved by drugs. Investigation is performed prior to this by means of angiography. If the function of the heart is adequate then one of the two following operations are possible.

Coronary angioplasty is a relatively recent technique. A catheter is passed into the coronary artery up to the atheromatous blockage. A balloon at the end of the catheter is inflated to break down the atheroma. It has a risk of causing heart attack (2-4%) which may be fatal. Some one third of people reobstruct within 6 months[27] and a repeat operation is necessary.

The major operation is coronary artery bypass which has been performed for about 30 years. It is the most costly single surgical procedure in the US. This is the removal of a length of saphenous vein from the leg which is used to bypass the coronary artery blockage. There is a mortality from the operation of around 2% and symptom relief in around 80%. There is some debate in conventional circles as to whether the operation prolongs life[28]. There is a significant morbidity post-operatively

---

[27] Eur. Heart Journal 1992 Dec; 13(12): 1626-31.

[28] The long-term effects of coronary bypass surgery are very much open to debate. There have been conflicting results from trials. There have been three major trials comparing medical and surgical treatment. Two revealed no difference whilst one was equivocal. In the textbooks you see statements such as, "...but there is a general acceptance that surgery improves prognosis in the highest risk

with the immediate problems of a wound in the leg and the chest. The sternum is split to gain access to the heart and so many people experience pain in the chest for months.

Other problems include severe tiredness which may persist for many months. It is as if the pain is now not able to restrict the person's activity and so the weakness of the heart is exposed. The problem is essentially one of energetic deficiency and this is why the operation does not affect the long-term outcome.

Severe depression is only just beginning to be recognised by the conventional profession to be a problem after coronary bypass surgery. This can be extreme in its manifestation and reflects the deep significance of the heart and chest. The lungs are typically associated with grief and the heart with joy and it takes no great leap of the imagination to see how physical manipulation of this area may disturb the energies to the extent that depression results. The picture in these people is one of extreme grief and it can be very difficult to obtain relief.

Alternative management:

The only point of the operation it would seem to me would be to in cases of severe pain with great limitation of activity where no other treatment is of help. I have treated people with Chinese medicine and it is certainly possible, with appropriate changes in lifestyle, for people to greatly improve even when taking large doses of drugs. These can be reduced as improvement begins and in selected cases stopped altogether.

Surgery is an extremely expensive procedure and is greatly invasive. The term heart bypass is a useful one because this is the effect of the surgery - it bypasses the problem. Then it returns at some later date either requiring the same operation or the imbalance has now entered another organ or level.

Recently, trials have been published showing that other methods may be used to treat severe heart disease. These take several approaches of dietary change, exercise and visualisation.[29] They have shown that such methods are more effective than conventional methods. It would seem that the only reasons that they are not taken up enthusiastically by the conventional profession is these ideas do not fit easily into the accepted medical model and it is impossible to earn large amounts from such drug-free methods.

CASE OF ANGINA PECTORIS

A man of 54 years came for treatment with tight pains in the centre of his chest on exertion. The pains radiated to the inner aspect of the left arm and into the back. He could only walk 100 yards before the pain appeared and then would have to stop and rest. These symptoms were much worse in cold weather. He had a heart attack some 6 months before and was found to be anaemic. This was presumed to be the cause of the heart attack although no cause was found for the anaemia. His work was very stressful and he was currently unable to work.

---

groups." *If* they are 'effective' then this only seems to be so in cases of severe disease where there is blockage of the left main coronary artery or distally of the three main coronary arteries. Of course, there have been no double-blind controlled trials of their effectiveness. Long-term some 80% of bypasses are blocked ten years later when a saphenous vein is used. It is more effective to use the internal mammary artery.

A study published in 1979 by Dr Eugene Braunwald of Harvard Medical School showed that although 12 out of 23 bypass patients experienced a significant improvement in their symptoms although angiography revealed that their grafts had obstructed. "Will to be Well" by Neville Hodgkinson (Rider, 1984).

A survey at the University of North Carolina revealed that 83% of a group of people who had received bypass surgery some 2 years previously were unemployed. Over half had impairment of sexual function. A large number had poor self-images. "Will to be Well" by Neville Hodgkinson (Rider, 1984).

[29] A landmark trial was carried out in the US partly funded by the National Institute of Health. Dr Dean Ornish, an associate professor at the University of San Francisco developed a programme of diet, relaxation with visualisation and exercise. 82% of the treated group improved within a year as evidenced by symptoms and high-tech cardiac investigations. The people in the control group who continued to have conventional drug treatment deteriorated in almost half of cases. As Dr Ornisch states it the presence of loneliness and separation which is responsible for the genesis of heart disease. Lancet 1990; 336: 129-33.

His medication was:

- Ranitidine 300mg each night - used in the treatment of gastric and duodenal ulcer
- Atenolol 100mg daily - betablocker
- Glyceryl trinitrate 1mg when required for pain - symptomatic nitrate vasodilator
- Isosorbide dinitrate 20mg three times daily - prophylactic nitrate vasodilator
- Ferrous sulphate one three times daily - iron supplementation

He was due to have investigations with a view to bypass surgery in the next few months. This is clearly a serious case as evidenced by comparing the information here with that in Table 7.8. I discussed dietary changes with him of reducing fatty and sweet foods together with a wholefood diet eaten regularly throughout the day and taking regular gentle exercise. I gave him information about the bypass operation being a pain-reliever rather than a prolonger of life. I suggested that he could wait and see how the treatment progressed before making a decision.

He received regular acupuncture treatments and started to notice more energy together with an ability to walk further before developing chest pain. After this initial improvement he stopped the ranitidine as there was never any evidence of an ulcer. He also stopped the iron supplements as there are less harsh ways to obtain this. As he continued to improve he was able to reduce his betablocker gradually over the period of several months. It must never be stopped suddenly since this may cause a heart attack. He moved onto the isosorbide dinitrate finally and after about 1 year of treatment was able to walk 5 miles with no problems, rarely had any chest pain and felt well. He had decided to give up his previous stressful occupation.

During the course of the treatment he was called for coronary angiography investigation. He decided to go as he wanted to know how severe was any blockage in the coronary arteries. After the investigation he had some tiredness and increased chest pains for about 4 weeks before it settled down. There was evidence of 2 blockages in his coronary arteries - one severe and one mild. He was told that he would need a bypass operation by his surgeon although his physician said that he did not require surgery. He decided to defer the operation as he was doing well with the acupuncture.

This case reveals that alternative treatment is a perfectly valid option for heart disease even if severe at the time of presentation. There is often a divergence of conventional opinion and in my experience surgeons usually advise surgery (as physicians usually advise medicines, acupuncturists acupuncture, herbalists herbs and so on!). As the person improves it is possible to reduce medication although this must be done slowly[30] over several months. It is essential to monitor closely the person's symptoms whilst this is done.

In terms of Chinese medicine, angina pectoris usually corresponds to Heart Qi or Yang deficiency. There may be some Stagnation of Heart Blood which develops as a result of this deficiency or as a consequence of long-term emotional stagnation which disturbs the mind.

Betablockers have common side-effects as mentioned above. They would seem to deplete Heart, Liver, Spleen, Lung and Kidney Yang. In people whose Yang is already markedly depleted, there may be the appearance of Water Overflowing as the Yang then fails to dominate the Yin. An example of this is the precipitation of cardiac insufficiency.

In cases of Lung Yang or Qi deficiency the use of betablockers may initiate wheezing and some people die due to collapse of Lung Yang. It is interesting to note that betablockerss are used in painful conditions such as migraine and angina pectoris. In the case of migraine, it is effective in those cases due to Liver Yang Rising or Heat in the Gall Bladder/Stomach. This effect on Liver Yang is the explanation for the relief of tremor by betablockerss. In the case of angina pectoris, the effect would be due to a general weakening of Yang so that Stagnation syndromes are no longer seen. In the long-term, you would expect to see more cases of cardiac insufficiency as the Heart Yang is weakened.

Calcium antagonists seem to act in similar ways to betablockers but they are relatively new and many effects have not been identified yet.

Nitrates are vasodilators and this is a Yang action. They produce side-effects including sensations of heat, throbbing headache and facial flushing. They particularly affect Heart and Liver.

Another way of describing angina pectoris is to say that there is too much energy in the chest due to stagnation. If this energy can be regulated then the symptoms will be alleviated. Heart attack is merely a more severe form of this stagnation with consequent collapse of Yang (shock).

---

[30] "Prescribed Drugs and the Alternative Practitioner" by Dr S Gascoigne (Energy Medicine Press, 1992) gives detailed advice on the management of prescribed drug withdrawal.

HEART ATTACK (ACUTE MYOCARDIAL INFARCTION)

This is the death of heart muscle due to an inadequate blood supply. The usual cause is obstruction of the coronary artery due to atherosclerosis as outlined above. The condition may occur suddenly or with a history of angina pectoris. It is the most common cause of death in the Western world although it was rare before 1910.

Some people have little evidence of an actual blockage and the assumption is that spasm of the coronary artery is responsible. This is especially likely to occur with extreme stress or violent activity. The squash court is a familiar venue for such occurrences.

Symptoms:

There is pain in the chest which may be of a similar nature to that of angina pectoris although stabbing pain is more likely with this condition. It is severe and may come on at rest or wake the person at night. It is not relieved by rest. It lasts for anything between 30 minutes and 2 days but may be less severe in the elderly. Palpitations are common. There is great anxiety during the attack and fear of death may be extreme. Heart attack may be fatal and if the person survives then it will probably be the closest they come to death without dying. A comparison of angina pectoris and heart attack is summarised in Table 7.9 below.

Some anxiety may develop in the post-attack phase with people becoming worried about the least activity because of the fear of another attack. Such 'cardiac neurosis' can be very debilitating but can be minimised by appropriate mobilisation and reassurance.

There are associated signs of shock so the person is pale, cold, sweaty with a low blood pressure and rapid, thready pulse. If there is associated cardiac insufficiency, and there is some in virtually all cases, there may be cough, breathlessness and so on as seen in this condition.

Gastrointestinal symptoms are common particularly nausea and vomiting. There may also be diarrhoea and flatulence. The existence of such symptoms may lead to confusion with indigestion.

Pericarditis may develop in the days after the attack. In one quarter of severe cases there is also deep venous thrombosis because of the decreased mobility leading to sluggish circulation.

When considering the outcome of heart attack, it is clear that there is a great mortality rate. The greatest risk is in the first two hours after the attack and as time passes more and more survive. Half of the deaths which occur, do so in the first 2-3 hours and three quarters in the first 24 hours. Two thirds of people with this condition are alive after 5 years and over half live 10 years.

SYMPTOM	ANGINA PECTORIS	HEART ATTACK
Chest pain - severity	Variable	Severe
Chest pain - modalities	Worse for exercise, cold, meals, emotion. Better for rest or nitrates	Not better for rest or nitrates
Chest pain - duration	Few minutes	15 minutes or longer
Associated symptoms	Pallor, slight sweating	Cold, clammy, nausea, vomiting

TABLE 7.9: COMPARISON OF ANGINA PECTORIS AND HEART ATTACK

Investigations:

The ESR is raised to 70mm and there is an increase in the white cell count.

Cardiac enzymes are increased as they are released at the time of the damage to the heart muscle. Creatine kinase (first 24 hours), aspartate aminotransferase (formerly serum glutamic oxaloacetic transaminase - 24-48 hours) and lactic dehydrogenase (3-4 days) are all raised. They are usually performed daily for the first three days and the first test is often normal.

The ECG shows typical features[31] but may take 48 hours to become apparent. They include Q wave development, ST segment depression or elevation and T wave inversion. Q wave development is a permanent feature of the ECG and provides past evidence of a heart attack. Several people have

---

[31] This is rather technical information and is provided for the sake of completion to those who are interested in such matters.

such ECG evidence yet with no history of chest pain. This group forms 20% of the total number of heart attacks counted in the statistics.

Treatment:

This is primarily hospital-based with the use of intensive care or coronary care units despite the fact that there is no convincing evidence that such treatment is advantageous.[32] In fact, one could argue that travel to hospital at such a vulnerable time for the heart in a speeding ambulance, the stress of hospital admission, the constant observation and general urgent atmosphere may be harmful. Certainly, the major problem is the development of abnormal cardiac rhythms which may be fatal. Some people may be treated, post-heart attack, at home if the attack is mild and there are no complications.

In hospital, people are closely observed with continuous ECG monitoring. The main treatments are supportive with relief of pain, circulatory support to minimise the development of shock, use of antiarrhythmic agents, treatment of any complicating cardiac failure.

After the immediate post-attack stage, there is gradual mobilisation until full mobility is attained after a week to ten days. After about 3 months the person should be back to their normal level.

People are often given betablockers long-term in the belief that this may prevent a further heart attack[33]. Aspirin (150mg daily) is also administered as a long-term prescription to reduce the risk of heart problems.[34] [35] If people develop angina pectoris subsequently, the treatment is as indicated for that disease.

Alternative management:

This is a more extreme form of ischaemic heart disease than angina pectoris and so the comments I made there are relevant also. With heart attack, however, the situation is more serious and most people will be treated in hospital. There are clearly advantages in alternative treatment before admission if there is time or whilst an in-patient. This would be especially helpful to prevent and treat arrhythmias which are so common. When I was training in acupuncture in China, it was an integral part of the management of people with heart attack in the hospital. Treatment in the post-heart attack phase will take a similar form to that of angina pectoris. It is important that you know the features of chest pain and particularly how to recognise a serious condition.

In terms of Chinese medicine, heart attack usually corresponds to Stagnation of Heart Blood with Collapse of Yang.

---

[32] The mortality rate after heart attack is dependent upon the speed of access to full resuscitation measures. If so, then survival is increased. If not then selection as to hospital admission can be made for those with cardiac insufficiency and arrhythmias. Otherwise home is a valid option and it is certainly far cheaper.

[33] The use of betablockers does seem to reduce the possibility of a further heart attack although only by a small degree. There are a large number of side-effects and they are depleting to the general energy of the body. This may lead to more serious conditions of the heart such as cardiac insufficiency.

[34] The use of aspirin after a heart attack seems only to help those with unstable angina. This would be those people with severe chest pains after small amounts of exercise or at night. It is considered that 75mg per day is the optimum dose to ensure adequate thinning of the blood whilst producing a low incidence of side-effects. Lancet Oct. 6th 1990, Page 827. Conversely, a trial in the UK showed that long-term aspirin had no effect on the incidence of stroke or heart attack. BMJ 1988; 296: 313-6.

[35] A letter in the Lancet of Feb. 24th 1990 suggested that the use of aspirin given at the onset of chest pain of a heart attack made no difference to mortality. If it is of use then it needs to be used long-term in cases of angina pectoris. This will lead to a risk of blood disorders as well as analgesic nephropathy. The replacement of a heart disease by kidney failure is, of course, suppression.

- DIFFERENTIAL DIAGNOSIS OF CHEST PAIN -

In all cases of pain there are questions to ask in order to elicit as much information as possible. This will ensure that the diagnosis is as accurate as possible. There are considered to be 9 questions to ask about pain. These are:

MAIN SITE

The most important question to ask is, "Where is the pain?" Do not just accept a vague wave of the hand but ask exactly. Make sure that the terms used are understood by you and the person consulting you and ask for confirmation by being shown.

RADIATION

The pain may be felt in places in addition to the primary site. This is typical of certain conditions and certain processes.

CHARACTER

It can be difficult to describe the particular quality of pain but certain conditions are associated with characteristic types, e.g. burning, stabbing, aching. Some people merely describe pain as being severe but with encouragement will offer terms to describe quality. It may be necessary in some cases to suggest a list of choices from which one is selected.

SEVERITY

Pain can be of any severity according to the cause or it can vary from person to person. The pain of heart attack, for example, is usually particularly severe.

DURATION

Ask how long the pain has been present, not only this attack but also the whole process. Is this a recent event or have there been repeated attacks in the past?

FREQUENCY

How often does the pain recur?

TIME OF OCCURRENCE

At what time does the pain appear?

MODALITIES

This term is applied to situations which make the pain worse or better. It is better to ask an open question first such as, "Does anything relieve or worsen the pain" before moving onto more closed questions in an attempt to confirm a particular diagnosis.

ASSOCIATED PHENOMENA

You should take note of any symptoms which appear with the pain. These may be nausea, cough, sputum and so forth.

From the questioning above, done in a careful and orderly way, most cases of chest pain can be diagnosed. Confusion can occur from the history, as with differentiating some cases of angina pectoris from reflux oesophagitis but precise history-taking will minimise this. The most important questions are site, radiation, modalities and associated symptoms. These four are the most helpful in the differentiation of disease states.

QUESTION	CARDIAC	OESOPHAGEAL	PULMONARY 1	PULMONARY 2	MUSCULO-SKELETAL
Main site	Central chest	Central chest	Central chest	Axilla/scapula	Any site
Radiation	Jaw, neck, inner aspect of arms (L>R), back	From epigastrium up to throat	None	None	None
Character	Tight, burning, gripping, heavy	Burning	Sore, scratchy	Sharp	Sharp
Severity	Variable	Mild	Mild	Variable	Variable
Duration	Variable	Some minutes	Several days	Several days	Several days
Frequency	Recurrent	Recurrent	One attack	One attack	One attack
Timing	See modalities, possibly night	Night	None	None	None
Modalities[36]	< exercise, meals, cold, emotion, < rest, nitrates	< meals, lying down, bending, > sitting up, nitrates	< coughing, > supporting chest	< coughing, respiration, > shallow breathing, supporting chest	< coughing, respiration, > shallow breathing, supporting chest
Associated symptoms	Sweating, palpitations, pallor, nausea, vomiting	Nausea, vomiting, acid regurgitation	Cough, sputum, fever	Fever, cough	Painful and tender area on the chest wall
Conventional diagnosis	Angina pectoris, heart attack	Reflux oesophagitis	Acute bronchitis	Pleurisy	Injury to chest wall

TABLE 7.10: DIFFERENTIATION OF CHEST PAIN

Table 7.10 is a summary of the commonest types of chest pain. The details of each may be found in their relevant Chapter. It can be seen from this Table that cardiac and oesophageal chest pain have some similarities as do pleurisy and musculoskeletal problems. It is useful to ask about previous history as musculoskeletal chest pain may have a history of trauma. Such pain may, however, develop after an episode of coughing and this can confuse the issue slightly. The most important thing is take a careful history and especially take heed of site, radiation, modalities and associated symptoms.

- CARDIAC INSUFFICIENCY -

This is also known as cardiac or heart failure and these terms may be confused with heart attack which has been described in the section on ischaemic heart disease. Cardiac insufficiency is preferable as it implies that there is insufficient blood leaving the heart for the needs of the body. It is a relative term and does not mean that the heart has stopped or failed completely. There is a weakness of the cardiac muscle. As a result there is less blood pumped out of the heart into the arterial system and a consequent build-up of blood in the venous system. Therefore symptoms are worse on exertion, at the end of the day or in the presence of other disease such as respiratory problems.

It occurs in about 10 people per 1000 over the age of 65 years. It is frequently a serious condition with 50% of people alive one year after diagnosis and 30% 2 years after. Treatment makes no difference to this prognosis and the use of powerful diuretics is associated with great tiredness and the development of kidney failure.

---

[36] For ease I use the following convention - > means better for and < means worse for.

The main symptom of cardiac insufficiency is oedema. The mechanisms of oedema production and its differentiation are detailed on Page 103. It is useful to study cardiac insufficiency by looking at left ventricular and right ventricular types separately. In reality, the picture is usually a mixed one. The combination of left and right sided failure is known as congestive cardiac failure.

LEFT HEART (VENTRICULAR) INSUFFICIENCY

This is the commonest type and is usually due to a weakness of the left ventricle. The mechanics of the disease is weakness either due to prolonged effort to push against an obstruction or due to inadequate blood supply for its needs. This may follow a long history of high blood pressure, poor blood supply to the heart muscle as in long-standing ischaemic heart disease or heart valve disease. In Western clinical practice it is the first two cases which are the commonest.

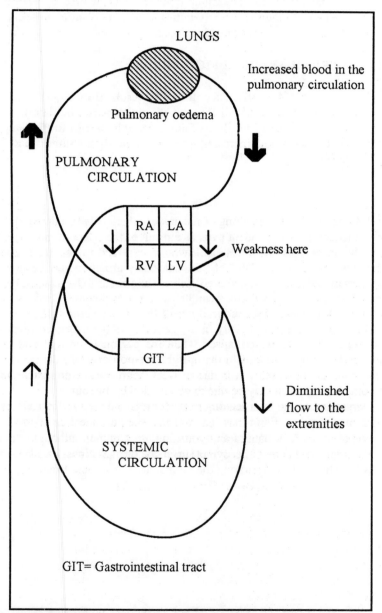

FIGURE 7.3: DIAGRAMMATIC REPRESENTATION OF LEFT VENTRICULAR INSUFFICIENCY[37]

As left ventricular function becomes insufficient for the needs of the body, less blood is ejected and there is a resultant build up of pressure in the left atrium. Increased left atrial pressure is then

---

[37] RA = right atrium, RV= right ventricle, LA = left atrium, LV = left ventricle.

passed onto the pulmonary circulation. Increased pressure in the pulmonary veins results in the "leaking" of fluid into the lungs - pulmonary oedema. The main symptoms of this condition are as a result of this process.

Symptoms:

In left ventricular insufficiency, the oedema is not obvious as it collects in the lungs. There is cough and breathlessness especially on exertion and when lying flat (orthopnoea). In more severe cases the person wakes in the night at around 12-1am. Breathlessness forces them to sit up or even get up to gasp at an open window. There may also be a cough or wheeze. Pinkish frothy sputum may be produced. This picture is known as cardiac asthma or paroxysmal nocturnal dyspnoea.

Other symptoms include palpitations, tiredness, faintness, pain in the chest, sweating. The person looks cold, pale and cyanosed. The symptoms are made worse by effort, emotion and respiratory problems. The lack of blood to the extremities results in nocturia, muscle fatigue which is worse with exertion, cold and pale extremities and peripheral cyanosis[38].

RIGHT HEART (VENTRICULAR) INSUFFICIENCY

This is less common than left-sided insufficiency. It usually results from chronic lung disease where the heart has to work harder to push blood through the pulmonary circulation. It may develop secondary to the pulmonary oedema of left heart failure. In right-sided insufficiency, less blood is ejected by the right ventricle and so the increased pressure in the right atrium is passed backward to the hepatic and systemic veins.

Symptoms:

Oedema is peripheral in site. There is swelling of the ankles which is worse at the end of the day and after exercise. The oedema affects dependent parts as a result of the effect of gravity. The feet, ankles and lower legs are the usual sites but in a person who is confined to bed the sacrum needs to be checked. The oedema is pitting in type. Weight gain and scanty urination may be apparent before the noticeable development of oedema because around 10lb of fluid needs to be retained before it becomes clinically apparent. Other fluid accumulations can be manifest as pleural effusions or ascites. Deep venous thrombosis is a risk because of the reduced rate of flow in the veins of the legs.

Distended veins are apparent especially in the neck due to the increased pressure in the right atrium. In health, the neck veins are collapsed when the person is upright and distended when horizontal. If you see the veins distended in the upright position or when the person is reclining it indicates raised pressure. In this disease it is due to weak heart muscle and back pressure into the venous system. In other situations it may be due to obstruction by tumour.

There is enlargement of the liver leading to tenderness and pain in the right hypochondrium. Eventually jaundice may develop. Fluid may leak out into the peritoneal cavity and lead to ascites. Gastrointestinal symptoms such as nausea and vomiting are common although the drugs used for cardiac failure can be implicated here. Other symptoms include palpitations, breathlessness, pallor and cyanosis as there is insufficient blood entering the pulmonary circulation, tiredness, pain in the chest and sweating.

---

[38] Cyanosis is a blue appearance of the skin due to an inadequate amount of oxygen in the blood. In conventional medicine, it is differentiated into central - tongue and peripheral - lips and extremities. Central cyanosis is due to cardiac or pulmonary disease. Peripheral cyanosis is due to cardiac disease or may occur in normal people with sluggish circulation particularly in cold weather.

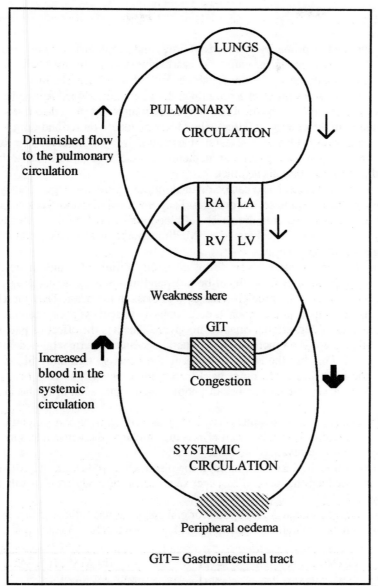

FIGURE 7.4: DIAGRAMMATIC REPRESENTATION OF RIGHT VENTRICULAR INSUFFICIENCY[39]

A comparison of left and right heart insufficiency is summarised in Table 7.11. In clinical practice, it is usual to see a combination of these.

SYMPTOMS	LEFT HEART INSUFFICIENCY	RIGHT HEART INSUFFICIENCY
Oedema	Pulmonary - breathlessness, orthopnoea, cough with pink, frothy sputum, paroxysmal nocturnal dyspnoea	Peripheral - swelling of ankles, lower limbs, sacral oedema if in bed
Palpitations	Yes	Yes
Gastrointestinal symptoms		Nausea, vomiting, anorexia, right hypochondriac pain, jaundice
Symptoms due to decreased blood leaving the heart	Cold extremities, tiredness, cyanosis, sweating	Breathlessness

TABLE 7.11: COMPARISON OF LEFT AND RIGHT HEART INSUFFICIENCY

---

[39] RA = right atrium, RV= right ventricle, LA = left atrium, LV = left ventricle.

Treatment:

The conventional approach is primarily by means of drugs and people may also be given advice about diet and exercise. If there is a recognised cause e.g. heart valve disease this may be treated surgically.

Digoxin was originally derived from foxglove, a plant which has the function of making the heart beat stronger. This is an example of a prescribed drug being developed from a herbal remedy. It is given in drug form as a purified chemical and in relatively high dosage and so it is easy to produce toxic effects especially in the elderly. It is the only widely available prescribed drug which increases the force of heart contraction. This is as a result of its action as a cardiotonic. The toxic effects are more likely to develop in cases of potassium depletion and so special care has to be taken when people are given diuretics and digitalis together.

Diuretics are commonly used and can be divided into three groups. High potency ones are used in acute situations or when there is severe oedema. They invariably lead to the loss of potassium so should be given with supplements. Regular checks of blood urea and electrolytes should also be made but this is rarely the case in clinical practice. Medium potency and low potency diuretics are correspondingly weaker in their actions.

Vasodilators are used in more severe forms of cardiac failure although, increasingly, may be given early. They may dilate arteries, veins or both depending upon the actual drug given. They do nothing to remedy the cause of the problem, that is, weakness in the heart. They merely move blood from one side of the circulation to the other. If cold limbs and tiredness are a problem due to lack of blood supply to the extremities, arterial dilators are given. This has the effect of placing more blood in the periphery and so there is an increase in peripheral oedema. If peripheral oedema is a problem, venodilators are given. This has the effect of opening the veins so that more blood sits inside the veins. Therefore, the heart has to do more work and symptoms such as cold limbs and tiredness become more marked. A significant number of people cannot take such drugs because of the side-effects produced.

ACE inhibitors are given in some cases. They act by causing vasodilatation due to their inhibition of vasoconstrictor substances. Their effects are similar to the vasodilators mentioned above. The drugs and their use are summarised in Table 7.12.

Other treatment may be instituted through the diet such as reduction of sodium to around 1-1.5G daily. This may reduce the amount of water retained in the body. Added salt is stopped and salty foods are avoided.

Cardiac transplantation may be an option for end-stage cardiac failure or in younger people. If there is careful recipient selection then 1 year survival is 85% and 78% at 3 years.

TREATMENT	TREATMENT LEVEL
Digoxin	1
Diuretic • low potency • medium potency • high potency	2
Vasodilator or ACE inhibitor	3
Cardiac transplantation	4

TABLE 7.12: CONVENTIONAL TREATMENT OF CARDIAC INSUFFICIENCY

Alternative management:

It is unusual to see people with cardiac failure in the clinic. This may be because they do not know that alternative medicine may help or perhaps because of the relative severity of the condition. In terms of Chinese medicine, this condition is usually due to Heart and Kidney Yang deficiency with Water overflowing. There is a lack of energy in the chest and is, therefore, the opposite of angina pectoris where the energy is stuck in the chest. This difference is reflected in the prognoses of the two conditions.

The essential point of treatment is to tonify the Yang by means of warming foods, specific treatment and the avoidance of cold foods. Adequate rest is important but regular, gentle exercise can strengthen the function of the heart.

Digoxin, as it is derived from a herbal remedy, is probably the appropriate energetic remedy in some cases but causes problems because of the dosages used. It would appear to tonify Heart Yang and lead to control of Water so that the oedema lessens.

Diuretics act by causing the kidneys to let go of water and so do nothing to treat the cause. They are cold in nature and long-term use leads to damage to Kidney Qi and Yin deficiency. It is common after some years to see a situation where there is Yin deficiency yet fluid accumulation so the person still has oedema with thirst and dry mouth.

- HOW TO RECOGNISE SERIOUS CONDITIONS OF THE CARDIOVASCULAR SYSTEM -

Diseases of the cardiovascular system are common in our society and the symptoms listed below are extremely common. It is important to know how to recognise if a symptom arises from a serious situation. You can use Table 7.13 below as a guide to refer to when faced with a person who has one or more of these symptoms. I make no mention of disease labels in the column on the right as I would not expect you to be able to diagnose conventionally. Seriousness can be assessed merely by reference to symptom pictures. However, you will be able to recognise that there are clinical appearances which would be diagnosed as a particular disease. For example, if you look at chest pain and its seriousness, you will see that this is the appearance of heart attack.

SYMPTOM	COMMENTS
CHEST PAIN	severe long duration (over 20 minutes) at rest with vomiting with rapid pulse, low blood pressure, sweating and pallor increased frequency of attacks occurring at night
BREATHLESSNESS	severe acute progressive with confusion with cyanosis pulse rate > 120 per minute paroxysmal attacks occurring at night
PALPITATIONS	pulse rate > 120 per minute pulse rate < 50 per minute with chest pain with oedema with loss of consciousness
OEDEMA	acute unilateral severe progressive with cardiac symptoms with renal symptoms
CYANOSIS	central - tongue peripheral - lips and extremities (unless due to cold)
LOSS OF CONSCIOUSNESS	on exercise
COUGH	with pink frothy sputum
DISTENDED VEINS	in an abnormal site, e.g. neck when sitting up, over the chest or abdominal wall

TABLE 7.13: HOW TO RECOGNISE SERIOUS CONDITIONS IN CARDIOVASCULAR DISEASE

- DISEASES OF THE LYMPHATIC SYSTEM -

INTRODUCTION

In conventional medicine, the lymphatic system has two main functions. It drains excess fluid from the intercellular spaces and returns it to the cardiovascular system. It also has a function in the production and maturation of lymphocytes and so plays an important role in the deeper workings of the immune system. There is a close relationship between the lymphatic system and the blood which is reflected in their similar function of fluid movement . The basic anatomy and physiology which it would be useful to know is listed in Table 7.14.

As a preliminary to study of disease of the lymphatic system you are able to:

List the main structures of the lymphatic system

State the main groups of lymphatic glands in the body

Describe the areas of the body which are drained by these main glands

Describe the function of the lymphatic glands as related to the immune system - lymphocyte production and development

---

TABLE 7.14: OBJECTIVES FOR ANATOMY AND PHYSIOLOGY AS PREREQUISITE FOR STUDY OF DISEASE OF THE LYMPHATIC SYSTEM

There are certain diseases affecting the blood, for example, which have associated lymphatic gland enlargement and certain lymphatic system diseases which may exhibit changes in the blood. The diseases of the lymphatic system can be classified as in Table 7.15.

There are interesting interconnections between these illnesses. Removal of the tonsils, a common treatment for recurrent tonsillitis increases the risk of Hodgkin's disease by a factor of three. Glandular fever may be the precursor, some years later, of Hodgkin's disease. Some people develop syndromes with or without lymphatic gland enlargement but do have some blood changes and there is doubt about the diagnosis - could it be leukaemia or lymphosarcoma or whatever?

MILD CASE

Acute inflammatory disease, e.g. tonsillitis
Chronic inflammatory disease, e.g. glandular fever
Lymphoma
• Hodgkin's
• Non-Hodgkin's
Lymphosarcoma
Leukaemia

SEVERE CASE

TABLE 7.15: CLASSIFICATION OF LYMPHATIC SYSTEM DISEASES

A clinical situation may help to explain what I mean. Someone came to see me who had developed an acute fever with sweating and malaise. It lasted for several weeks and there was no firm conventional diagnosis. After a series of blood tests it was concluded that he may have lymphoma. There was no lymphatic gland enlargement but one was removed from his neck to investigate its appearance. After this operation his fever returned to normal and his symptoms subsided. The biopsy was negative but further study of the blood tests had led to a diagnosis of leukaemia. He was to attend for chemotherapy the next week. Before he received his first course of treatment, he had repeat blood tests performed which were now normal. He was now told that he did not have leukaemia. The diagnosis now was probably glandular fever or a related viral illness for which he required no treatment.

This strange story does not reveal that conventional doctors misdiagnosed the case. What it does show is that as the level of imbalance changes then so do the symptoms and the investigations will show different results. In terms of Chinese medicine, he had an attack of heat which had descended deep into the body. This had resulted in fever and malaise. As it descended deeper it disturbed the blood and revealed abnormal blood results. The operation on his neck gland had the effect of bleeding him which is an old treatment for fevers and still used by practitioners of Chinese medicine. Bleeding relieves heat and so his condition improved. Subsequently, the blood tests had returned to normal and the doctors, no doubt, were confused about the course of events. To a conventional mind this sequence is impossible as you either have a disease or you do not. The idea of dynamic movement is not accepted.

Heat descending into the body can, therefore, result in symptoms such as fever, lymphatic gland enlargement and eventually organ damage. If the blood is affected then symptoms such as bleeding occur (leukaemia), convulsions (meningitis) or hallucinations (delirium). The actual pattern seen will depend upon the person, the preceding state of health and the particular circumstances.

LYMPHATIC GLAND ENLARGEMENT

There are four main conditions to consider here. You can get a good idea of the situation from the clinical appearances. Biopsy is often performed in people with persistent lymphatic enlargement of a localised nature especially if one of the more serious causes is suspected. The main thing to consider is whether the problem is acute or chronic and whether the enlargement is localised or generalised. The main situations can be summarised as in Table 7.16.

LOCALISED		GENERALISED	
ACUTE	CHRONIC	ACUTE	CHRONIC
Local inflammation[40], e.g. tonsillitis, skin infection	1. Local inflammation which is chronic, e.g. tuberculosis, fibroadenosis of the breast, malignancy[41] 2. Secondary malignancy[42]	Glandular fever,	Lymphoma[43], leukaemia[44]

TABLE 7.16: DIFFERENTIATION OF LYMPHATIC GLAND ENLARGEMENT

It can be seen from this Table that there are widely differing causes of lymphatic gland enlargement. It is important to ask about duration of the swelling, progression, associated symptoms and to check on the area drained in the case of localised enlargement. In this way an assessment about severity can be made. I would refer you to Chapter 6 - Cancer for a discussion about lumps - benign and malignant.

- DISEASES OF THE BLOOD -

INTRODUCTION

In conventional medicine, the blood is seen as a collection of cells and fluid which have a physical function. In terms of Chinese medicine, Blood is Yin and Yin is to do with receptivity, sensitivity and the emotions. There is a very close relationship, therefore, between the function of the Blood and our emotional state. There is a rather old term, sanguine, which means optimistic and confident. It was applied to one of the humours of Greek philosophy which corresponds to blood. Exsanguination is loss of blood. If the Blood is weak or disturbed, people feel generally sad and may have specific symptoms such as anxiety or depression. This is often the causation of post-natal depression where

---

[40] There will be the appearances of inflammation as described in Chapter 3 - Basic Pathological Processes in the local area with lymphatic gland enlargement in the group of glands which drain that area. The term lymphadenitis is applied to this situation.

[41] Lymph glands may become enlarged when draining an area containing a malignant tumour but they may merely be affected by an inflammatory process. Enlargement in this case then does not always mean that they are involved in the malignant process.

[42] The appearances of glands will be dependent upon whether the underlying process is benign or malignant. This was discussed in detail in Chapter 6 - Cancer.

[43] The lymph glands are described as being rubbery on palpation and larger than is the case with diseases such as tonsillitis or glandular fever.

[44] There will be the associated symptoms of leukaemia which are bleeding, pallor (due to anaemia) and sore throats (increased likelihood of infection).

the Blood has been depleted by pregnancy and childbirth. The situation will be exacerbated by blood loss at the time of delivery. Conversely, long-term worry, anxiety and depression will damage the Blood. I describe a case of a person with anaemia below which illustrates these connections.

In Chinese medicine, Blood has functions to do with cooling and moisturising. If the Blood is weak there can be symptoms such as feelings of heat, flushes, dry skin, thirst and general dryness, constipation, muscle and joint aches and pains, tingling, numbness and tremors. It is the Yin aspect of the body which balances the Qi or Yang aspect. Disturbances in the Blood can correspond, in conventional medicine, to anaemia, psychological disorders, multiple sclerosis, Parkinson's disease, arthritis and so forth. This is a much wider idea of Blood than the conventional one.

The manufacture, storage and function of Blood in energetic medicine depends primarily upon the functions of the Spleen, Heart, Liver and Kidney. Disturbances in any of these organs can lead to Blood imbalances.

Conventional diseases of the blood may be classified as in Table 7.17. The more superficial levels of the blood involve the red blood cells. Deeper disease will affect white blood cells and the worst situation here is total collapse of the blood where no cells of either type are produced - pancytopenia.

MILD CASE
Anaemia Thrombocytopenia Leucopenia Agranulocytosis Pancytopenia
SEVERE CASE

TABLE 7.17: CLASSIFICATION OF BLOOD DISEASE

- BASIC ANATOMY AND PHYSIOLOGY -

The blood in conventional medicine is seen as comprising of fluid and cells. The fluid, plasma, is a transport medium for nutrients and waste products. The cells are of different types and deal with transport of oxygen (red blood cells), immune system function (white blood cells) and prevention of haemorrhage and abnormal clotting (platelets). There is a connection with the bone marrow where the cells are manufactured and the kidney which secretes a hormone which stimulates red blood cell production.

There are several basic facts of anatomy and physiology which it is useful to know. I have listed the objectives which I consider useful to achieve as a preliminary to study of blood diseases. These are detailed in Table 7.18.

As a preliminary to study of disease of the blood you are able to: List the main constituents of blood Explain how they are produced and factors which influence this Describe the functions of plasma, red blood cells, white blood cells (5 types) and platelets

TABLE 7.18: OBJECTIVES FOR ANATOMY AND PHYSIOLOGY AS PREREQUISITE FOR STUDY OF DISEASE OF THE BLOOD

- ANAEMIA -

This is a common condition and is seen in the UK mainly in children under 5 years of age, pregnant women, social classes 4 and 5[45] and the elderly. It is considered to be present when the level of haemoglobin in the blood is decreased. This is a laboratory definition but I would consider the symptom picture to be most important to alternative practitioners.

The type is differentiated in conventional medicine according to the appearance of the red blood cells - small, normal or large. Each of these appearances tend to be related to a particular causation. For example, iron deficiency anaemia is associated with red blood cells which are paler and smaller in size.

The classification below takes account of the site of abnormality, e.g. inadequate intake, inefficient production. It is important to bear in mind that several factors operate in chronic disease. Treatment would need to be directed at all of them to be effective. Those in italics are the most important in outpatient practice.

IMPAIRED PRODUCTION OF HAEMOGLOBIN AND RED BLOOD CELLS

Iron deficiency anaemia: the main causes are inadequate intake, malabsorption or excessive loss of blood. Such anaemia is commoner therefore in women who menstruate. The commonest situations are poor diet, gastric disease, intestinal malabsorption, parasites, pregnancy, menorrhagia and haemorrhage. The appearance of an anaemia in a person in middle life with no previous problems suggests the possibility of a hidden blood loss. The condition which must be considered is cancer of the colon as blood loss here can be unrecognised.

Folic acid deficiency anaemia: The main causes are pregnancy, diet, malabsorption and drugs phenytoin, primidone, methotrexate and trimethoprim.

Vitamin B[12] deficiency anaemia: the major cause is pernicious anaemia which is a disease of autoimmune origin affecting the stomach leading to reduced secretion of intrinsic factor - essential for Vitamin B[12] absorption. Other situations include gastrectomy, intestinal malabsorption and poor dietary intake.

Vitamin C deficiency anaemia: this occurs due to dietary lack or after bleeding.

Thyroxine deficiency anaemia: reduced secretion of thyroxine leads to an reduced red blood cell production. It is part of the clinical picture of hypothyroidism as described in Chapter 15 - Endocrine System.

Protein: the structure of red blood cells is made of protein and so may deficient in malnutrition or intestinal malabsorption.

BONE MARROW DISEASE

If bone marrow function is disordered in some way there is a reduction in some or all of the cells produced there. Diseases include:

* aplastic anaemia
* leukaemia
* myelomatosis

---

[45] The association of social class with disease seems to be a particularly British institution. When I speak to people from mainland Europe they comment on its strangeness. My personal view is that disease is clearly associated with certain lifestyles, e.g. respiratory disease is commoner is miners but this is a consequence of their work rather than their social class. Medical labels are frequently used as a form of social control and when combined with comments about class can only lead to more stereotypical behaviour on behalf of the medical profession. Consequently, I avoid using social classification throughout this book.

EXCESSIVE DESTRUCTION (HAEMOLYSIS) OF RED BLOOD CELLS

In severe cases there is the appearance of jaundice. If the red blood cells are broken down quicker than their usual 120 days of life, the circulating level of haemoglobin is reduced in amount. Causes include:

- *autoimmune*
- infection or toxin
- overactive splenic function
- drugs, e.g. sulphonamides

DEFECTIVE HAEMOGLOBIN PRODUCTION

There are uncommon causes of anaemia where abnormal types of haemoglobin are produced. The important situations clinically are thalassaemia and sickle cell disease. It is out of the remit of this book to discuss these but they are important in their particular racial groups. Sickle cell disease affects those of African origin and thalassaemia affects several groups but particularly those of Mediterranean descent.

General symptoms of anaemia:

These are indicative of the interference with the normal functioning of haemoglobin and the red blood cell and is common to all the anaemias, whatever the cause. There is tiredness and pallor. The pulse may be rapid with palpitations, shortness of breath, light-headedness, fainting, anxiety or depression. Some people complain of floaters in the field of vision. Fever is present in severe cases.

Iron deficiency anaemia may also present with spoon-shaped fingernails (koilonychia) and dysphagia.

Vitamin B^{12} deficiency anaemia may also present with a smooth, sore tongue and an enlarged spleen. There is a typical nerve condition - subacute combined degeneration of the cord - which leads to pins and needles, ataxia, muscular weakness and eventually paralysis. It is classified as a type of neuropathy and these are discussed in Chapter 14 - Central Nervous System.

Complications

COMPLICATION	SYMPTOMS TO LOOK FOR
Left ventricular insufficiency	Breathlessness, cough with frothy sputum, palpitations
Right ventricular insufficiency	Peripheral oedema, palpitations
Angina pectoris	Central chest pain on exertion radiating to neck, jaw, inner aspect of arms but especially the left

TABLE 7.19: COMPLICATIONS OF ANAEMIA

Investigations:

These will vary according the suspected cause or they may be done altogether to investigate an anaemia of unknown cause.

Full blood count will reveal a reduced haemoglobin level and changes in red blood cell colour and shape. Iron deficiency anaemia is characterised by red blood cells which are paler and smaller than normal. In folic acid and Vitamin B^{12} deficiency anaemia the red blood cells are larger than normal. Serum iron, folic acid and Vitamin B^{12} may be reduced depending upon the cause.

Treatment:

The correct treatment of anaemia in conventional medicine hinges upon the diagnosis. If there is a lack of a specific factor then this is given as supplementation. In clinical practice this means replacement of iron, folic acid or Vitamin B^{12}. Dietary advice will be given to maximise intake of the relevant factor.

Iron is particularly found in liver, green vegetables, eggs, meat and milk. Foods such as green vegetables, liver and kidney are rich in folic acid. Vitamin B^{12} is particularly found in animal products such as meat, fish, eggs and milk. Vegans, therefore, have to be careful about their intake of this vitamin.

Other causes of anaemia are more difficult to treat and the success is largely dependent upon the severity of the original condition.

Many people who have an anaemia, and most cases clinically are due to a multiplicity of factors, are given iron in the assumption that this "is good for anaemia". As described above, the causes are many and varied. It is not enough in most situations to only consider iron intake.

Alternative management:

Anaemia is common and the common situations are dietary lack (either quantity or quality), blood loss and chronic disease. Most cases are treated conventionally with iron although this should be reserved for those with proven iron deficiency. Iron is hot energetically and usually causes constipation as it dries the motions. In some people who have Spleen deficiency perhaps with Damp accumulation, there may be diarrhoea instead. It is a harsh drug and disturbs absorption of other minerals such as zinc. I think that it is better to obtain iron from foods such as liver or green vegetables. Herbal remedies are excellent at strengthening the blood. In chronic cases be aware of the relationship between the blood and the emotions mentioned above. Flareups of the emotions may have to be dealt with carefully along the way.

The causes of anaemia in conventional medicine are fine as far as they go but the one important factor which is missing is energy. It is possible to have an adequate diet in terms of nutritional components but if the energy of the digestion, for example, is depleted then the body will not be able to make blood. Alternative medicine gives further insights into the causes and treatment of anaemia.

In terms of Chinese medicine, the counterpart of anaemia is usually Blood deficiency. Its actual manifestation depends upon the particular organ primarily involved. If it is the Heart then the main symptoms are palpitations, anxiety, insomnia, dreams disturbing the sleep. This is a clinical picture which is diagnosed as neurosis in conventional medicine and this is discussed in Chapter 16 - Psychological Disorders. If the Liver is involved then there are symptoms such as blurred vision, numbness and tingling, depression. This clinical picture may be diagnosed as neurosis as with Heart Blood deficiency or a central nervous system disorder such as repetitive strain injury or multiple sclerosis. These situations are discussed in Chapters 10 - Musculoskeletal System and 14 - Central Nervous System, respectively.

CASE OF ANAEMIA

A woman of 35 years came for treatment after she had a ruptured ectopic pregnancy some 4 months before. She had lost so much blood that she received 9 pints of transfused blood. Since then she had developed symptoms of weeping, palpitations, general shaky sensation and tiredness. Her blood count was now 12.8G which is almost normal but it was the emotional symptoms which were the most difficult. In addition to any problems with the blood there would also be the loss due to a bereavement.

She was reassured when I explained how these symptoms were interconnected and related to the loss of blood. She was treated with Chinese herbs to strengthen the Blood and given advice as to diet. Her basic constitution was quite sound and she improved within a couple of months. Her energy returned and the emotional symptoms resolved.

In cases of more chronic blood deficiency, it will take a long time to resolve any emotional state. I find that a combination of acupuncture and Chinese herbs together with counselling or psychotherapy to be a potent combination for health. The person is supported as well as having the opportunity to resolve old emotional patterns.

LEUCOPENIA

This is a low white cell count and may occur on its own or as part of aplastic anaemia. It is due to factors such as infection, toxins and drugs.

AGRANULOCYTOSIS

This is a lack of granular white cells and is severe. Its causes include radiation and drugs such as gold, phenylbutazone, chloramphenicol, thiouracil, imipramine, cancer chemotherapy and sulphonamide antibiotics. It may worsen and involve all the elements of bone marrow and then become aplastic anaemia.

Symptoms:

There is fever with sore throat as there is a reduction in white cells to fight infection. Septicaemia may result.

Treatment

This is similar to that of aplastic anaemia.

APLASTIC ANAEMIA (PANCYTOPENIA)

This is a collapse of bone marrow function leading to anaemia, leucopenia and thrombocytopenia. The commonest causes are direct damage to the bone marrow by radiation or by drugs such as sulphonamide antibiotics, gold, chloramphenicol, cancer chemotherapy and immunosuppressants.

Symptoms:

These are the classical triad of pallor and tiredness due to anaemia, sore throat due to infection as a consequence of leucopenia and bleeding/bruising due to thrombocytopenia. It is clearly a serious condition and 50% die within 1 year.

Treatment

There is little treatment available other than stopping the drug and supportive transfusions. In some there may be the option of bone marrow transplantation[46]. All people who take drugs with this side-effect must be told to report a sore throat as a blood count will be necessary.

- HOW TO RECOGNISE SERIOUS CONDITIONS OF THE BLOOD AND LYMPHATIC SYSTEM -

It is important to know how to recognise if a symptom arises from a serious situation. You can use Table 7.20 below as a guide to refer to when faced with a person who has one or more of these symptoms. I make no mention of disease labels in the column on the right as I would not expect you to be able to diagnose conventionally. Seriousness can be assessed merely by reference to symptom pictures.

---

[46] Bone marrow transplantation is indicated for bone marrow disease where there is no or little cellular production or as a result of the chemotherapy treatment of leukaemia. There is a mortality rate of 25% from this procedure alone which increases with age or if there is infection. The original disease may increase this rate depending upon the case and the person.

SYMPTOM	COMMENTS
Pallor	Severe With fainting With marked light-headedness or dizziness
Bruising	Severe Spontaneous
Bleeding	Severe Persistent Recurrent With pallor, sore throat and lymphatic gland enlargement
Lymphatic gland enlargement	With pallor, bleeding and sore throat Progressive Moderately enlarged

TABLE 7.20: HOW TO RECOGNISE SERIOUS CONDITIONS OF THE BLOOD AND LYMPHATIC SYSTEM

- SUMMARY -

Disease of the cardiovascular system is common.

Most of this disease will be chronic and degenerative in nature.

The main cause of heart disease in the West is disturbance of the emotions.

Serious heart disease can be clearly identified in most cases by attention to the symptom picture.

Alternative methods of treatment are very effective for cardiovascular disease especially when incorporated with visualisation and relaxation techniques.

Diseases of the blood are frequently associated with emotional changes.

Know the indications of a serious condition thoroughly.

8 RESPIRATORY SYSTEM

OBJECTIVES:

At the end of this Chapter you will be able to:
Describe the differences between the alternative and conventional views of the respiratory system.
List the symptoms attributable to disturbances of the respiratory system.
State when a symptom(s) would indicate a serious underlying condition.
Describe the main symptoms of diseases covered in this Chapter.
Explain the relevant management by an alternative practitioner of each disorder.

- INTRODUCTION -

The respiratory system can be usefully divided into the upper and lower respiratory tracts. The upper portion contains the nose, sinuses, naso-pharynx and larynx whilst the lower portion contains the trachea, bronchi and major airways, bronchioles, alveoli and alveolar-capillary membrane. The pleura lines the lungs and the inside of the chest wall and is included in this system.

The function of the respiratory system can be summarised as the maintenance of a normal level of oxygen and carbon dioxide in the blood. There are structures to filter and warm air as it enters the lungs but this is the essence. If there is interference with the functional unit of the lungs - the alveolar-capillary membrane - breathlessness will occur. Conversely, if a person complains of breathlessness, this is an indication that the lung is affected at a deep level.

There are several basic facts of anatomy and physiology which it is useful to know. I consider that most courses in these subjects are over detailed and reflect orthodox thinking rather than the particular needs of the alternative practitioner. I have listed the objectives which I consider useful to achieve as a preliminary to study of respiratory disease. These are detailed in Table 8.1.

As a preliminary to study of disease of the respiratory system you are able to:
Identify the surface anatomy of the lungs
Identify the structures contained in the respiratory system
Describe the functions of these structures
Describe the mechanisms of inspiration and expiration especially with regard to gaseous exchange
Explain the carriage of oxygen and carbon dioxide in the blood
Describe the control mechanisms of respiration

TABLE 8.1: OBJECTIVES FOR ANATOMY AND PHYSIOLOGY AS PREREQUISITE FOR STUDY OF DISEASE OF THE RESPIRATORY SYSTEM

Here again we see the physical view of the human body with no correlation between this and the mental or emotional sphere. The information in Table 8.2 reveals the associations which are made through a knowledge of vitalistic principles. The comments on the right of the Table are to explain these associations. The information in this Table is derived from Chinese medicine and will be most familiar to practitioners of this. However, the underlying energetic principles are common to all methods of alternative medicine and so there will be glimpses of recognition for other practitioners.

In Chinese medicine there is an association with the emotion of sadness in the form of grief. We know from our experience of treating patients that people who suffer from a loss or bereavement may then develop a pneumonia or an acute chest problem. This connection of the emotional or the mental with the physical is missing. The conventional view of respiratory disease is seen purely in terms of the physical descriptions .

ASSOCIATION	COMMENTS
Rules Qi[1]	Qi is sometimes translated as breath[2] and is the counterpart of the conventional idea of lung function.
Function of descending and dispersing	The energy of the Lung goes down and out. This can be likened to the direction of the bronchial tree.
Dominate the Water passages	The Lungs have a function of controlling the movement of water in the body, particularly the upper body. There is no equivalent in conventional medicine but does explain the often-noted observation of upper body oedema in chronic lung disease.
Rules the exterior of the body	Protection of the outer levels of the body against pathogenic influence is a function of the Lung. This organ, therefore, has a major role to play in the immune system.
Paired organ is Large Intestine	This connection explains why lung pathology may be reflected in the bowels. Constipation may due to a lack of Lung energy, smoking stimulates the action of the Large Intestine, colonic irrigation may weaken Lung energy[3]
Opens into the nose	This is recognised in conventional medicine and the nose is considered to be the opening of the respiratory system.
Dominates skin	Diseases such as eczema may be due, in part, to a Lung imbalance.

---

[1] All organs which are capitalised, e.g. Blood, Lung, Kidney indicate that I mean the energetic view of that organ and not the narrowly defined physical structure of Western science.
[2] As is the Ayurvedic *prana* and the Tibetan *rlung*.
[3] Aspects relating to the Large Intestine are covered in detail in Chapter 13 - Gastrointestinal System.

Colour - white	This is the colour of grief although we now use black. This is due to suppression, I believe, as in the West death is denied in many instances. Black is the colour of the Kidney which is the deepest organ. A person with lung disease may have a white nose or face.
Taste - pungent	An excess of pungent (acrid) taste may damage the Lungs.
Season - autumn	The energy of autumn is harvesting and reaping. It is a time of making ready for the coming winter. It is collection and maturation for the coming quiet, cold time.
Element - metal	The nature of metal is not holding or letting go. This is connected to the Lungs and Large Intestine by their function of elimination. If the metal element is disturbed, we have difficulty in letting go and this leads to grief, loss, constipation and so on.
Time - 3am to 5am	Lung problems which are characterised by an excess of energy are worse at this time, e.g. whooping cough. Asthma in patients with weak Lung energy may be worse around 3-5pm.
Emotions - grief, sadness	This is linked to the function of letting go. If this is incomplete or interrupted then grief or a sense of loss may result.
Mental aspect	Sensibility, sensitivity, compassion and attitude. Vulnerability.

TABLE 8.2: HOLISTIC ENERGETIC VIEW OF THE LUNG

- CLASSIFICATION OF RESPIRATORY DISEASE -

Diseases of this system can be categorised into those which occur in the upper respiratory tract and those which occur in the lower respiratory tract. Therefore, the seriousness of a disease can be assessed according to its chronicity, its depth and the rate of its progression. Table 8.3 is a classification which may be applied to respiratory disease.

MILD DISEASE

Common cold
Influenza
Sinusitis
Tonsillitis
Scarlet fever
Allergic rhinitis
Laryngitis
Acute bronchitis
Pleurisy
Pneumothorax - depends on severity
Pneumonia
Asthma - depends on severity
Bronchiectasis
Pulmonary embolism
Chronic bronchitis and emphysema
Tuberculosis
Cancer of the lung

SEVERE DISEASE

TABLE 8.3: CLASSIFICATION OF RESPIRATORY DISEASE

- UPPER RESPIRATORY TRACT DISEASE -

Upper respiratory tract infections in general, and the common cold in particular, offer an opportunity to explain disease in principles of energetic medicine without resorting to a discussion of organisms. The energetic view of such disorders is that they manifest on the external surfaces of the body. The symptoms will vary according to the depth to which they descend. These ideas were introduced in Chapter 2 - Philosophy and Chapter 5 - Infectious Disease.

The usual description of these diseases in conventional textbooks deals with a variety of syndromes associated with organisms. They can, in fact, be differentiated clearly using information from energetic medicine and studying the symptom picture. The causative factors of course, are not organisms but changes in the energetic balance usually as a result of climatic factors, emotional states and so forth. In Chinese medicine emphasis is placed on the climatic factors of cold, heat, wind, damp, dryness and summer heat since Chinese philosophy seeks to observe nature in its entirety. Treatments exist to remove these 'temporary guests' from the body.

In general, patients with acute upper respiratory tract infections can be divided into three groups depending upon the strength of their energy. The stronger their energy then the stronger the symptom picture. This is summarised in Table 8.4.

ENERGY OF PERSON	CONVENTIONAL LABEL	COMMENTS
Strong	Common cold	My description below does not match those in the conventional texts
Weak	Common cold which descends	When the Qi is weak the pathogenic factor descends into the Lungs leading to deeper disease.
Weak	Influenza	When the Blood is weak then the main symptoms are in the muscles, i.e. aching.

TABLE 8.4: UPPER RESPIRATORY TRACT DISEASE CLASSIFIED ACCORDING TO PERSON'S ENERGY

COMMON COLD - STRONG ENERGY

This is the commonest of all upper respiratory tract infections. It is associated with a virus. Immunity is short-lived and specific only for that particular virus. There are many viruses which can lead to this illness. The syndrome I describe here occurs in people with strong energy. It is quite an unusual manifestation as most people today do not have sufficient energy to produce these symptoms.

The view in Chinese medicine is that when a pathogenic influence such as wind or cold enters the body, the defensive energy tries to prevent further entry and closes the pores. There is then a struggle between the energy of the pathogenic influence and the energy of the person. The stronger the energy then the greater the symptoms.

Because the pores are closed there is high fever with no sweating. There is stiff neck and occipital headache as this is where the pathogenic influence enters the body. The person is averse to cold temperature. The Lungs are affected and so there are symptoms of a tickling sensation in the nose and sneezing. The throat is dry and sore, the head feels "stuffed" and there is a profuse, watery nasal discharge. Symptoms last one to two days.

COMMON COLD - WEAKER ENERGY

Many of the comments I made above are relevant here. The symptom picture is somewhat different because the person's energy is not so strong. The Qi of the person is not able to close the pores in this case and so sweating occurs with a lower fever.

The complexion is pale and there is aversion to cold. There is fever with chills and the chills predominate. Tightness in the chest with phlegm are seen indicating that the pathogenic influence has descended deeper into the body. There may be diarrhoea and scanty urination for the same reason. In severe cases there may be shortness of breath and this picture would more resemble severe acute bronchitis.

INFLUENZA

This is associated with a virus. It occurs in epidemics and occasionally pandemics. There are 3 viruses, A which is the main one, B and C. Immunity is short-lived and type specific. Major epidemics occur every few years. The epidemic of 1918/19 killed more people than had died during World War I and confirms the observation that such a disease only attacks the weak and debilitated. The incubation period is 24-48 hours long.

Symptoms:

These are more systemic than those of the common cold. Malaise is usually extreme with pains and aching in the back and limbs. The skin is greyish and the person is often thin. There is irritability. Fever can be marked with chills but fever is predominant. There is little or no sweating.

Recovery takes place within three to five days but it can take longer to regain full activity. Influenza is a severe illness in some and most people with this condition will not be able to go to work at least for a few days. It is a deeper disease in energetic terms and so should be treated with respect.

UPPER RESPIRATORY TRACT INFECTION - GENERAL COMMENTS

Complications:

COMPLICATIONS	SYMPTOMS TO LOOK FOR
Sinusitis	Pain in the face particularly under the eyes, yellow nasal discharge, headaches
Tracheitis	Retrosternal pain, dry cough, pain worse for coughing
Acute bronchitis	As above with progression to cough with sputum which is yellowish
Pneumonia	Cough with brownish sputum and the development of breathlessness
Post-attack debility	Prolonged attack, tiredness and debility, depression
Post-influenzal encephalitis	Occipital headache, photophobia, neck stiffness

TABLE 8.5 : COMPLICATIONS OF UPPER RESPIRATORY TRACT INFECTION

The respiratory complications of all the above are more common in patients with pre-existing disease such as chronic bronchitis, diabetes mellitus, asthma or in the old and frail. Clearly, the weaker the energy then the more likely are there to be complications. Influenza, for example, regularly leads every winter to deaths especially in the elderly and debilitated. There are often cases of post-influenzal depression and weakness which may be severe. It usually lasts 1-2 weeks but in some may merge with M.E.-like syndromes.

It can be seen from the above descriptions that the usual label of cold is nothing of the sort. Any mucus discharge or cough is so described. If there are not the signs of an acute exterior syndrome such as fever and/or chills or occipital headache I would be reluctant to call it a cold. These situations are usually reflections of an inner imbalance. Mucus collections in the body may discharge through the nose or lungs and be due to an internal, chronic condition. Such people would invariably be given antibiotics by conventional practitioners. With an understanding of depths of disease it is possible to differentiate. In clinical practice, I always suggest to patients that they stop the antibiotics particularly if I am giving them an alternative form of treatment. The antibiotic use can only lead to further depletion of energy and more mucus formation. In these situations, the antibiotics will deplete Lung energy further with consequences for the immune system as a whole.[4]

Treatment:

This is largely symptomatic and there are many proprietary medicines available for the relief of symptoms. It can be safely assumed that, as with any condition in conventional medicine, the effectiveness of remedies is in inverse proportion to their number. The main emphasis is on relief of fever and nasal symptoms. There are dangers with medications such as nose drops as they can be

---

[4] See energetic view of the Lung at the beginning of this Chapter.

addictive and harm the mucous membrane of the nasal cavity. It is much better either not to treat and just rest or to use simple natural remedies.

Rest is much more important if the illness is more systemic and deeper. If adequate rest is not obtained or not maintained then post-attack debility may occur as the pathogenic influence remains in the body. Antibiotics are given for the complications of upper respiratory tract infections. Conventionally, vaccination is advised for health workers and for patients who suffer from chronic ill-health. I have discussed vaccination issues fully in Chapter 5 - Infectious Disease. The vaccine changes from year to year according to which virus is around at the time. It reputedly gives 70% protection and is given to patients with diabetes and pulmonary, cardiac or renal disease. There are the usual problems after vaccination such as fever and debility and of course you must consider the effects on the vital force of these procedures. In conversations with workers in old people's home, it is clear that influenza vaccination has a great effect on people's vitality. Those who receive the vaccination seem to be more likely to be ill, have increased health problems and some die later in the winter.

Alternative management of upper respiratory tract infection:

The "cold" may be an indication of a chronic condition clearing its way out of the body and in this case then you may not wish to interfere with this process. Suppression of the symptoms at this stage will serve to exacerbate the chronic condition. Antibiotics are the classical way to do this but any therapy has this capability. Simple supportive measures may the best way to approach this situation.

In the case of an acute condition, it is helpful to treat if there are indications of depleted energy, the illness begins to progress into the interior or if the symptoms become 'stuck' at the exterior level. The energy of the person is the key to deciding whether to intervene or not. There may be no need to treat in cases where the condition is resolving,

I nearly always discuss with patients the option of stopping antibiotics in these cases as they are unnecessary and harmful. It is important that you know the indications of a serious condition as listed at the end of the Chaopter.

In terms of Chinese medicine, these diseases fall into the category of External Pathogenic Invasion. The precise pathogenic factor involved is determined by the symptoms. Cold, damp, wind, dryness and heat may all invade the body and cause problems. Essentially, Wind-Heat is present if fever predominates and Wind-Cold is present if there chills predominate. Wind-Heat occurs in those of strong constitution and if the Blood is deficient and Wind-Cold occurs in those with Qi deficiency.

The usual conventional drug, aspirin, is derived from willow bark and pretty close to the appropriate energetic remedy. This drug will relieve fever by releasing the exterior of the body, opening the pores, dispersing the energy and causing a sweat. It is warm in nature. It works to relieve the pain of arthritis by the same means. Long-term usage will deplete the energy, damage the Blood and weaken the Kidneys. This and related drugs, the non-steroidal anti-inflammatory agents, are the cause of a significant number of cases of analgesic nephropathy. This is drug-induced kidney damage which may lead to kidney failure.[5]

SINUSITIS

This is inflammation of the sinuses which are air-filled cavities in the head. They form part of the respiratory system and have a function in warming and moistening inhaled air. They are affected as a consequence of an upper respiratory tract infection or in cases where mucus is a predominant symptom. The mucus tends to collect in the sinuses and may flare up from time to time as an inflammation. Alternatively, it may cause long-term symptoms of congestion in the head, nasal obstruction and nasal discharge. In some people there is an allergic component.

Symptoms:

The symptoms are centred around the head and nose. There is blocked nose, nasal discharge which is usually yellow or green and a frontal headache. The symptoms can be severe with extreme pain in some cases particularly if the mucus is thick and doesn't move. The sinuses are tender to palpation. There may be a feeling of 'muzziness' in the head especially in the mornings.

---

[5] There are variable numbers of people with kidney failure resulting from analgesic use. In Australia, for example, this is 20% of kidney failure cases.

Complications:

COMPLICATIONS	SYMPTOMS TO LOOK FOR
Nasal polyps	Chronic nasal obstruction. The polyps may be visible in the nostril
Laryngitis	Hoarse voice, dry and sore throat
Tracheitis	Retrosternal pain, cough, pain worse for coughing
Acute bronchitis	As tracheitis with progression to cough with sputum which is yellowish

TABLE 8.6: COMPLICATIONS OF SINUSITIS

Investigations:

X-ray of the sinuses may show them to be filled or partially filled with fluid (mucus).

Treatment:

The conventional treatment of sinusitis is not especially effective and people receive a variety of things over the years. Analgesics and decongestants are the mainstay of treatment. Drugs such as ephedrine, an example of the sympathomimetic group[6], are used to dry up secretions. They are stimulant in nature and any effect is suppressive in nature. Therefore, withdrawal or reduction of dosage may result in a flare-up of symptoms. This can be interpreted as another attack and another course of treatment instituted so that the person becomes locked into a cycle of continuing drug-use.. Antibiotics are invariably given for severe attacks and for nasal discharge which is yellow or green in colour. .

Surgical treatments include sinus washout which is a singularly unpleasant procedure. Local anaesthetic is used and a probe inserted into the maxillary sinus. Water is washed around the sinuses to remove mucus collections. This operation is of short-term benefit only as the cause of mucus production is not addressed.

Polyps are removed surgically. Both operations are often repeated until either the person wearies of the process or the condition is suppressed, usually into the lungs. I describe such a situation in the discussion of asthma.

Alternative management:

In terms of Chinese medicine this usually corresponds to a combination of Lung Qi deficiency, Spleen Qi deficiency and Damp accumulation which collects in the sinuses. Alternatively, Fire in the Liver and Gall Bladder may ascend to the head. An acute flare-up is often a result of a Wind-Cold invasion attacking the Lungs.

In energetic terms this is a relatively minor condition as the Lung Qi is strong enough to hold the imbalance in the upper respiratory tract. This is why persistent suppression is hazardous as it weakens Lung Qi and may eventually drive the Damp deep into the Lungs.

The Damp (mucus) is produced by the Spleen and so dietary advice is paramount. The general advice for someone with Spleen Qi deficiency is covered in Chapter 13 - Gastrointestinal system. Exercises to strengthen to Lung Qi are helpful as is specific treatment for the particular individual.

---

[6] The sympathomimetics are those chemicals which 'mimic' the sympathetic nervous system. Adrenaline and noradrenaline (epinephrine and norepinephrine in the US) are the main examples of this group but others include ephedrine, pseudoephedrine, phenylpropanolamine, phenylephrine. They are stimulatory in action and have related effects to other groups of drugs such as antidepressants, bronchodilators, appetite suppressants and amphetamines.

TONSILLITIS

This is inflammation of the tonsils and is associated with either a bacterium or a virus. There is no difference, clinically, between the two types and so to automatically prescribe antibiotics on the basis of appearance makes no sense at all. A throat swab will delineate the bacterium (if any) present in the throat but these may be found in people with no symptoms. The relationship between symptoms and bacteria is not absolute. A severe tonsillitis with pain in the throat which lasts for longer than normal may be glandular fever. A related condition is enlargement of the adenoids which I discuss in Chapter 19 - Children's Health.

Symptoms:

Children are more commonly affected than adults. The main symptom is sore throat. There is associated difficulty in swallowing and fever. The lymph glands in the neck are swollen and tender. The tonsils themselves are enlarged and red, with white or usually yellow discharge on their surface. The tongue is coated and the person feels generally ill.

Investigations:

In normal clinical practice, there is usually no investigation performed. A throat swab can reveal evidence of bacteria.

Complications:

COMPLICATIONS	SYMPTOMS TO LOOK FOR
Otitis media	Pain in the ear, discharge from ear in severe cases
Acute glomerulonephritis	Pain in the loin, haematuria, oedema
Rheumatic fever	Palpitations, malaise, joint pains, skin rashes
Quinsy (tonsillar abscess)	*Pain* in the throat (rather than soreness), severe tonsillar swelling on one side

TABLE 8.7: COMPLICATIONS OF TONSILLITIS

Treatment:

This is invariably with antibiotics despite my comments above about the associated organism. Attacks are frequently recurrent and antibiotics may be used each time. If the attacks are frequent then tonsillectomy[7] will be performed.

Alternative management:

In terms of Chinese medicine, this is usually due to Heat in the Lung or Stomach which flares up into the throat when there is an acute attack of Wind-Cold or Wind-Heat. It is important to treat constitutionally between attacks in order to minimise the chance and number of repeat attacks. To remove the tonsils, an essential part of the immune system, is to weaken the general immunity. Some children have problems in the stomach or lungs after tonsillectomy as this line of defence has been removed. Alternative treatment on a regular basis is an effective option to prevent such an operation. As with any problem in the throat, it is useful to think of this area and its role in communication. The throat chakra is where energy becomes blocked if speech is suppressed or emotion is held. I discuss this again in Chapter 15 - Endocrine system in relation to goitre and thyroid disease.

Some people get recurrent attacks of sore throat which are not associated with tonsillar enlargement or discharge. If it is mild in its manifestation then it is almost certainly not tonsillitis. Energetically, Kidney or Liver energy can flare up to the throat and cause mild discomfort, dryness,

---

[7] The numbers of tonsillectomies performed have declined in recent years with a corresponding increase in the number of operations for grommet insertion to drain fluid in the middle ear - see Chapter 19 - Children's Health for more details.

soreness and redness. This may also be treated conventionally by antibiotics. Such an event is, however, not an acute attack affecting the tonsils but a manifestation of deeper organ imbalance.

SCARLET FEVER

This is an acute tonsillitis due to streptococci in association with the typical rash. The incubation period is 2-7 days.

Symptoms:

These are mostly mild now although in the past it has been a great problem. It seems to have undergone quite a change in the last 50 years so that now most cases are minor. Energetically this can be interpreted as a weakening of the general energy of the population so that the symptoms are weaker. The conventional explanation is that the organism has become weaker.

There is an acute onset of fever which becomes high. Vomiting commonly occurs also. On examination the tonsils are very red with swelling. There may be yellow discharge from the tonsils. There is associated lymph gland enlargement. The rash appears within 24 hours as a fine red rash. It soon becomes generalised although it is more marked at the flexures such as the elbow, axilla and groin and it is less marked around the mouth - the classical circumoral pallor.

The tongue undergoes typical changes also with white fur on the first day. On days 2 and 3 the papillae are seen to be larger than usual and the coat starts to peel at the tip and sides - "white strawberry" tongue. On days 4 and 5 the peeling continues until the tongue is clean, red and shiny - "red strawberry" tongue.

Complications:

COMPLICATIONS	SYMPTOMS TO LOOK FOR
Acute glomerulonephritis	Loin pain, haematuria, oedema
Rheumatism	Pain and swelling in the joints
Rheumatic fever	Palpitations, pain in chest, tiredness

TABLE 8.8: COMPLICATIONS OF SCARLET FEVER

Investigation:

The characteristic organisms are found on a throat swab. The presence of rising antibody levels confirms the diagnosis. There is no clinical difference between a tonsillitis caused by streptococci and one caused by viruses. In the case of scarlet fever, the presence of the rash is often enough to confirm the diagnosis. It is useful to be aware that many throat swabs in people with no symptoms may also show streptococci.

Treatment:

Penicillin is always given and quickly eradicates the bacteria from the throat and renders the person non-infective within 24-48 hours.

Alternative medicine:

This condition is not common these days but can be dealt with in the same way as tonsillitis. Treatment in the acute phase will minimise the occurrence of complications. Complications are when the pathogenic heat descends into deeper levels in the body. Early treatment where this is released will therefore prevent progression.

ALLERGIC RHINITIS

There are similarities between symptoms of this disease and those of the common cold. Allergic rhinitis is chronic in nature in that it recurs and indicates a deeper pathology. It is the appearance of upper respiratory symptoms when in contact with a variety of factors. It is usually divided according to these factors and either seasonal - classical hay fever - or perennial - symptoms appear regularly.

It is considered to be due to a hypersensitivity reaction of the nasal mucosa to specific substances. The seasonal types are caused by the pollens of grasses, flowers, trees and, very commonly, nettles. Contact with oil seed rape is becoming a common problem especially in the UK . These are the 'hay-fevers' you see in the summer. The perennial types are caused by many factors often undiscoverable. House dust and house dust mite are common causes as are the products of hydrocarbons such as traffic pollution leading to poor air quality, perfumes, sprays etc. Animals such as cats, dogs, and horses commonly cause these reactions also.

Symptoms:

Frequent, sudden attacks of sneezing with a profuse watery nasal discharge and nasal obstruction are the usual features. They last for a few hours and are often associated with itching, watering and red eyes. There may be itching of the roof of the mouth. In the perennial types the attacks are more continuous and less severe. More chronic cases are characterised by nasal obstruction rather than the acute symptoms of sneezing with watery discharge.

There may be a feeling of heat, especially in the head although there may not be a fever to be detected by a thermometer. The sensation of heat due to exposure to hay (although often other substances) gives this its usual name. Some patients develop cough and wheezing. These cases are then similar to asthma.

Treatment:

Conventional medicine is at a bit of a loss when it comes to the treatment of many allergic disorders and this is no exception. The usual treatment is by drugs and the following are employed in turn if there is little effect from the preceding drug:

TREATMENT	TREATMENT LEVEL	COMMENTS
Antihistamine	1	The stock response to any allergic disorder and causes tiredness and drowsiness. They are of variable effectiveness.
Decongestant nasal spray	1	Used if there is a great problem with a runny or a blocked nose. Discharges from the body are a method of elimination. Stopping up a discharge by external means such as drugs or surgery prevents this route and the consequences can be severe. In the case of nasal problems the likely result is the development of lung disease such as asthma or bronchitis.
Sodium cromoglycate nasal spray	2	Stabiliser of mast cell membranes in an attempt to stop the release of histamine. Its exact method of action is unknown in conventional medicine. Of variable help in allergic disorders. It is also used in asthma. In an oral form it is used for patients who suffer from bowel disorders due to food intolerance.
Corticosteroid nasal spray	3	Reduces inflammation in the nose and so the amount of discharge and obstruction. The same comments are applicable here as above but of course to a much greater degree because corticosteroids are so powerfully suppressive. Despite this comment, these drugs are commonly used as the drug-of-choice.
Systemic corticosteroids	4	The most powerful in their effect. Corticosteroids are described in detail in Chapter 10 - Musculoskeletal system.

TABLE 8.9: TREATMENT OF ALLERGIC RHINITIS

Prevention:

Attempts are made to 'desensitise' patients to the external factor by sequential injections of increasing strength of the relevant allergen. They can cause anaphylactic shock and have led to sudden death in patients. They should nowadays only be given in hospital with resuscitation equipment to hand. The same criticism can be applied here as in the case of vaccination in that this is the deliberate injection into the blood-stream of the offending antigen. This is the very thing which the body tries to prevent. Why else produce such strong symptoms in the nose and throat and eyes? This is the defence mechanism in operation. The last thing to do is to bypass it in an attempt to "treat" the condition. In my experience, such treatments are frequently of minimal effectiveness.

Alternative management:

In energetic terms, although the acute manifestations are due to an external factor, the chronic cause is due to an internal condition. In Chinese medicine, this is often DampHeat Accumulation which flares up into the Lungs when conditions are right. Many people report that there is a poor association with pollen counts. More important factors are diet, levels of emotional stress, heat and damp. There may be an element also of Kidney not grasping Lung Qi particularly in those with wheezing and cough. Others have Liver Blood deficiency as is evidenced by eye symptoms.

  The most effective approach to take is to begin treatment before the pollen season in the case of the seasonal type and there may not be much improvement the first year. Emphasis outside of the season should be placed on resolving the underlying imbalance. Only by the second or third summer after treatment has begun will you notice the main benefits of treatment.

LARYNGITIS

This is an inflammation of the larynx. It is usually a consequence of an upper respiratory infection which has descended into this area. It may be the precursor to deeper symptoms such as cough, sputum and breathlessness.

Symptoms:

There will be the symptoms of the original condition with the development of hoarse voice. This may become so severe that the person may only be able to emit a scratchy whisper. It lasts for several days and then begins to recover. Complete recovery is the rule.

  It may become recurrent in singers, smokers and those who use their a voice excessively, e.g. public speakers. The symptom of hoarseness may be the first sign of a tumour of the vocal cords. In this situation, the hoarseness is long-lasting (more than three weeks). In this case it is important for the vocal cords to be examined by an ear, nose and throat specialist (otorhinolaryngologist).

Treatment:

This is merely symptomatic including resting the voice. Underlying causes such as smoking need to be addressed. Public speakers and singers may benefit from voice-training.

Alternative management:

The comments I made with regard to upper respiratory tract disease are applicable here. In terms of Chinese medicine, it is usually part of the picture of an attack of WindCold or WindHeat descending into the Lungs. As mentioned in the description of tonsillitis, Liver or Kidney energy may involve the throat and cause soreness. Hoarse voice may be part of such an energetic pattern.

- LOWER RESPIRATORY TRACT DISEASE -

Diseases in this part of the respiratory system necessarily indicate that there is a more serious imbalance in lung energy. If the Lung Qi is strong enough, the problem is held in the superficial levels. The diseases below occur in those people who have such conditions as part of their general state of health or they may be the result of suppressive treatment. In clinical practice, there are many people who develop lower respiratory tract disease secondary to suppressive treatment of upper respiratory tract disease. As you treat such diseases, you may see the reappearance of symptomatology in the more superficial levels.

ACUTE BRONCHITIS

This is an acute inflammation of the trachea and bronchi and is often associated with bacteria. It can develop after upper respiratory problems in which instances it is an example of the pathogenic influence descending into the lungs. It may also occurs in patients with chronic bronchitis as an acute exacerbation of the chronic condition. Predisposing factors are cold, damp and foggy weather, dusty atmospheres and smoking.

Symptoms:

The symptoms of the original condition are present which then develop into a dry, irritating cough with retrosternal discomfort. This is the cough of acute tracheitis where the pain is sore and scratchy, it is felt behind the sternum and the person will sit up to cough and hold the chest. There is tightness in the chest with a low fever. Breathlessness is unusual unless there is wheezing or an associated chronic lung disease.

Sputum is scanty, white and thick at first. It then develops into more copious, yellow or greenish sputum. There is usually a fever. Most patients recover in four to eight days without any problems.

Investigations:

There is an increase in the white cell count. Chest X-ray is normal.

Treatment:

Antibiotics are usually given as indeed they are for any discharge which is yellow or green in colour. It is often said that acute bronchitis lasts around 7 days without the use of antibiotics and one week with them! Steam inhalations are helpful to relieve cough and soreness. This condition reveals the importance of correct treatment of acute illnesses such as influenza, measles and the regular treatment of patients suffering from chronic conditions such as chronic bronchitis.

Alternative management:

In terms of Chinese medicine this usually corresponds to PhlegmHeat Retention in the Lungs. It may be a consequence of an acute pathogenic influence or of an internal condition where Dampness and Phlegm collects in the Lungs. The use of antibiotics will clear any Heat but do nothing about the underlying Phlegm condition and will actually make that worse as the Lung and Spleen Qi will more depleted.

PNEUMONIA

In conventional medicine, pneumonias are classified according to the causative organism. This is in line with the usual conventional methods of classifying infectious disease I discussed in Chapter 5 - Infectious disease. Table 8.10 classifies pneumonia according to the clinical appearances and so is more useful for the alternative practitioner.

TYPE OF PNEUMONIA	ASSOCIATED ORGANISMS	COMMENTS
MILD DISEASE		
Lobar	Pneumococcus, Mycoplasma (occasionally)	Affects 'healthy' adults. Strong symptoms reflect the relatively strong level of energy.
Bronchopneumonia	Mycoplasma, Haemophilus influenzae, Chlamydia psittaci[8], Staphylococcus aureus, Legionella pneumophilia[9], Pneumocystis carinii[10]	Affects debilitated people and may be a terminal event. Mild, vague symptoms reflecting the depleted energy.
SEVERE DISEASE		

TABLE 8.10: CLASSIFICATION OF PNEUMONIA ACCORDING TO CLINICAL APPEARANCES

LOBAR PNEUMONIA

This, as its name suggests, is usually restricted to one lobe of the lung and so is a fairly localised phenomenon. It is an illness of young, 'healthy' adults. As indicated in Table 8.10, the usual causative organism is the pneumococcus - a type of streptococcus.

Symptoms:

There is a sudden onset of fever with chills and shivering. The temperature is high at around 40°C (104°F) and continues to be so. The face is flushed. The pleura is usually involved and so there is a typical pleuritic pain - a sharp pain in the axilla or around the scapula which is worse on respiration and coughing. The respiration is shallow and rapid. There is often an attack of herpes simplex ("cold sores") on the lip.

These days most people are given antibiotics and there will be an improvement in the condition within 48 hours. Before these were available there would be a "crisis" around the seventh day when the fever would suddenly remit and the person would either start to recover or they would deteriorate.

Investigations:

Clinical examination of the chest shows the typical signs of pneumonic consolidation. These are a pleural rub, dullness to percussion and coarse crackling over the affected area. Chest X-ray will reveal shadowing over the affected lobe of the lung due to the inflammatory process and serves as a confirmation.

Complications:

Lobar pneumonia usually ends in resolution and the person recovers. The occurrence of problems such as lung abscess or empyema are rare.

---

[8] An organism present in birds, particularly parrots.
[9] The organism of Legionnaire's disease.
[10] The organism affecting people with severely depleted immune system such as those with AIDS or receiving immunosuppressive corticosteroid or cancer chemotherapy medication.

Treatment:

This is universally with antibiotics to which the organism is sensitive. In a case of lobar pneumonia in a young, fit person recovery may be complete.

Alternative management:

Before the advent of antibiotics, homoeopathic and herbal remedies were the only way that people could obtain help. The homoeopathic texts abound with examples of patients who recovered in a few days with the appropriate remedy. There is no reason to suppose that this cannot be the case today but there are factors to take into account such as the support the person has at home and the actual condition of the person. Whilst few of us have access to residential care we have problems in caring for people who are too ill to be treated on an out-patient basis. Having said all that, people can be treated with early signs of a pneumonia and this will probably remove the need for antibiotics. You should assess carefully the condition of the person, give the appropriate treatment and you should review regularly. If the person's condition starts to deteriorate then a reappraisal is essential. You must be familiar with how to recognise a serious condition.

In terms of Chinese medicine, pneumonia usually corresponds to Phlegm-Heat congesting the Lungs. The cause of this in the acute phase is Wind-Heat or Wind-Cold attack but there will be an underlying Lung imbalance as a predisposing factor.

BRONCHOPNEUMONIA

This is a more generalised disease and is associated with organisms which are normally present in the respiratory tract or which are usually successfully resisted. It occurs in the very young, the elderly and the debilitated. This is clearly more a case of weak defensive energy and this type of pneumonia is seen after other respiratory infections. In this category would be included diseases such as Legionnaire's disease, pneumonias occurring in people with AIDS and so forth.

Symptoms:

These are much more vague than with the classical picture of lobar pneumonia. For example, the fever is mild with malaise, aching in the head and limbs and perhaps low spirits. The person will feel generally unwell and after a couple of days a cough will appear with the typical pain of pleurisy. These symptoms are in keeping with the view that intensity of symptoms is a reflection of the strength of the person's energy and weak people exhibit very few and diffuse symptoms.

In the case of people with AIDS or other severe disease, a pneumonia may only be recognised by the existence of breathlessness. The person may be too weak to even produce a cough or sputum. The acute onset of confusion, particularly in the elderly, may be the first indication of pneumonia.

Investigations:

Chest examination shows only minimal signs such as an area of decreased air entry with crepitations or occasionally bronchial breathing and dullness on percussion. The Chest X-ray reveals diffuse shadowing over the bases of both lungs reflecting the more widespread nature of the disease.

Complications:

COMPLICATIONS	SYMPTOMS TO LOOK FOR
Chronic 'infection' - persistent inflammation	Persistent cough, sputum and breathlessness
Lung abscess	Symptoms of pneumonia worsen and persist, large amounts of foul sputum
Cardiac insufficiency	Oedema, breathlessness worse for lying and at night

TABLE 8.11: COMPLICATIONS OF BRONCHOPNEUMONIA

Treatment:

This is with the particular antibiotic appropriate for the causative organism. Many people continue to have chronic respiratory problems. In some people who develop these pneumonias when they are debilitated, the pneumonia would normally be a terminal event and antibiotics may prevent death. The person then partially recovers to succumb at some later date from another attack of pneumonia or perhaps cardiac insufficiency.

TUBERCULOSIS

I have included this disease as it is of some importance to homoeopaths who regard suppressed tuberculosis, in the person's medical or family history, to be an important cause of disease. It is true that there are similarities between tuberculosis and cancer and it may be true that we have replaced one disease by the other. Both diseases are often associated with wasting and there are areas of the body which are affected by destructive lumps.

Tuberculosis is a specific type of respiratory problem which is unusual in the UK but is becoming commoner. It can affect virtually any organ and tissue in the body but here I want to discuss pulmonary tuberculosis.

It is considered to be due to infection with the tubercle bacillus. In the West, it is the human type which is more common and is spread through droplets (cough, sneeze). In less 'developed' countries you see the bovine bacillus which is spread through drinking contaminated milk. In the UK there is a system of accrediting herds as being free of tuberculosis. Therefore, it does not enter the milk supplies. In addition, most milk is still pasteurised as a hangover from the days when tuberculosis was present in cattle.

It is a disease of poor conditions of housing, sanitation, food and this is the reason why tuberculosis is now increasing in the UK. Over the past 10 years or so there has been a general increase in poverty, particularly in inner city areas and especially amongst more deprived social groups. The death rate formerly had declined steadily since the introduction of effective legislation governing public health and, as I discussed in Chapter 5 - Infectious Disease, there is no evidence that any difference to the pattern of the disease has been made by either vaccination or antibiotics. This is summarised in Table 8.12.

YEAR	DEATH RATE/10000	EVENT
1812	700	
1882	370	Isolation of TB bacterium by Koch
1910	180	Opening of first sanatorium
1945	48	Antibiotics not yet widely available

TABLE 8.12: EFFECT OF CONVENTIONAL MEDICINE ON THE DEATH RATE FROM TUBERCULOSIS[11]

Tuberculosis may present in one of two forms.

PRIMARY TUBERCULOSIS

This is the first infection. It mainly shows itself as enlargement of certain lymph nodes.

Symptoms:

In the primary form there is a small lesion in the lung and the local lymph nodes are enlarged. There is a small shadow on X-ray and there will be evidence of lymph gland enlargement. The Mantoux reaction[12] is positive. General symptoms are minimal and around 95% of people will recover on their own. Many people have had such events in the past and are unaware of this until it is revealed by a

---

[11] Data is extracted from "Medical Nemesis" by Ivan Illich (Bantam, 1976) and relates to New York.
[12] The Mantoux reaction is an intradermal injection of tuberculin protein. If there is a reaction, the person is considered to be positive. Those who are negative are given B.C.G. whilst those who are positive are checked by chest X-ray. A common test which is based on the same principles but simpler to administer is the Tine test.

routine chest X-ray. Occasionally, this condition may lead to bronchiectasis, tuberculous bronchopneumonia and tuberculosis in other sites such as bone, joints, kidney and so on.

POST-PRIMARY TUBERCULOSIS

This is a subsequent infection with the tubercle bacillus or, more likely, a reactivation in someone with a depleted immune system. It is invariably pulmonary in site and usually in the upper lobes. The infected area breaks down, a cavity forms in the lung and infected sputum is produced. Infection may occur in other parts of the lung from this sputum. Pleurisy may develop if the periphery of the lung is involved and blood is coughed up when blood vessels are eroded.

The rate of progression of the disease is variable and clearly depends on the strength of the individual person. In some there is slow deterioration and the illness may in fact be arrested by the healing process of fibrosis and calcification. In others there is a steady and at times rapid progress into ill-health and death.

Symptoms:

In the early stages there may be minimal symptoms and the coughing up of blood can be the first sign. Typically there are the appearances of night sweats, tiredness, progressive weight loss and loss of appetite. Eventually the person will waste hence the old name of consumption. There may also be the symptoms of tuberculous infection elsewhere such as the larynx (laryngitis), trachea (tracheitis) and ileum (ileitis).

Examination will reveal persistent crepitations at one apex of the lung and later dullness to percussion, bronchial breathing and crepitations over a wider area. If there is any degree of fibrosis then there may be evidence that the mediastinum has shifted over and the trachea will no longer be central.

Investigations:

Chest X-ray shows signs of shadows in the upper lobes, fibrosis and possibly cavities. Bacteriological examination of the sputum reveals the causative organism - Mycobacterium tuberculosis. Biopsies of the pleura and lymph glands may be performed to confirm the diagnosis.

Treatment:

Conventionally, this is by means of antibiotics. They are given for one or two years and in combinations so that two or more drugs are usually given together. Attention is made to general health such as adequate diet, rest and convalescence although not as much emphasis is placed on this as in the days of sanatoria. Vaccination is given by means of the B.C.G.[13] for everyone in this country who is Mantoux negative.

Alternative management:

It is not likely that people with tuberculosis will present for alternative treatment. They usually seek conventional advice. There are treatments which exist in Chinese medicine and homoeopathy but I would view the management of TB to be similar in many ways to that of cancer. There needs to be a multiple approach with a greater commitment from the person. An added factor is that of transmission to susceptible people[14]. People with tuberculosis may cough sputum which contains tubercle bacilli.

In terms of Chinese medicine, tuberculosis corresponds to two main patterns. It may be due to Deficiency of Yin where Fire damages the fluids. The other type is due to Deficiency of Yang especially of Lung, Spleen and Kidney. Both of these syndromes may also be responsible for what may be diagnosed in conventional medicine as cancer. This would seem to underline any connection between the two diseases.

---

[13] B.C.G. is the Bacille Calmette-Guérin vaccination which has been given in the UK since 1954.
[14] Studies have shown that tuberculosis is more likely to occur in those people who have suffered a loss of bereavement recently. "Emotional Factors in Pulmonary Tuberculosis" by David M Kissen (London, 1958) and "Diseases of Civilisation" by Brian Inglis (Paladin, 1981).

SARCOIDOSIS

This is a multiple system, inflammatory disease which has many characteristics in common with tuberculosis. When I was at medical school and studying respiratory diseases, I always believed that they were the same disease but one had bacteria and the other did not. I now find that energetically this is the case.

There are collections of inflammatory tissue which can collect in any organ but commonly the lungs. The cause is unknown in conventional medicine. It mainly affects young people and is commoner in women. It occurs in the UK at the rate of 19 cases per 100,000.

Symptoms:

Sarcoidosis may affect many organs and the clinical picture is dependent upon the exact sites involved. The lungs are a common site. The symptoms are similar to those of tuberculosis and may include tiredness, weight loss, lymphatic gland enlargement and fever. There will be a cough with or without sputum.

In 10% of cases the skin is involved with the occurrence of erythema nodosum. This is the appearance of painful lumps on the shins. They fade to a bruised appearance over several weeks. Other causes include sulphonamide antibiotics, oral contraceptives, inflammatory bowel disease and streptococcal infections. Other skin problems include chilblain-like areas and nodules.

Around one quarter of people develop an anterior uveitis. This is described in Chapter 12 - Special Senses. Conjunctivitis may also occur in people with sarcoidosis. The eyes may be dry due to decreased tear production.

The central nervous system is involved in only about 2% of cases but it can be severe. It leads to weakness, tingling and numbness.

Investigations:

Lung biopsy is the usual method of diagnosis. It is obtained via bronchoscopy. Lung function tests reveal decreases in function.

Treatment:

Corticosteroids may be given especially if the symptoms are severe or vital tissue such as eyes or nervous system are affected. Otherwise there is little which can be offered conventionally. In some cases, there is resolution of the disease particularly in those with localised lung disease - 60% of the mildest cases to only 30% if there is more widespread lung involvement.

Alternative management:

This is a severe condition which would benefit from a multiple approach. In terms of Chinese medicine, it usually corresponds to the same patterns as described under tuberculosis. Corticosteroids may help the symptoms in the short-term but eventually the person's health will be worse as they erode the vital energy.

BRONCHIECTASIS

This is an unusual condition of chronic infection in the lungs where there is a persistent dilatation of the airways. It is rare nowadays. It begins with an obstruction to an airway so that secretions collect in the air passages. Infection supervenes and the inflammatory and infective process leads to widening of the bronchioles and smaller bronchi. Usually a small segment of lung tissue is involved distal to the obstruction although in extreme cases there can be most of one lung affected. The presence of large amounts of infected material in the lungs leads to the classical symptoms of this condition.

It usually occurs after an acute childhood respiratory infection which is why there is so much emphasis placed on the prevention of whooping cough. Obstruction of an airway such as by peanuts or other inhaled object, carcinoma, pulmonary tuberculosis and the thickened secretions of cystic fibrosis can lead to distal infection which becomes chronic unless the obstruction is relieved.

Symptoms:

The main feature is of copious amounts of sputum. There are large amounts coughed up each day in the order of several cupfuls. The sputum is often green or dark green. There is offensive breath because of the purulent material in the lung. Haemoptysis can occur as the continuing infective process erodes into blood vessels. Breathlessness, cyanosis and finger clubbing is seen if the illness is fairly severe.

Treatment:

Daily physiotherapy using postural drainage is the main measure utilised by conventional medicine. It is essential to clear sputum out of the chest and antibiotics are administered for acute exacerbations. Surgery may be an option if the area of bronchiectasis is clearly defined and relatively small.

Alternative management:

This is a chronic infective condition where there are large amounts of infected material in the lungs. There are problems of general debility as well as the issue of lung symptoms. Any measure which will lead to a reduction in the amount of infected sputum is important. Here postural drainage is useful and should continue regularly. A diet which will lead to the production of less mucus will help. Also, specific therapy will help clear the lungs and also to strengthen them. Breathing exercises are especially beneficial in tonifying the lungs.

You would expect to treat a person for a considerable length of time and 'cure' may not be something to realistically expect. However, there is a lot we can do for such people especially in the area of self-help with regard to diet, exercise and breathing. You would hope to help the general health so that the infective area became less active and acute flare-ups, as the infection "spills over" into other areas of the lung, less frequent.

- WHEEZING DISEASES -

INTRODUCTION

Wheezing is a specific musical sound produced by the small airways of the lung when they are narrowed. This narrowing may be the result of spasm of the muscle surrounding the airways, mucus partially obstructing the airways or disease which damages the lung tissue. Wheezing may be diagnosed as asthma but this is merely one situation. I shall discuss the three diseases of asthma, chronic bronchitis and emphysema together with ideas gathered from alternative medicine. In this way, you will then have a clear idea of the common patterns of chest disease characterised by wheezing and how they can be differentiated.

I prefer to differentiate asthma and the other wheezing diseases according to their clinical appearances. Therefore, the descriptions I give below may not completely match those given in conventional textbooks.

ASTHMA

This is common and becoming more so with the general deterioration in the immune system and the increasing levels of atmospheric pollution. It is uncommon in 'developing' countries. There are over 2 million cases in the UK with 1 in 10 being children. The disease consumes 8% of the NHS drug budget. Asthma may be severe and can kill although it was rarely fatal before 1900. There are around 3 deaths per 100,000 cases in some countries now.

Asthma is a disease which is characterised by episodic attacks of reversible wheezing and breathlessness. The key term here is "reversible wheezing". The airways of the lungs are constricted by muscular spasm - bronchospasm - and so this can come as well as go. The transient nature of the spasm and its response to the commonly used group of drugs (bronchodilators) accounts for the reversibility.

The disease is divided conventionally into extrinsic and intrinsic types. Extrinsic asthma is usually first seen in childhood and there is often a family history of allergies. This occurs in the so-called atopic type of individual. The person may also have other conditions such as eczema, hay fever or migraine. The intrinsic type is seen in adult life and there is not such an emphasis on allergy either in the family or personal history. This type has more in common with the clinical picture which I describe under chronic bronchitis. Overall, there are more children affected with asthma than adults and it occurs more commonly in males than females.

Symptoms:

There is tightness in the chest which develops before the wheezing. The difficulty with respiration and wheezing is always described in conventional texts as being worse on expiration. In clinical practice it depends upon the individual and inspiration *or* expiration may be more troublesome. As the wheezing develops there is breathlessness. The severity of attacks are variable with some being mild with only wheezing whilst others develop with severe breathlessness.

A cough is common which is usually dry. Any sputum produced is scanty, white but can be yellowish. The yellowish appearance is almost always due to allergy rather than infection. Eosinophils, white blood cells produced in allergic situations, impart a yellow colour to discharges.

There is a rapid pulse which can be quite high. At a level of 120 per minute it indicates a severe attack and at 140 per minute a life-threatening situation.

Acute attacks of wheezing can be precipitated by several factors including allergens[15], exercise, excitement, cold environment and respiratory infection. Attacks are episodic and will occur at intervals dependent on the particular person and the presence or absence of precipitating factors. Important precipitators of attacks are drugs particularly aspirin, non-steroidal anti-inflammatory drugs, betablockers[16], acetylcysteine[17], betahistine and the female sex hormones of oral contraception and hormone replacement therapy. Tranquillisers, sleeping tablets and morphine derivatives, which includes codeine, may suppress respiration to a dangerous degree in people with asthma and it is dangerous to prescribe them.

At the end of an attack, when the bronchospasm releases, more sputum may be produced which can take the appearance of "casts" - plugs of mucus which take the outline of the bronchiolar wall.

Emotional symptoms are the norm in attacks of asthma with anxiety and fear particularly of suffocation. People may feel that they are taking their last breath.

Investigations:

Chest X-ray is a common first test and is unremarkable except for showing hyperinflation of the lungs. Lung function tests can show the amount of bronchospasm present in a quantitative way. An easy test is the peak flow meter which measures the force of expiration. This may be used to monitor progress during treatment. Do not rely too much on this alone and allow it to determine interventionist treatments such as drugs. It is preferable to decide upon treatment on the basis of symptoms and use such tests as a guide. Medical treatments such as corticosteroids may be given solely on the basis of an investigation revealing reduced air flow. This is a prime example of treating the investigation rather than the person.

Skin hypersensitivity tests are performed in cases of suspected allergy. These are notably unreliable since a positive response on the skin has a poor relationship to respiratory symptoms.

Treatment:

The main aim in conventional medicine is to prevent wheezing to minimise long-term lung damage. Therefore, medical practitioners are keen to use treatments regularly and long-term in an attempt to achieve this result. Corticosteroids are increasingly likely to be used as a first choice.

Precipitating factors are avoided if known and exercise is helpful to strengthen the lungs[18]. Physiotherapy and breathing exercises are underused in the context of general practice.

---

[15] Salbutamol bronchodilators can produce allergic wheezing attacks and some deaths have occurred.
[16] Some betablockers are denoted as being cardioselective, that is, they are reputed not to affect the lungs. This is not true and it is dangerous for any patient with a history of wheezing to take any betablockers. Deaths have resulted from such a prescription.
[17] This is a constituent of cough medicines.
[18] One study showed that blowing up a balloon ten times a day was as effective a treatment in the long-term as bronchodilators.

Allergic cases may be given courses of desensitising injections which are discussed in relation to allergic rhinitis. They are more hazardous in cases of asthma because of the risk of precipitating a severe attack. Deaths have occurred due to overwhelming allergic reaction - anaphylaxis.

The mainstay of treatment is through drugs and especially with bronchodilators. There are several on the market but they have a similar action in that they have adrenaline-like effects. The commonest one is salbutamol which is given either as an inhaler or tablets. It is moderately effective as a dilator of bronchi but there are problems with cardiac effects such as tremor and rapid pulse and the lungs start to rely on the stimulant effect. Certainly people should only take such a drug when necessary and not "just in case".

If the disease fails to respond and an allergic component is present or suspected, sodium cromoglycate is taken as an inhaler. It is recommended to be taken every day three or four times. Its action is to stabilise the membrane of the mast cell and so stop the release of histamine in an allergic reaction. It is of variable effectiveness and I have known people use it for an acute attack since it can relieve wheezing. The conventional view is that this drug has no bronchodilatory activity.

If the person continues to get attacks despite these drugs, corticosteroids will usually be given. They are administered orally in severe cases or inhaled in less severe cases. The inhaled form will certainly have less side-effects than the oral form but it is still suppressive and you will need to take the same general approach to corticosteroids as outlined in the Chapter 10 - Musculoskeletal System.

TREATMENT	TREATMENT LEVEL
Bronchodilators • inhaled • oral	1
Sodium cromoglycate	2
Corticosteroid • inhaled • oral	3
Bronchodilator • nebulised • injected	4
Corticosteroid • injected	5

TABLE 8.13: TREATMENT OF ASTHMA

People with a severe attack of asthma will be admitted to hospital. They will be given oxygen as well as intravenous bronchodilator and corticosteroids. Bronchodilators may also be given in nebulised form. This can be administered at home for some people and their prescription indicates a relatively severe case. Nebulisation is a method of applying the drug in the form of a fine spray.

Antibiotics are invariably prescribed in an acute flare-up of asthma. This is an invidious practice to say the least as there is rarely evidence of bacterial infection. In my days as a hospital doctor, I had the opportunity to work for 6 months on an asthma ward. We never used antibiotics in an acute flare-up and they were considered to be unnecessary. The correct management, conventionally, is to use a combination of bronchodilators and corticosteroids.

CHRONIC BRONCHITIS

The formal definition is of a daily cough, productive of sputum for three months a year for at least two years. It leads to around 30,000 deaths per annum in the UK. The definition above is mainly for studies of its incidence but it does serve as a guide to indicate a chronic overproduction of bronchial mucus.

It is considered to be caused by smoking and air pollution and it is true that these can lead to the accumulation of mucus in the lungs. As I explain in the section on alternative management there is a collection of mucus and the disease is associated with damp and cold weather. Therefore, smoking which heats the lungs will help to relieve the symptoms. Smoking may be the result rather than the cause of the underlying imbalance. The use of a drug regularly, of course, does serve to deplete the body's energy and lead to more ill-health but in the short-term there can be symptom relief.

Symptoms:

In the early stages, it is merely a morning cough with sputum as is seen in many smokers. Then breathlessness develops with wheezing as the lung is increasingly affected. The cause of wheezing here then is partly due to mucus collections, spasm of bronchi and destruction of lung tissue by the inflammatory process. The key feature to distinguish this situation from asthma is that in chronic bronchitis the wheezing is usually more constant and bronchodilators are of variable benefit.

The sputum is usually white but, typically, there are episodes of yellow sputum with perhaps increased breathlessness and cough. Haemoptysis is an occasional associated symptom. This may occur due to a rupture of small blood vessels as they are damaged by the coughing. It usually takes place during an acute exacerbation of the chronic condition. Such an event is more common in the winter months or in cold, damp weather. It is more likely to occur if the person smokes or if the atmosphere is smoky or dusty. Each acute infective episode will further damage the lungs and so there is a gradual deterioration in lung function. The end result is either respiratory failure or cardiac insufficiency.

The term 'blue bloater' has been used to describe people with chronic bronchitis. They may be overweight and as the disease progresses there is the development of oedema. Due to the interference with pulmonary function, there may be blueness (cyanosis). The general appearance is of dampness, mucus, sluggishness, coldness. This may be the reason why smoking is associated with this disease. If you are cold and wet (mucus) then smoking, which is heating, will tend to dry up the secretions and warm the energy. Smoking is more likely then to be the *result* of the preceding energetic condition rather than a *cause* of this disease.

Investigations:

The chest X-ray in this condition is usually normal and so is only of use if the existence is suspected of another condition such as cancer, pneumonia or lung collapse. Lung function tests in an acute episode are often abnormal and ECG examination will reveal the presence of right ventricular enlargement[19]. Sputum may be taken for culture of the infective organism and its sensitivity to antibiotics determined.

Treatment:

This disease is considered to be incurable in conventional medicine and so people are advised to do things which will minimise the rate and the amount of lung damage. They are advised to stop smoking and to be in clean air whenever possible. Antibiotics are used for acute exacerbations. The long-term management includes the use of bronchodilators if wheezing is a large problem although in this disease they are of variable effectiveness. Physiotherapy to the chest aids the removal of secretions and breathing exercises strengthen the chest. They are of definite benefit and should play a part in the correct management of the disease.

EMPHYSEMA

Emphysema is the term used to describe abnormal distension of tissues with air. This can occur in several sites but here we are talking about pulmonary emphysema. The distension occurs in the alveoli and there is gradual destruction of lung tissue leading to the development of enlarged air spaces. This is represented in Figure 8.2. The distension occurs because the lungs are dry and lacking in moisture leading to lung tissue being traumatised.

Smoking is the commonest association and is the disease to be feared by smokers because of its severely debilitating effects. The occupations which may lead to emphysema are those involving dust such as coal mining, quarry workers and those involving heat such as glass blowers.

---

[19] In cases of chronic lung disease, there is increased strain on the right side of the heart which has to push blood through the diseased organ. This is the reason why respiratory disease is a cause of right-sided cardiac insufficiency.

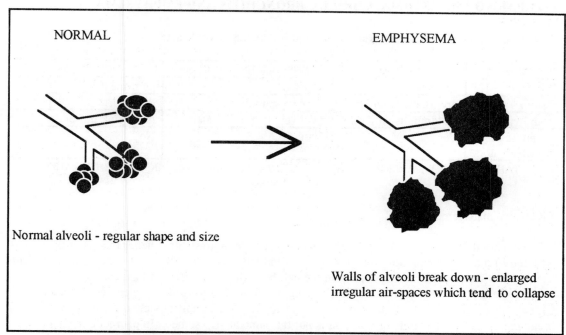

FIGURE 8.2: EMPHYSEMA AND CHANGES IN LUNG STRUCTURE

Symptoms:

The main symptom is breathlessness. It can be severe and is responsible for severely restricting the activity of the person. The process of alveolar wall destruction described above leads to a great reduction in the area of lung tissue available for gaseous exchange. There is associated wheezing which in this case is due to destruction of lung tissue. It is therefore permanent and does not vary.

Upper chest breathing develops and a barrel-chested deformity is seen. Accessory muscles of respiration are used, e.g.. sternocleidomastoid, intercostals. The expiratory breath is done through pursed lips and leads to the description of such people as 'pink puffers'. There are rapid, puffing respirations and the person is usually pink and thin. People do not become cyanosed as in chronic bronchitis since the rapid respirations wash carbon dioxide out of the blood.

Complications:

COMPLICATION	SYMPTOMS TO LOOK FOR
Right ventricular insufficiency	Peripheral oedema, palpitations, nausea, anorexia
Pneumothorax	Sudden worsening of breathlessness, pain and reduced movement on the affected side of the chest
Respiratory failure	Increasing breathlessness, confusion

TABLE 8.14: COMPLICATIONS OF EMPHYSEMA

Treatment:

Emphysema is seen as being progressive and incurable in conventional medicine. Oxygen is administered if there is severe breathlessness and disability. An acute infective situation is treated with antibiotics. Smoking is advised against as this only leads to further lung tissue destruction. Breathing exercises are useful to try to improve the function of the lung. There is a pessimistic view that people will inevitably deteriorate.

Bronchodilators may be given in some cases but there is little relief as the narrowing of the airways is due to a destructive process.

COMPARISON OF ASTHMA, CHRONIC BRONCHITIS AND EMPHYSEMA

A summary of the three diseases I have discussed is detailed in Table 8.15.

SYMPTOM	ASTHMA	CHRONIC BRONCHITIS	EMPHYSEMA
Wheeze	episodic	variable	permanent
Cough	dry, scanty sputum	profuse sputum	dry
Body type	children, usually thin	overweight, 'blue bloater'	thin, 'pink puffer'
Response to bronchodilators	Yes	Variable	No

TABLE 8.15 : COMPARISON OF THE DISEASES OF ASTHMA, CHRONIC BRONCHITIS AND EMPHYSEMA

Alternative management:

It is recognised in conventional circles that in cases of asthma, fresh air is better treatment than drugs with the former improving lung function by 30% and latter only 5-10%. Fresh air also reduces drug use by 60%. Despite this, most people you see will be taking some form of medication.

Whenever you see a person with wheezing it is important to come to an energetic diagnosis. In Chinese medical texts, the term asthma is used to describe conditions characterised by difficult breathing and so the meaning of the term is not the same as its use here. In energetic medicine, it is clear here asthma is made up of several discrete entities. One key question is whether the wheezing and breathlessness is worse for expiration or inspiration. Expiratory difficulty indicates a disharmony in the Lungs and inspiratory difficulty is due to a Kidney disharmony.[20]

The descriptions I have given above may be related to several syndromes in Chinese medicine. Asthma commonly corresponds to Lung Qi Deficiency and Kidney Not Grasping Lung Qi. The Chinese medical counterpart of chronic bronchitis is commonly Spleen Qi Deficiency with DampCold Accumulation and Lung Qi Deficiency. Emphysema usually corresponds to Lung and Kidney Yin Deficiency.

Breathing exercises are extremely helpful for tonifying the chest and lungs and should be given to every person to practice at home[21]. Gentle exercise such as swimming, walking or cycling is very beneficial and should be encouraged. With these measures many people can be benefited and you will probably find that the dose of drugs can be reduced or often stopped completely.

Bronchodilators are related to the chemical ephedrine. This is related to adrenaline and share many effects. These latter two are grouped together as sympathomimetics. Ephedrine is derived from the herb ephedra (Chinese - Ma Huang). In Chinese medicine, this herb is used, always in a balanced formula with other herbs, to release the exterior and induce a sweat. It is warm in nature and is used in External Pathogenic Invasion which affects the Lungs.

Its action, therefore, is to disperse Lung Qi to relieve symptoms such as cough and wheezing. In an acute situation this may be the appropriate treatment. In conventional medicine, it is used in a purified form, in high dosage (compared to herbal dosages), for chronic conditions and for many years. The results of this will be weakness of Lung Qi, Lung Yin Deficiency and ultimately Kidney Yin Deficiency. This explains the common observation that bronchodilators are ineffective for emphysema as it is already a case of Lung Yin Deficiency.

Asthma is a potentially serious condition depending upon the severity of the attack. In the 1950's, adrenaline itself was used to treat asthma but it was discovered that the mortality rate from

---

[20] As I mention in Chapter 9 - Urogenital System, one of the energetic functions of the Kidney is to grasp Qi from the Lungs. If the Kidney cannot do this there will be respiratory symptoms such as wheezing, breathlessness and cough.

[21] Yoga exercises are particularly helpful. A study was reported which revealed that after yoga breathing exercises there was an increased resistance to allergic factors. This was a double-blind study. Lancet 1990; 335: 1381-83.
Yoga breathing exercises have the effect of increasing lung function. Indian J. Physio.Pharmacol. 1992 Apr; 36(2): 105-8.
Yoga breathing exercises led to a significant improvement in lung function, decreased symptoms and decreased drug requirements in children with asthma. This beneficial effect was present some 2 years later. J.Asthma 1991; 28(6): 437-42.

asthma was related the number of prescriptions of adrenaline inhalers. They were withdrawn from the market and the drugs used now are milder in their action. There are still some doubts about their safety however and fenoterol, a common bronchodilator, was banned in Australia and New Zealand in 1990[22]. It is still widely used in the UK and USA. Salbutamol is a related drug.

It would seem clear, from a knowledge of Chinese medicine, that long-term use of such drugs will deplete the Lung Qi to such a point that it may collapse. This is particularly likely to happen when a sudden strain is placed on the person such as stress, sudden allergic load or an infection. As the Lung and Heart Qi are closely related in the chest, any drug which depletes Lung Qi is also likely to deplete Heart Qi. Certainly bronchodilator use causes palpitations in some people. They are strong drugs and need to be approached with care.

Corticosteroids are widely used for asthma. They are being prescribed as a first line treatment in increasing numbers. I discuss their energetic actions more fully in Chapter 10 - Musculoskeletal system. They are hot in nature and provide energy from the Kidney to support other organs. In this case they stimulate Lung Qi strongly to relieve wheeze and their hot nature will dry Phlegm and Dampness in the Lungs. Sudden withdrawal must be avoided as the Lung Qi is in danger of collapsing. Gradual withdrawal whilst alternative treatment is progressing is definitely possible. This is described in Case Two below.

CASES OF WHEEZING DISEASE

CASE ONE

A woman of 44 years came for treatment who had an episode of acute bronchitis some 2 years previously. After that attack she developed wheezing with breathlessness. She had a cough and occasionally produced sputum either white or yellow. She had about 2 severe attacks each year. The symptoms were always worse in cold and windy weather. There were associated symptoms of tiredness, weak legs, poor appetite and a weight loss of 7lbs over the past 2 years.

In terms of Chinese medicine this was a case of Lung Qi deficiency which explained the persistent symptoms after an initial problem with acute bronchitis. There was Spleen Qi deficiency which had led to poor appetite and loss of weight. She was treated with Chinese herbal medicine to strengthen Lung and Spleen. She responded well and after a month of herbs had no symptoms and had regained her 7lbs in weight. I was surprised by her rapid response to treatment but her constitution was basically sound. The asthma had developed after an acute illness and so the case was clearly defined. These types of cases are relatively easy to treat.

CASE TWO

A man of 52 years came for treatment of his chest condition. Some 8 years previously he had 4 operations in a year for sinusitis and nasal polyps. After the last one he developed congestion in his chest which had lasted ever since. His symptoms were severe and consisted of breathlessness and cough with profuse white sputum. He wheezed occasionally but his chest rattled all the time due to retained phlegm. His chest was worse in cold weather and alcohol made his nose run continuously. His general energy was quite good but exercise made him breathless.

His medication consisted of:

- Salbutamol inhaler
- Salbutamol nebulised daily
- Corticosteroid inhaler
- Corticosteroid orally - prednisolone 20-30 mg daily

---

[22] It has been suggested that the increasing illness and death rate associated with asthma may be related to the use of such drugs. They have an effect on opening up the airways but also have a suppressive anti-inflammatory mechanism in the lungs. This may have the effect of causing *increased* levels of inflammation in lung tissue. Lancet 1991; 337: 717-20.
Also see a discussion of the adverse effects of bronchodilators in asthma - Br.J.Clin.Pharmacol. 1992 Feb; 33(2): 129-38.

He varied his dose of oral corticosteroid depending upon his symptoms but was never able to get below 20mg. This is a high dosage of this drug and was responsible for him gaining 28lb in weight over the past few years.

This is clearly a problem of overproduction of mucus which collects in the lungs. It is as a direct result of the surgery to his nose and sinuses. The mucus was not allowed to collect there and so it was suppressed into the lung. This is a common scenario and illustrates the great danger in localised forms of treatment.

In terms of Chinese medicine, his diagnosis was Spleen Qi deficiency with Damp accumulation and Lung Qi deficiency. After treatment of acupuncture and herbal medicine, his sputum decreased in amount resulting in less breathlessness, reduced cough and little or no phlegm in the mornings. He was able to stop his nebulised bronchodilators and found that 20mg of prednisolone was fine to manage his symptoms.

After he had received treatment for some 6 months he is now taking 15mg of prednisolone daily with no flare-up in symptoms and his treatment is continuing. It is important for people to reduce their corticosteroid medication slowly. Sudden withdrawal after long-term use leads to collapse as the adrenal glands have been suppressed for a long time. With slow reduction, the adrenals recover and there will be less likelihood of a flare-up of the condition you are treating.

His conventional diagnosis was asthma which reveals the impreciseness of this term. His condition actually had more in common with the chronic bronchitis picture described earlier.

The main treatment which is affecting this man is the corticosteroid prescription. It is hot in nature and so dries the Damp in the Lungs. If he stopped these suddenly his chest would just fill up with mucus and he would be severely breathless. The corticosteroids also stimulate the Lung Qi to help his breathing. I decided to reduce the drugs when his mucus was much improved and to do so slowly so that any release of mucus could be dealt with and stabilised before going on to further reduction.

- CANCER OF THE LUNG -

This is a major cause of disease in the UK and there are 35000 deaths each year. Over half of cases will occur in people over the age of 65 years. It was rare before the 1940's. Over three times more men are affected than women.

There has been a well documented connection made between cigarette smoking and lung cancer. In fact, one in ten smokers develop this disease and smoking is more likely to lead to heart disease and stroke. However, continual irritation of the lungs is a risk as is pollution of the atmosphere. Other factors include radiation, contact with chromium, arsenic or asbestos.

Symptoms:

There is almost always a history of smoking. If you refer back to Chapter 6 - Cancer, the key features which may indicate cancer are short history and progression of symptoms. In the case of lung cancer, there is a persistent cough, haemoptysis on several occasions and the recent development of other symptoms such as breathlessness. Pain is unusual and occurs late in the disease. Pain due to cancer is invariably dull and constant in nature. It does not change with respiration or movement. If it is due to the invasion of bone by secondary deposits it can be severe. There may be symptoms of a general nature such as anorexia and weight loss.

There may well be signs of the spread of the disease at the time of diagnosis. These include lymphatic gland enlargement in the supraclavicular region on the affected side, hoarse voice[23] and distended veins in the neck and chest.[24] Secondaries in the liver, bone, brain and skin may give rise to pain, nodules or symptoms specific to that organ. The exact symptoms are similar to those detailed

---

[23] The recurrent laryngeal nerve dips into the chest and up again to supply the larynx. If the cancer presses on the nerve it can lead to hoarse voice. The causes of some symptoms in conventional medicine require some detailed knowledge of anatomy or physiology. Whilst I have tried to keep these to a minimum, I mention them for the sake of completeness and to connect with more conventional textbooks.

[24] Pressure on the superior vena cava, the main vein draining blood from the head and neck, may become compressed and so flow is slowed or prevented completely. The appearance is of many distended veins over the chest wall and a congested appearance to the upper body.

under cancer of each organ in the relevant Chapter.

Diagnosis:

Chest X-ray will show the tumour in most cases although it may fail to pick up very small growths. Tomography will reveal more detail. Sputum examination may reveal the presence of cancerous cells. Bronchoscopy is frequently used to look directly at the tumour and to take biopsy material.

Treatment:

It is said conventionally, that surgery "offers the only cure". Certainly, only 15-20% of cases at the time of diagnosis are operable as it has spread too far by that time. Of these who have surgery, only 30% survive 5 years[25]. That is, over 90% of people diagnosed with lung cancer are dead within 5 years. Radiotherapy and chemotherapy are considered to be merely palliative.

Alternative management:

The issues involved for the alternative practitioner in the treatment of cancer are discussed in Chapter 6 - Cancer.

- PNEUMOTHORAX -

This is the presence of air in the pleural cavity. The resultant clinical appearances are due to compression of the lung on the affected side, with collapse of the lung occurring in severe cases. The air is the result of a connection either with the outside as via a perforating chest injury or with the internal air spaces of the lung. The latter can be the result of an injury or due to rupture of air spaces as in emphysema or asthma. I mention this condition, not because it is common (it is in fact quite unusual) but because of the importance to acupuncturists.

It can occur in young people, men more than women, for no apparent reason - spontaneous pneumothorax or as a complication of lung diseases such as asthma, emphysema, tuberculosis, pneumoconiosis. A perforation injury such as by fractured rib, knife etc or the insertion of a needle may pierce the lung.

Symptoms:

There is the sudden appearance of pain in the side of the chest which is affected and breathlessness. The severity of the clinical picture is variable depending upon the amount of air in the pleural cavity and the general condition of the person. Those with pre-existing lung disease may be severely affected and death can occur. There may be breathlessness and in severe cases, cyanosis and confusion.

Occasionally the air in the pleural cavity can continue to build up through a valve-like mechanism. Such a *tension* pneumothorax is characterised by increasing breathlessness and more discomfort. These cases are a medical emergency.

Diagnosis:

Clinical examination reveals reduced chest expansion, resonant percussion over the affected area and absent breath sounds. Chest X-ray confirms the diagnosis.

---

[25] The use and meaning of 5 year survival rates by conventional medicine is interesting. They are usually see as being the same as 'cure' in the conventional sense of the word. I treated a woman once who had a malignant melanoma diagnosed and removed surgically. She was well for 4 years and 11 months and then developed symptoms of secondaries. Another month and she would have been classified as a 'cure'. This is why you have to be very careful with statistical statements of survival and 'cure' rates. What is of over-riding importance is the quality of life of the person not the duration and the individual circumstances regarding life-style, emotional state, relationships and so forth.

Treatment:

The air is drained from the pleural cavity by means of a tube inserted through an intercostal space. This necessitates a stay in hospital of several days.

POINT NUMBER	POINT NAME	POINT NUMBER	POINT NAME
Lung 1	Zhongfu	Urinary Bladder 11	Dashu
Lung 2	Yunmen	Urinary Bladder 12	Fengmen
Large Intestine 16	Jugu	Urinary Bladder 13	Feishu
Large Intestine 17	Tianding	Urinary Bladder 14	Jueyinshu
Stomach 12	Quepen	Urinary Bladder 15	Xinshu
Stomach 13	Qihu	Urinary Bladder 16	Dushu
Stomach 14	Kufang	Urinary Bladder 17	Geshu
Stomach 15	Wuyi	Urinary Bladder 18	Ganshu
Stomach 16	Yingchuang	Urinary Bladder 43	Gaohuangshu
Stomach 18	Rugen	Urinary Bladder 44	Shentang
Spleen 17	Shidou	Urinary Bladder 45	Yixi
Spleen 18	Tianxi	Urinary Bladder 46	Geguan
Spleen 19	Xiongxiang	Urinary Bladder 47	Hunmen
Spleen 20	Zhourong	Urinary Bladder 48	Yanggang
Spleen 21	Dabao	Pericardium 1	Tianchi
Heart 1	Jiquan	San Jiao 15	Tianliao
Small Intestine 14	Jianwaishu	Gall Bladder 21	Jianjing
Small Intestine 15	Jianzhongshu	Gall Bladder 22	Yuanye
Kidney 22	Bulang	Gall Bladder 23	Zhejin
Kidney 23	Shenfeng	Gall Bladder 24	Riyue
Kidney 24	Lingxu	Liver 14	Qimen
Kidney 25	Shencang	Extra point M-BW-1	Dingchuan
Kidney 26	Yuzhong	Extra point N-CA-8	Ganshi
Kidney 27	Shufu	Extra point M-BW-12	Yishu
		Extra point N-CA-7	Xiongdaji

TABLE 8.16 ACUPUNCTURE POINTS OVERLYING OR ADJACENT TO LUNG TISSUE

Alternative management:

The main issue for alternative practitioners is for acupuncturists who must be aware of back and chest points which overlie the lungs. This is more important in those with hyperinflated lungs such as occurs in emphysema, asthma and in thin people. It is impossible to perforate the lung if a needle is inserted correctly in terms of depth and angle. Table 8.16 is a list of the acupuncture points which overlie lung tissue.

- PLEURISY -

This is inflammation of the pleura. The two pleural layers rub together and leads to the classical pain of this condition. With a stethoscope you can hear a coarse crackle - the pleural rub.

The inflammation may be a localised affection of the pleura or part of a wider problem, e.g. pneumonia or pulmonary embolism. The main thing to consider is whether the pleurisy has occurred following an upper respiratory tract infection. These cases are relatively straightforward. More serious situations are present if more severe respiratory symptoms are associated with it.

Symptoms:

The primary feature of pleurisy is pain in the chest. This is sharp in nature and commonly felt in the axilla or around the scapula. It is worse for movement, coughing and respiration. There may be a low grade fever and a dry cough.

The differential diagnosis of chest pain is considered in Chapter 7 - Cardiovascular System. The main differentiation here is from musculoskeletal conditions.

Complications:

COMPLICATION	SYMPTOMS TO LOOK FOR
Pleural effusion - fluid in the pleural cavity	Pain disappears but there is the development of restricted breathing, breathlessness
Empyema - pus in the pleural cavity	Similar symptoms to the above but with fever, malaise

TABLE 8.17: COMPLICATIONS OF PLEURISY

Treatment:

Antibiotics are invariably given for this condition. The majority of associated infections are viral. Rest and painkillers are advised. Investigations such as Chest X-ray and tomography will be performed if a serious underlying cause is suspected.

Alternative management:

In most cases, there is no need to worry about this condition in that it is mild and self-limiting. You need to know the symptoms which are indicative of a serious condition so there is more concern if breathlessness or haemoptysis is present.

- PULMONARY EMBOLISM -

This is an obstruction of the pulmonary artery by a clot which has usually become detached from a deep vein thrombosis.

Symptoms:

These are of sudden development due to the underlying process. If a large artery is obstructed then sudden death may result. In milder cases there is appearance of breathlessness, pleuritic chest pain and haemoptysis. There may be fever also. Most people are acutely ill and require hospitalisation for pain relief.

Investigations:

An ECG is normal in most cases besides an increase in heart rate. In severe cases there may be tall P waves with evidence of enlargement of the right ventricle. A Chest X-ray may be normal in the early stages but later shows, in severe cases, a wedge-shaped area of affected lung. More sophisticated techniques such as radioisotope scans and angiography will confirm the diagnosis. The diagnosis can usually be made, however, on the basis of the history.

Treatment:

This is similar to that of deep venous thrombosis particularly with regard to anticoagulation.

Alternative management:

The main issue for alternative practitioners is around the use of anticoagulants. This is discussed in Chapter 7 - Cardiovascular System in relation to deep venous thrombosis.

- REVIEW OF SYMPTOMS -

COUGH

This is exceedingly common and many people suffer from it at some time or another. It may be such a feature of someone's life that they can deny a cough even when you can hear it during the consultation. It will have passed out of awareness because it has been around for so long.

In general, conventional medicine sees cough as important in terms of three factors:

1. *The degree of disturbance to the person.*

If the disturbance is great then suppressants will be given for dry coughs and expectorants for a productive cough. There is little evidence to suggest that either are effective and certainly not more so than honey and lemon as a hot drink or a steam inhalation and this is the view of most respiratory specialists. Most proprietary cough medicines contain lots of sugar and suppressants are usually based on codeine or its derivatives. Codeine is methylmorphine and as such will produce addiction if taken for long periods and will also cause constipation and drowsiness. Expectorants usually contain anti-histamines and/or amphetamine-like compounds, e.g. ephedrine which dry mucus but can lead to agitation and insomnia. Suppression of any cough may be harmful as it is a natural defence mechanism aiming to discharge problems from the body although there is no fault with taking soothing, non-toxic substances. Honey is a lubricant and so will aid dry coughs. It should not be taken in large quantities if there is a lot of mucus.

2. *Presence or absence of bacterial infection.*

Any cough or sputum which seems to indicate a bacterial infection will be treated with antibiotics. The dividing line is the colour of the sputum and if this is white (mucoid) then no bacterial infection is considered to be present and if it is yellowish (mucopurulent) or greenish (purulent) bacterial infection is assumed. Even conventionally, these drugs should not be given unless there is bacteriological evidence for infection but in general practice the routine is to give antibiotics on the clinical evidence. The other reason for waiting for bacteriological evidence is that the wrong antibiotic may be prescribed. The organism responsible may be resistant to that agent and only laboratory investigation will reveal the correct drug to be taken.

This reflex attitude to the colour of the sputum leads to large quantities of antibiotics being prescribed during winter episodes of upper respiratory tract infection whether or not they are actually indicated. It is worth noting that green or yellow sputum can be seen in certain allergic disorders such as asthma where it is due to the presence of eosinophils and it cannot be differentiated on naked-eye appearances from sputum where bacteria are present. I made this point in relation to the treatment of an acute asthma attack where antibiotics are not required as the problem is inflammatory, not infective.

In energetic terms the colour of the sputum is to do with the amount of Heat present. White means Cold and yellow means Heat, not necessarily the presence of bacteria. If yellow sputum is examined bacteriologically then not all the samples will show bacterial infection.

3. *Presence of serious underlying disease.*

There are some people with cough who have severe pathology. These cases will be investigated with at least a chest X-ray.

SPUTUM

The colloquial term for this is catarrh or phlegm but you must always check with people what they mean by various terms. Medically, mucus describes the substance produced from the respiratory system and sputum refers to mucus which is coughed up. In terms of conventional medicine, the distinction is of sputum which is white or yellow.

Mucoid sputum is white or colourless and is due to an overproduction of bronchial mucus. Purulent sputum is yellowish or greenish and may be indicative of a bacterial infection (see above).

The consistency of sputum can be helpful in aiding the diagnostic process and should be enquired about. It is certainly true that the British are extremely reticent when it comes to discussing their bodily functions and discharges. It is helpful to explain the importance of asking these questions and to do so with tact..

TENDENCY TO CATCH COLDS

This is a symptom which is not given much emphasis in conventional circles but is very important from the point of view of alternative medicine. It gives an indication of the state of the defensive system in warding off attack from the outside in general and the strength of the lungs specifically.

HAEMOPTYSIS

This is the appearance of blood in the sputum ranging from faint streaking to obvious blood. You should first ensure it is in the sputum from a respiratory origin as bleeding gums, nose or mouth may lead to blood appearing in material which is coughed up and spit out.

The symptom of bleeding, wherever it occurs, should always be viewed seriously. What action is taken subsequently is then between you and the person consulting you but it is sensible to consider making an assessment of the source of the bleeding. If the symptom is associated with an acute bronchitis in a young person then perhaps there is no cause to worry. However, the situation in a 55 years old smoker who perhaps coughs blood on several occasions is a different proposition. In the case of haemoptysis, only 40% of cases have a demonstrable cause in conventional medicine.

CHEST PAIN

This was discussed in Chapter 7 - Cardiovascular System. I would remind you that dull, constant pain in the chest pain can be indicative of serious disease such as lung cancer. In general, pain of this type is seen in people with severe conditions where the energy is quite weak. In conventional terms it is often associated with cancer. It is more worrying to see pain of this type than sharper pain which changes in response to posture, respiration and so on.

BREATHLESSNESS

This symptom has been discussed in relation to some diseases in Chapter 7 - Cardiovascular System. Breathing is a complex act and related to many areas of the body and mind. Emotional disturbances are very often reflected in changes in the breath and some psychotherapeutic procedures, especially the newer bodywork therapies, utilise the breath to release emotional, mental and physical energies which have become fixed. The Hindu word *prana* is sometimes translated as breath and is the ayurdevic equivalent of Qi in Chinese medicine. This translation serves to indicate the close link between these energies and the mind.

This is a vast subject and certainly beyond the scope of this book but the whole area is accessible through some schools of psychotherapy and some religious traditions. I would mention here that unskilful use of the breath by practitioners, particularly utilising hyperventilation, can lead to the release of emotional states which can overwhelm the person. This is especially true of rebirthing where such a catharsis can present many powerful emotions into the person's conscious mind and lead to severe problems. Transformative practices are much gentler and allow people time to adjust to altered states.

CYANOSIS

This symptom was discussed in Chapter 7- Cardiovascular System. It indicates a severe situation unless it is the extremities in cold weather (poor circulation).

WHEEZE

This is a high-pitched musical sound which is heard during respiration. It may be present during inspiration, expiration or both. It is an indication of an obstruction to the airflow in the smaller airways of the lungs. The main thing to consider is the degree of interference with respiratory function. Breathlessness is the key issue to take into account when presented with someone who is wheezing.

STRIDOR

This is obstruction of a major airway and is a crowing noise mainly heard during inspiration. It is seen in obstruction by an inhaled object and in some infectious disorders of childhood, e.g. whooping cough.

FINGER CLUBBING

This is thickening at the base of the finger nails. It may also be seen in the toes. There is normally an angle between the nail and the finger at the nail-bed. This disappears in finger clubbing. In extreme cases the end of the finger or toe becomes bulbous. It occurs in several diseases and they include tuberculosis, bronchiectasis, lung abscess, empyema, lung cancer, congenital heart disease, liver cirrhosis and inflammatory bowel disease.

In terms of Chinese medicine, it is due to Phlegm which collects in the ends of the digits as the flow of Qi is obstructed.

- HOW TO RECOGNISE SERIOUS CONDITIONS OF THE RESPIRATORY SYSTEM -

SYMPTOM	WHEN TO WORRY
COUGH	persistent with blood with breathlessness
CHEST PAIN	constant dull
BREATHLESSNESS	severe acute progressive with confusion with cyanosis pulse rate > 120 per minute paroxysmal attacks occurring at night
HAEMOPTYSIS	recurrent older person, smoker
SPUTUM	copious green/yellow blood stained frothy
WHEEZING	if accompanied by breathlessness (see above)
TENDENCY TO CATCH COLDS	not serious
STRIDOR	always
CYANOSIS	central - tongue peripheral - lips and extremities (unless due to cold)
HOARSENESS	persistent (more than three weeks)
FINGER CLUBBING	always

TABLE 8.27: HOW TO RECOGNISE SERIOUS CONDITIONS IN RESPIRATORY SYSTEM DISEASE

Diseases of the respiratory system are common in our society and the symptoms listed below are extremely common. It is important to know how to recognise if a symptom arises from a serious situation. You can use Table 8.27 as a guide to refer to when faced with a person who has one or more of these symptoms. I make no mention of disease labels in the column on the right as I would not expect you to be able to diagnose conventionally. Seriousness can be assessed merely by reference to symptom pictures. However, you will be able to recognise that there are clinical appearances which would be diagnosed as a particular disease. For example, if you look at breathlessness and its seriousness, you will see that this is the appearance of a severe asthma attack.

- SUMMARY -

The lung is known as the 'tender organ' as it is vulnerable to attack by external climatic factors.

The respiratory system can be divided into an upper and lower part. The depth and progression of symptoms is directly related to the state of the person's energy.

Many respiratory conditions are treated with antibiotics which are overused and frequently unnecessary from a conventional viewpoint.

Chronic lung diseases are common, especially in cold, damp and polluted climates. Alternative medicine is an effective option to deal with them.

In cases with mucus collections, it is useful to remember that this substance has emotional overtones. What I mean by this is that mucus is Yin as are emotions. Emotional states may be manifest as such or held in the body. Mucus is a typical way in which they may be stored. An example of this is when people stop cigarette smoking. They may develop emotional discharges of vulnerability, weeping, feeling sensitive and so on or develop a cough with mucus. Such releases of suppressions may, therefore, present in several ways and it is important for the practitioner to recognise this. I deal with emotional releases in Chapter 16 - Psychological disorders.

9 URINARY SYSTEM

OBJECTIVES:

At the end of this Chapter you will be able to:
Describe the differences between the alternative and conventional views of the urinary system.
List the symptoms attributable to disturbances of the urinary system.
State when a symptom(s) would indicate a serious underlying condition.
Describe the main symptoms of diseases covered in this Chapter.
Explain the relevant management by an alternative practitioner of each disorder.

- INTRODUCTION -

In conventional medicine, the functions of the kidney primarily deal with the regulation of water and electrolyte balance. There are additional functions which deal with acid-base balance, maintenance of blood pressure, stimulation of red blood cell production and Vitamin D metabolism. This is clearly a dynamic process in order to retain essential substances and allow unwanted materials to be excreted. In conventional clinical practice however, the kidney is likened to a filtration system and from this view arises the concept of 'flushing', taking large quantities of water. With conditions such as urinary infections or kidney stones, people are advised to drink 5 or 6 pints of water (minimum) each day. The aim is to flush the system out and remove any impurities or organisms.

This view denies the existence of energetic factors and sees the kidney merely as a physical filter. Energy is needed to drive the system and the energy will be swamped if excessive amounts of fluid are taken. Long-term this will lead to depletion of kidney energy and the development of urinary symptoms such as tiredness, frequent urination, backache and oedema. In conventional physiology, there is acknowledgement that the processes of water and electrolyte balance are active and dynamic. This is not often recognised or dealt with by conventional clinicians.

The information in Table 9.1 reveals the associations which are made through a knowledge of vitalistic principles. The comments on the right of the Table are to explain these associations. The information in this Table is derived from Chinese medicine and will be most familiar to practitioners of this. However, the underlying energetic principles are common to all methods of alternative medicine and so there will be glimpses of recognition for other practitioners.

ASSOCIATION	COMMENTS
Stores Jing	Jing is a fundamental substance of Chinese thought and is associated with birth, reproduction and maturation. On a narrow, physical level it may be likened to ideas of genetics in Western science.
Root of Yin and Yang	These principles have no counterpart in conventional thought. The Kidneys provide the basis of Yin and Yang for the whole body. Kidney function is therefore reflected in the whole person and long-term disease will lead to depletion of Kidney Yin or Yang or both. The decline in constitutional energy over the past few generations can be viewed in one way as a general decrease in Kidney function.
Rules Water[1]	This is done by the Yang aspect of the Kidney. People who retain fluid and become overweight easily may have a deficiency of Kidney Yang (Fire) not ruling Water. This is why large intakes of water lead to fluid retention as it damages the Kidney Yang.
Rules Bones	In conventional medicine, vitamin D metabolism is influenced by the kidney. Vitamin D has an effect on calcium metabolism.
Rules grasping of Qi	The Kidneys pull qi down from the Lungs and aid in respiration. Some lung disorders such as asthma, therefore, may be due to a Kidney imbalance. This has no counterpart in conventional medicine.
Generates Marrow, Fills up the Brain	This is an interesting connection. The Chinese understood that the Kidneys have a role in making marrow and thence Blood several centuries before such a connection was made in conventional medicine. In addition, the Brain is described as the 'Sea of Marrow' and so Kidney function is reflected in thought, memory and concentration. This is why dementia is more common now at younger ages as the Kidney energy is becoming depleted.
Paired organ is Urinary Bladder	This is comparable with the conventional view that the bladder stores urine produced by the kidney.
Opens into the ear	Many ear problems are considered to be due to Kidney imbalance in Chinese medicine. In conventional medicine it is recognised that administration of certain drugs in kidney disease may cause deafness.
Colour - black	This is the colour of Yin, Water (see below). It also corresponds to the deep unconscious.

---

[1] All organs which are capitalised, e.g. Blood, Heart, Kidney indicate that I mean the energetic view of that organ and not the narrowly defined physical structure of Western science.

Taste - salt	Each major organ has an associated taste. In this case excess salty food can damage the Water element.
Season - winter	The energy of winter is quiescent, drawn deep within the body, descending. This can be compared to the kidneys in that they are hidden deep within the body, difficult to palpate[2].
Element - Water	The Element correspondence reveals the connection of Chinese medical theory to nature. Each Element is connected to the others to provide, in health, a harmonious balance.
Time - 5 pm to 7 pm	The 'time' of an organ is when its energy it at its maximum. This explains why most people die in the early hours of the morning - time of deficient Kidney symptoms. Also, asthma caused by a Kidney weakness in grasping the qi will be worse at 5 am.
Emotions - fear	This association explains why extreme fear can affect the Kidneys. There may be increased urination, for example, at such times.
Mental aspect	Intellect, intelligence and wisdom, insight and quality of intelligence. Will power and ambition depend upon Kidney function.

TABLE 9.1: HOLISTIC ENERGETIC VIEW OF THE KIDNEY[3]

There is a tradition of urine therapy[4] in Ayurvedic medicine where the washing of affected parts in urine or the drinking of urine is used to treat many conditions. There have been many documented cases treated by such methods and emphasises that urine is not only a waste product.

- BASIC ANATOMY AND PHYSIOLOGY -

As stated above, the functions of the kidney are seen as being physical in nature by conventional medicine. In clinical practice, it is essential to view the kidney as a dynamic, energetic entity and to give information to people on this basis. There are several basic facts of anatomy and physiology which it is useful to know. These are detailed in Table 9.2.

As a preliminary to study of disease of the urinary system you are able to:
State the main structures of the urinary system
Identify the main features of the kidney
Describe the appearance of the basic functional unit of the kidney - the nephron
Discuss the function of the nephron
Describe the endocrine functions of the kidney - erythropoeitin and red cell production, renin-angiotensin and maintenance of blood pressure, Vitamin D metabolism
Identify the main features of the testes and prostate
Discuss the functions of the testes and prostate

TABLE 9.2: OBJECTIVES FOR ANATOMY AND PHYSIOLOGY AS PREREQUISITE FOR STUDY OF DISEASE OF THE URINARY SYSTEM

I have included the male organs of testes and prostate since their function, in Chinese medicine, is dependent upon Kidney energy. Also there is no study of male disease (andrology) in conventional medicine and so it seems helpful to put it here. In women, disorders of menstruation, fertility and childbirth are often related to the function of the Kidney (as well as other organs) but all these are discussed separately in Chapter 17 - Pregnancy and Childbirth and Chapter 18 -

---

[2] It is interesting that the conventional classification of kidney keeps changing and there are many aspects of physiology which are still not understood. This is a reflection of the nature of the kidneys. They are hidden from view and are the deepest level of the physical body.

[3] An excellent source for information about the energetic organ systems of Chinese medicine is "Between Heaven and Earth" by Beinfield and Korngold (Ballantine, 1991). I mention the main points here to perhaps shed some light on a wider view of the organs. Homoeopaths may recognise remedy pictures in these descriptions as these are merely another way of describing the same energetic entity.

[4] Books which describe urine therapy include, "Shivambu Kalpa" by Arthur Lincoln Pauls (Ortho-Bionomy Publishing, 1978), "Water of Life" by J W Armstrong, "Manar Mootra - Auto-Urine Therapy" by RM Patel (Bharat Serak Samaj Publications, 1987).

Gynaecology.

- CLASSIFICATION OF URINARY SYSTEM DISEASE -

The conventional classification of kidney disease is confusing since it changes every few years. This reflects the confusion in conventional circles as to the physiology of the kidneys. The reasons for this are discussed above.

MILD DISEASE		
INFLAMMATORY		INFECTIVE
		Sexually transmitted disease • gonorrhoea • non-specific urethritis Prostatitis (including prostatic enlargement) Cystitis
		Acute pyelonephritis
Acute glomerulonephritis		
Proliferative aka nephritic syndrome aka Ellis Type I aka Bright's disease	Minimal lesion/membranous aka nephrotic syndrome aka Ellis Type II	
Renal stones Cancer		
		Chronic pyelonephritis
Chronic glomerulonephritis		
End-stage kidney disease		
SEVERE DISEASE		

TABLE 9.3: CLASSIFICATION OF RENAL DISEASE

Table 9.3 reveals the main differentiation between infective and inflammatory kidney disease. I discuss these in detail below and how to analyse relative severities. The main thing to consider is the site of the problem. If the disease affects the deeper organs such as the kidney, then it is clearly more serious than disease which affects superficial areas such as the urethra. When comparing infective with inflammatory, any condition with bacteria indicates stronger energy. Therefore, acute glomerulonephritis is more serious, i.e. affects weaker people, than acute pyelonephritis.

- CYSTOSCOPY -

This is a specialist investigation of the urinary tract. It is a form of endoscopy and I would refer you to Chapter 4 - Investigations for comments on these. Cystoscopy allows examination of the bladder wall and urethra. It is done under either local or general anaesthetic.

The indications for its use are haematuria and urinary tract infection. Diagnosis can be made of stones, tumours, prostatic enlargement. Stones may be removed by the instrument and biopsy can be performed.

The complications include haemorrhage, perforation of the bladder, urinary retention and infection.

- INFECTIVE DISEASE OF THE URINARY SYSTEM -

This is a major category of disease of the urinary system. Infections of this area are very common and can occur in the kidney, ureters, bladder or urethra. The urinary system may be divided at the level of the bladder into the upper and lower urinary tracts. Most lower urinary tract infections will not lead to infection in the upper urinary tract. This can be compared to the division of the respiratory system. As I discussed in relation to respiratory disease, infection in the deeper levels of a system only occurs if the energy of that system is markedly disturbed. If the energetic state of the person improves then the disease will move out into more superficial areas.

I would emphasise that organisms are not the cause of such disease but merely an associated occurrence. This idea is discussed fully in Chapter 5 - Infectious Disease. The presence of strong symptoms with a clearly identified organism indicates that the energy of the person is relatively strong.

GONORRHOEA

This is classified as a sexually transmitted disease. It is associated with a bacterium, Neisseria gonorrhoeae, and has an incubation period of 2-10 days. It is mainly an affection of the mucous membrane of the genital tract, rectum, pharynx and eyes.

The incidence increased rapidly in the 1970's, as a result of greater sexual freedom and the decline in use of barrier contraceptive methods. The risk of infection is different in males and females. 60-80% of women in contact with an infected man will develop gonorrhoea. This is in contrast to 20-30% of men who contract the disease when in contact with an infected woman. Discrepancies in infection rate are also noted with HIV. It seems that the *penetrating* partner is less likely to develop infection than the *penetrated* partner - male or female. There are large numbers of cases in the West and especially so in the United States. In 1985, there were 1 million reported cases in the US with an estimated similar number of others non-reported.

Symptoms:

The main symptoms in men are severe dysuria (likened to passing broken glass), frequency of urination and a yellow urethral discharge. There may be no or mild symptoms in a minority.

In women, the lower cervical canal is affected with the urethra and rectum in 50% of cases. In 50% of females and 10% of males there are no symptoms at all. Vaginal discharge is the common symptom with frequency of urination and dysuria. For this reason, the illness may not be recognised as such in women.

The pharynx is involved in a significant proportion of cases where there has been oral contact. There may be systemic symptoms of fever, muscle aches and pains, a diffuse rash of redness or pustules and a general feeling of ill-health.

Investigations:

These are performed if the diagnosis is clinically suspected. Swabs and culture are done using special media on which to grow the organism.

Complications:

COMPLICATIONS	SYMPTOMS TO LOOK FOR
Urethral stricture (narrowing) - this is rare now and was due to the use of caustic treatments	Urinary frequency, urgency, poor stream, dribbling urination
Epididymitis (males)	Swelling and pain in the testis
Prostatitis (males)	Urinary frequency, dark and strong smelling urine, dysuria, suprapubic tenderness, fever
Pelvic inflammatory disease (females)	Lower abdominal pain, fever, vaginal discharge
Neonatal conjunctivitis (rare)	Redness of the conjunctiva, yellow discharge

TABLE 9.4: COMPLICATIONS OF GONORRHOEA

Treatment:

This is with penicillin although some strains are resistant to this now (since 1976). Repeat cultures are taken until they are negative. Another part of treatment is the tracing of contacts and the offering of treatment to them.

NON-SPECIFIC URETHRITIS (NSU)

This is also known as non-gonococcal urethritis and is classified as a sexually transmitted disease. It was first recognised in the 1970's when people, who had been treated for gonorrhoea, returned with similar symptoms but no evidence of the gonococcal bacterium. The organism which is associated with this condition is an unusual one, Chlamydia trachomatis. It is also isolated from women with pelvic inflammatory disease. It is an interesting organism in that it is classified as being somewhere between a virus and a bacterium. In the UK, in men, urethritis is more often non-gonococcal than gonococcal.

Symptoms.

These are the same as gonorrhoea but milder. The urethral discharge is less yellow and profuse than that of gonorrhoea.

Investigations:

These are the same as for gonorrhoea.

Treatment.

This is with oxytetracycline as the organism does not respond to penicillin.

Complications:

These are the same as those of gonorrhoea.

Alternative management of gonorrhoea and non-specific urethritis:

This is the one situation in the UK which is governed by law. The Venereal Diseases Act of 1916 means, in effect, that gonorrhoea and syphilis must be treated by conventional medicine. Contact tracing by clinics are also an important aspect of management. There is no harm with treating at the same time as conventional practitioners but it is important not to put yourself in the position of threatening your practice.

In energetic terms, it is clearly suppressive to treat these conditions by means of antibiotics and if you read the accounts of the homoeopathic remedy, Medorrhinum[5] you will see the internal, mental and emotional disharmonies which are associated. In the end it is the person with the condition who must decide upon the course of action which is most appropriate.

In terms of Chinese medicine, the syndromes which correspond to disorders in this area are similar to those listed under the urinary disorders in general.

---

[5] There are several homoeopathic materia medicas available including "Materia Medica of Homoeopathic Medicines" by S R Phatak (Indian Books and Periodicals Syndicate, 1977). Medorrhinum is the remedy made from cases of gonorrhoea and is frequently indicated in cases of suppressed gonorrhoea. This may manifest as an infection in the person or it may be something in the family history.

PROSTATITIS

Prostatitis is an inflammation of the prostate. It commonly develops secondary to a urethritis, usually of a sexually transmitted origin. It may occur without evidence of infection but with identical symptoms. This type is of unknown cause in conventional medicine.

Symptoms:

There may be acute or chronic attacks. The acute types have stronger symptoms but most cases seen in the clinic are of the chronic variety which is described here. There are episodes of perineal pain with dysuria, frequency of urination, urgency and nocturia. Systemic disturbances are common with fever, general malaise and tiredness. There are acute flare-ups from time to time perhaps related to dietary factors, sexual activity, overwork and stress.

Treatment:

Antibiotics are invariably prescribed despite the poor penetrance of the drugs into the substance of the prostate. Relapses are almost universal. Non-steroidal anti-inflammatory agents are used in many situations especially if there is no evidence of infection. Conventionally, there is no long-term relief and some people may be given low dose antibiotics for continuously for years.

Alternative management:

In terms of Chinese medicine this usually corresponds to a condition of Dampness and Heat which collects in the Lower Jiao due to weak Kidneys. Such an event is also associated with the function of the Spleen. There may also be some Liver Qi Stagnation as the Liver Channel traverses this area.

CYSTITIS

This is inflammation of the bladder. It is rare in men and common in women where it is frequently associated with gynaecological symptoms. There are a variety of theories as to why this condition is commoner in women. They all revolve around the bacterial theory of disease causation despite a significant number of cases not having any demonstrable organism. The three main ideas are as follows. The area around the urethra is heavily colonised with bacteria although this is the same in both sexes. The urethra of women is shorter than men so infection can pass up it easier. I would think that *any* length of urethra is adequate and this may be a reference to the penis-envy theory of psychological thought. Lastly, if the bladder is not emptied properly, i.e. fully, there is residual urine which may serve as a reservoir for the growth of bacteria. It is suggested in some texts that women do not empty their bladders completely. The implication, of course, is that either there is an inherent design fault causing a loss of function or that women wilfully do not empty their bladders completely. These ideas reflect the strong sexist attitudes of conventional medicine and lead to treatments which are ineffective. I explore this view of women's health in Chapter 18 - Gynaecology.

There is a phrase in common usage, "pissed off" which suggests irritation or resentment. It is not surprising that the emotions closely associated with the bladder in Chinese medicine are suspicion and jealousy. In homoeopathy, the remedy Staphysagria has suppressed anger and resentment as a strong guiding symptom. It may be given for complaints of shame and mortification, for invasion by penetration. It is also indicated in cases of 'honeymoon cystitis' where sexual activity has led to the symptoms of cystitis. It is much more useful to look at symptoms from this perspective so that a deeper understanding of aetiology is gained which leads to more effective treatment. Men do not have the same symptoms as they are rarely 'invaded' in a similar manner. I have treated a number of women with recurrent symptoms of cystitis or burning pains in the vagina and there is almost always a history of a traumatic event, perhaps sexual, possibly emotional, leading to this clinical picture. Chapter 18 - Gynaecology describes several cases leading to gynaecological symptoms.

Symptoms:

Many women (50%) have the following symptoms at some point in their lives but usually as a single attack (90% of attacks are not repeated). The main symptoms are urinary frequency, dysuria and suprapubic pain. There is an intense desire to pass urine even if the bladder is empty (strangury). The urine may be of a strong colour, cloudy and with an unpleasant odour. Haematuria occurs in some. There is suprapubic tenderness on examination of the abdomen. There may be associated fever and chills although these symptoms are more typical of acute pyelonephritis.

In some people there is no culture of bacteria - about half of all cases. This is called the "urethral syndrome" and is ill-understood in conventional medicine for reasons stated above.

Around 1 in 20 pregnant women have evidence of bacteria in their urine and so all women who are pregnant have urine cultures as part of their antenatal care. The presence of such bacteria may be associated with pyelonephritis later in pregnancy, pre-eclamptic toxaemia and anaemia. It is indicative of an underlying kidney imbalance at least on the energetic level.

Investigations:

The correct management includes urinalysis with culture and determining the sensitivity of any organisms to antibiotics. On examination, the urine will contain bacteria and possibly pus cells. Dipsticks are available to detect nitrites which are produced by bacteria but they are unreliable. Blood tests reveal a raised white cell count.

Recurrent attacks (3 or more) of lower urinary tract infection in women (or in men and children after one attack) may be further investigated by means of cystoscopy and intravenous excretion urography. These are performed to detect predisposing factors such as structural abnormalities or kidney stones. Urinary tract infections are common when there are congenital defects of the kidney. From an alternative point of view this makes sense as an congenital structural defect means there must be a preceding energetic imbalance.

Treatment:

Antibiotics are the mainstay of treatment and these may be given long-term in some people. It is preferable to determine the presence of bacteria and their sensitivity to antibiotics before prescribing drugs but this is rarely done in clinical practice. Cultures should be repeated at the end of treatment to check that the bacteria have disappeared. There are some situations, particularly in the elderly, when there is 'asymptomatic bacteriuria'. This is the presence of bacteria in the urine with no symptoms. The correct conventional response is to observe since there is no problem in people with no symptoms. The same is true of women with asymptomatic bacteriuria unless pregnant (see above).

General advice includes drinking large amounts of fluid each day to 'flush' out the kidneys. People are advised to urinate frequently.

PYELONEPHRITIS

This disease is at the level of the kidney and so indicates a deeper, more severe situation. There are still the relatively strong symptoms associated with the presence of organisms but now revealing that the substance of the kidney is affected.

ACUTE PYELONEPHRITIS

This may occur secondary to infective disease in the urethra or bladder which has ascended into the upper reaches of the urinary tract. This may be due to associated factors such as catheterisation, obstruction to urinary flow by kidney stones, prostatic enlargement or urethral stricture, diabetes mellitus or if there is use of analgesics/non-steroidal anti-inflammatory agents. Some people develop pyelonephritis without an associated factor and this would represent an imbalance on the level of energy without detectable physical abnormality.

Symptoms:

There is the sudden onset of fever with chills, loin pain and vomiting. The person feels ill. As the inflammation affects most of the urinary tract there are associated symptoms of the frequent painful passing of small amounts of urine, painful desire to pass to urine but there is nothing there (strangury) and, in severe cases, haematuria.

Investigations:

The general approach is the same as described above for cystitis. A full blood count reveals increased numbers of white cells. Urinalysis is positive for protein and perhaps blood. Urine culture provides evidence of bacteria in many cases including their sensitivity to antibiotics.

Treatment:

This is invariably by means of antibiotics which may be given without evidence from urine culture.

Complications:

These are rare unless there is a structural abnormality of the kidney or a chronic disease such as diabetes mellitus.

COMPLICATIONS	SYMPTOMS TO LOOK FOR
Chronic pyelonephritis	Loin pain, frequent urination, tiredness, possibly dysuria
Renal papillary necrosis	Worsening symptoms, high fever, haematuria, the person is ill, deteriorating condition
Perinephric abscess	Fever, one-sided loin pain, recent history of urinary tract infection, relapsing fever
Kidney abscess	Fever persists or relapses

TABLE 9.5 COMPLICATIONS OF ACUTE PYELONEPHRITIS

CHRONIC PYELONEPHRITIS

This is persistent pyelonephritis. It occurs either in people who are not strong enough to throw off an acute attack or if there is a continuing underlying problem such as obstruction in the urinary tract (which includes multiple sclerosis as it leads to reduced urinary flow), the presence of stones, diabetes mellitus or analgesic/non-steroidal anti-inflammatory agent use.

Symptoms:

These are vaguer than those of the acute type, recur at intervals and tend to persist. The main symptoms are ill-health, tiredness and frequency of urination. Loin pain is universal and there may be episodes of dysuria.

Investigations:

These are as for acute pyelonephritis.

Complications:

COMPLICATIONS	SYMPTOMS TO LOOK FOR
Hypertension	Headaches, tinnitus, dizziness
End-stage kidney disease	Anorexia, nausea, vomiting, tiredness and others

TABLE 9.6: COMPLICATIONS OF CHRONIC PYELONEPHRITIS

Treatment:

This is as for acute pyelonephritis.

- INFLAMMATORY DISEASES OF THE KIDNEY -

Inflammatory conditions of the kidneys not associated with infection are probably much more common than is generally realised. Although the categories to follow are the definitive gross forms as recognised by conventional medicine it is important to remember that milder degrees do exist.

GLOMERULONEPHRITIS

This is a term which indicates inflammation of the functional unit of the kidney. It indicates a generalised affection of a deep level within the kidney. In conventional medicine, the underlying process is known to be one of immune damage where antibodies are formed which damage the kidney. This is an example of an autoimmune disease. I would refer you to Chapter 10 - Musculoskeletal System for details of others.

The precise cause for this dysfunction of the immune system is not known in conventional medicine although there are various substances which act as triggers. Some are external, e.g. bacteria and some are internal, e.g. DNA. There are varying clinical syndromes and these tend to be associated with particular cellular processes. Table 9.7 lists some of the known external events which may trigger these reactions.

There are two major clinical presentations of glomerulonephritis - nephritic syndrome and nephrotic syndrome. The exact terminology changes with time but I would refer you to Table 9.3 for a clear classification.

Bacteria:
•   Streptococcus
•   Staphylococcus - also causes boils, abscesses
Viruses:
•   Glandular fever
•   Hepatitis
•   Measles
•   Mumps
Other infections:
•   Malaria
Malignant disease
Drugs[6]
•   Antibiotics
•   Captopril
•   Gold
•   Hydralazine
•   Interferon
•   Lithium
•   Mesalazine
•   Non-steroidal anti-inflammatory agents but particularly ketoprofen
•   Penicillamine
•   Phenytoin
•   Practolol
•   Probenecid
•   Quinidine
•   Rifampicin

TABLE 9.7: KNOWN CAUSES OF GLOMERULONEPHRITIS

---

[6] "Textbook of Adverse Drug Reactions", Edited by DM Davies (Oxford Medical Publications, 1991)

NEPHRITIC SYNDROME (ACUTE PROLIFERATIVE[7] GLOMERULONEPHRITIS)

This was formerly known as Bright's disease. It may also be known as Ellis Type I nephritis. There is a classical picture of tonsillitis (streptococcal bacterial infection) which, some 1-3 weeks later, leads to the development of kidney symptoms. It is not that the infection directly affects the kidney. Rather that the body produces antibodies against the bacteria which also damage kidney tissue. This accounts for the delay in symptoms since the number of antibodies have to reach a certain level in the blood.

Symptoms:

Children are affected commonly. There is the acute development of haematuria, proteinuria and scanty urination. There is mild fever, general malaise, abdominal pain, nausea and vomiting. Since fluid is retained there is oedema and high blood pressure (which may give rise to headaches). The oedema classically occurs first on the upper body such as around the eyes, face and hands. Later as it worsens it is seen in the legs. There may be convulsions in severe cases.

After a period of 4-7 days, there is usually full recovery with profuse urination and the disappearance of oedema.

Investigations:

Urinalysis is positive for protein and blood. Red cell casts will be seen also. Full blood count reveals a mild anaemia. There is increased blood urea and ESR. In those who do not have an uncomplicated recovery (see below), annual checks of blood pressure and serum creatinine are advised.

Prognosis:

There is 'complete'[8] recovery in 90% of cases and this is especially true of children. The least favourable prognoses are in adults and in those without the specific trigger of a tonsillitis. Even in this 'recovered' group, 20-50% have mild raised blood pressure and impaired kidney function tests for some years. Others may have persistent haematuria and proteinuria for 2 years.

Less than 5% have scanty urination for more than 9 days. These have more severe kidney damage.

The remainder develop a rapidly progressive picture with persistent proteinuria. This develops into end-stage kidney disease in months or years.

Treatment:

There is no specific conventional treatment for this condition. The main aim is to prevent serious symptoms as recovery is the usual event. Uncomplicated and mild cases may be monitored at home but more severe attacks need to be dealt with in hospital. In extreme situations the use of dialysis is indicated. Penicillin is given if there is residual evidence of tonsil infection. The administration of antibiotics is widely advocated for tonsillitis and the occurrence of glomerulonephritis is stated as an indication. There is no evidence that the use of such drugs makes any difference to the occurrence or severity of post-streptococcal glomerulonephritis.[9]

---

[7] The term 'proliferative' applies to the cellular changes seen in the kidney cells. These changes are usually related to the nephritic syndrome but may cause nephrotic syndrome (see after). Whatever the term used for cellular changes, it is the clinical syndrome which is important.
[8] This is the conventional description despite the continuance of dysfunction in some people.
[9] "Cecil's Textbook of Medicine", Edited by Wyngaarden and Smith (W.B.Saunders, 1985)

NEPHROTIC SYNDROME
(MINIMAL LESION/MEMBRANOUS[10] GLOMERULONEPHRITIS)

This is a more severe type of acute glomerulonephritis. The trigger for the development of antibodies is unknown[11]. It is as if the body spontaneously produces antibodies which attack the kidney tissue. This would indicate the more serious nature of this condition. Any age may be affected rather than the predominance of children with nephritic syndrome.

Symptoms:

There is slow onset of symptoms. Protein is lost in the urine for some time before oedema develops. The cause of oedema in this case is low protein levels in the blood (hypoproteinaemia). The oedema is general in site. Fluid collects in the abdominal cavity (ascites) and causes discomfort and abdominal swelling. There is pallor and the continued loss of protein leads to ill-health and increased infections.

Investigations:

24-hour urinary loss of protein exceeds 3-5G/day in adults and may be as high as 40G/day. The serum albumin is low. Serum urea and creatinine are estimated as a check on renal function. Urine examination reveals red blood cells and red cell casts. Renal biopsy is performed in some cases when it is suspected that treatment with corticosteroids is applicable. It is not done in young children with no high blood pressure or blood in the urine (corticosteroids are given on the assumption that this is a type which will respond) or in those cases known to be caused by diabetes mellitus, metal toxicity, drugs and so forth.

Prognosis:

In case of the membranous type, 25% recover, 25% have persistent proteinuria with normal kidney function tests and 50% have a gradual deterioration of kidney function to end-stage kidney disease within 15 years.

In the case of the minimal lesion type, 33% have persistent proteinuria and haematuria, 33% have persistent nephrotic syndrome and 33% develop end-stage kidney disease within 6-10 years.

Treatment:

The use of antibiotics and improvements in general management have resulted in a decrease in the mortality rate from this disease over the years. The use of corticosteroids have never been shown to improve survival rates but despite this, they are frequently administered. They may have some symptomatic effect but long-term outcome is unaffected and side-effects are an additional burden.

Medium potency diuretics are administered to reduce the level of the oedema and corticosteroids are given in most cases. This is more effective, symptomatically, in those with membranous glomerulonephritis but this group of conditions does have a relatively high relapse rate. Immunosuppressants such as cyclophosphamide, chlorambucil or azathioprine may be given in addition to corticosteroids. If the glomerulonephritis is secondary to an autoimmune disorder or diabetes mellitus, the prognosis depends upon the severity of the original disease.

---

[10] The terms 'membranous' and 'minimal lesion' apply to the cellular changes seen in the kidney cells. These changes are usually, but not always, related to the nephrotic syndrome. Whatever the term used for cellular changes, it is the clinical syndrome which is important.
[11] In some it may be as part of an autoimmune disease (see Chapter 10 - Musculoskeletal System), diabetes mellitus, prescribed drugs (see Table 9.7), industrial metals such as mercury and cadmium or allergic reactions.

CHRONIC GLOMERULONEPHRITIS

This develops from acute glomerulonephritis which may or may not have been recognised. The type of acute glomerulonephritis is the nephrotic syndrome rather than the nephritic syndrome. End-stage kidney disease is the usual conclusion of this process.

Symptoms:

Chronic glomerulonephritis is a severe dysfunction and its clinical picture merges with that of end-stage kidney disease. There is progressive loss of kidney function with proteinuria, abnormal urinary sediments and diminishing kidney size.

Treatment:

This depends upon the clinical picture. Some cases have the features of nephrotic syndrome whilst others have more in common with end-stage kidney disease.

END-STAGE KIDNEY DISEASE

This, as its name suggests, is the final stage of degeneration of kidney function. It is placed in the context of kidney disease in general in Table 9.3.

Symptoms:

The clinical picture is due to increasingly severe biochemical abnormalities. There are disturbances of water, mineral and acid-alkaline balances. Abnormalities are seen in levels of calcium, magnesium phosphate, potassium and sodium.

There is a general feeling of ill-health with malaise. Nausea, vomiting and gastrointestinal bleeding are common. The person feels tired, irritable, depressed with insomnia and agitation. Twitching and restlessness of the legs are frequent associations. There is generalised itching which may be severe. Tingling and muscular weakness are experienced in the limbs. Loin pain is seen in everyone with this condition..

In the cardiovascular system, there is increased atherosclerosis, lipid (fat) levels are raised, blood pressure is high. There may be pericarditis as evidenced by sharp chest pain with palpitations.

Anaemia is universal leading to pallor and adding to the feelings of tiredness. Infections are more likely in people with end-stage kidney disease.

Treatment:

This is initially symptomatic with control of protein intake and the treatment of infection and hypertension. The end result is renal failure and transplantation or dialysis is the last resort.

ALTERNATIVE MANAGEMENT OF URINARY DISORDERS

In terms of Chinese medicine the conditions usually associated with these symptoms are DampHeat in the Bladder (Damp-Heat in the Lower Jiao) or Excessive Heat in the Small Intestine[12]. Urinary disorders with urinary frequency, urgency and pain are classified as Lin syndrome with five subtypes. There are Stone Lin (kidney stones), Lao Lin (chronic prostatitis), Milky Lin (diseases characterised by turbid urine), Heat Lin (acute infection of the urinary tract) and Blood Lin (tuberculosis, cancer or other tumour of the urogenital system, acute urinary infection).

The general principle of all the urinary disorders is that they indicate a systemic imbalance. The reasoning for such a statement is that an internal organ[13] is affected, they are usually recurrent and

---

[12] Energetically, the Small Intestine is paired with the Heart, and so anxiety and worry may lead to the symptoms of cystitis via this connection.

[13] Although the symptoms may arise from the bladder or prostate, for example, this whole area is governed, energetically, by the function of the Kidney.

are triggered by factors which lead to a flare-up of the underlying condition. The triggers are those things which, in terms of Chinese medicine, generate Heat, Dampness, Liver Qi Stagnation or Kidney depletion. These are listed in Table 9.8.

TRIGGER FACTOR OF URINARY DISEASE	COMMENTS
Alcohol, dehydration, irritants - perfumes, douches, 'feminine hygiene' products, spices, emotional stagnation including anger, irritation, "pissed off"	These generate heat which can lead to inflammatory reactions in the bladder and urinary tract.
Dairy products, greasy and fatty food	These lead to the formation of Dampness (mucus) which collects in the pelvic organs.
Sugar	This generates Dampness (mucus) as well as leading to Heat[14] stagnation.
Cold weather[15], fear/shock, sexual activity[16]	These tend to deplete Kidney energy and this adversely affects the functioning of other organs dependent on this energy.[17]
Constitutional factors	The constitution relies upon Kidney function. The strength of this has much to do with inherited factors.
Drugs - prescribed or social	The effect of these will depend upon their energetic quality. For example, antibiotics which are generally Cold and Damp in nature will deplete Kidney energy and lead to the collection of Dampness.

TABLE 9.8: IMPORTANT FACTORS IN THE DEVELOPMENT OF URINARY DISEASE

The most beneficial approach to urinary system disease is one which takes all these factors in into account. It is important to consider education, information, relaxation, resolution of emotional issues, diet and habits such as clothing and hygiene. I describe cases below which illustrate these.

CASE ONE

A man of 35 years of age came with pains in the knee after playing squash. It had been a recurrent problem over the past 6 months. On further questioning, he had a history of low back pain, recurrent attacks of dysuria, frequent urination with cloudy and smelly urine over the previous 3 years. It had been diagnosed by his doctor as prostatitis. He had 2 attacks of non-specific urethritis in the year prior to his first bout of prostatitis. He had always received antibiotics for his acute flare-ups.

In terms of Chinese medicine, his diagnosis was DampHeat Accumulation in the Lower Jiao with underlying Kidney Yang Deficiency. The Kidney governs the lower back and knees. I gave him advice about diet to reduce the foods which lead to Damp and Heat and to eat those which strengthen the Spleen (digestion). He went to see a food allergist some months later at great expense. He was

---

[14] For students of Chinese medicine it is necessary here to clarify my meaning. White sugar is Cold in energy and leads to the generation of Heat because the Cold causes Stagnation. This is more so in those with strong Qi. Brown sugar and malted products are Warm in nature and so lead to less problems although excess sweet taste from any source tends to deplete Spleen (digestive) energy.

[15] You may have heard comments from folk medicine of not walking in bare feet on a cold floor otherwise "you will get a chill in your kidneys". This is because the Kidney channel starts in the sole of the foot and cold can penetrate to travel up to the Kidneys.

[16] Sexual activity is not necessarily or inherently depleting of Kidney energy. There are methods for men and women of conserving energies during sexual intercourse. This belongs to the tantric aspect of spiritual traditions such as Buddhism, Hinduism and Taoism. The aim is to use the energy generated during sexual practice for higher spiritual practices. At the level of health, information about techniques in what could be called sexual yoga of the Chinese tradition can be found in the books of Mantak Chia. There are several including "Taoist Secrets of Love - Cultivating Male Sexual Energy" (Aurora, 1984).

[17] These are the organs in the lower part of the body and include the large intestine, bladder, prostate and the reproductive organs of the male and female.

most impressed that he was "allergic" to those foods which I had told him to avoid. I explore this idea more fully in Chapter 13 - Gastrointestinal System but it reveals that a knowledge of energetic medicine can lead to the same conclusions as whatever tests may be available.

I discussed relaxation with him as he had some stresses at home and his job was a high-powered position in the insurance world. He occasionally had flare-ups of his prostatitis symptoms along the way but these were managed by Chinese medicine rather than resorting to more antibiotics. In a woman, this imbalance would have led to recurrent vaginal discharge, pelvic inflammatory disease or similar.

It is an important part of the process to support people so that they can begin to have faith in the restorative abilities of their own body. Eventually, they will depend less on conventional medicine and drugs which can only make worse the underlying, chronic condition.

CASE TWO

This case connects with several areas including Chapter 10 - Musculoskeletal System. A woman of 55 years came for treatment of her joint problems. She had swelling, stiffness and pain in her hands, feet, elbows and knees. She felt generally hot with sweating. She urinated twice each night and had frequency of urination some 8 times or more during the day. Her urine would leak involuntarily on straining or physical exercise. Her energy was very low. Her skin was itchy and dry.

Her past medical history revealed a uterine prolapse followed by hysterectomy and bladder repair. A bladder repair is designed to reduce the amount of weakness at the bladder neck and so minimise leakage of urine and frequency. They are of variable effectiveness.

In terms of Chinese medicine, her diagnosis was Kidney Yang Deficiency with Blood Deficiency. Her pulses were extremely weak on her first visit and reflected a much depleted state of health. Her symptoms of heat, dry and itchy skin and joint discomfort were a consequence of the Blood Deficiency. Blood moistens, cools and nourishes and so heat may appear if it is lacking as well as symptoms in muscles and joints. The Kidney Deficiency was responsible for the urinary symptoms.

The aim of treatment was to gradually strengthen Kidney Yang and Blood. Her symptoms gradually improved over the next few months. She was working hard but her joints improved quite quickly. Her nightly urination declined to once and the frequency in the day became less. There was little leaking.

She was prescribed a homoeopathic remedy by a homoeopath and developed pain in her left loin radiating to the groin, bloated abdomen, alternating constipation and diarrhoea, painful urination and cloudy urine. These were bowel and bladder symptoms. She also experienced emotional symptoms similar to those she had some years before around the time of her hysterectomy. This release of old emotional states is typical of treatment by alternative medicine as the process of cure progresses. It is important to continue treatment, to deal with these flare-ups in a non-suppressive manner, to offer support to the person as they are experiencing these changes and to reassure them that this is a normal part of the healing process.

After a week or so of these symptoms, they settled and now, some 2 years after beginning treatment she is generally very well. There are few symptoms in any area and she manages a busy work schedule.

- INCONTINENCE -

This is the involuntary passage of urine. There are several causes of this in conventional medicine. The condition causes many problems for people not the least of which are embarrassment and inconvenience.

Stress incontinence:
Small amounts are passed upon straining, laughing, exercise and so forth. It occurs more commonly in women than men and is more likely with increasing age. It is unusual in women who have not had children. It is due to a weakness in the pelvic floor muscles.

Retention-overflow:

This is characterised by dribbling, pain in the pelvis and a palpable bladder. The bladder is full and urine leaks out intermittently. This type is seen in urinary outflow obstruction as with prostatic disease, with drugs such as anticholinergics, antidepressants, opiates and after the administration of anaesthetic agents.

Confusion:

This may lead to urination due to lack of awareness. A variable volume is passed depending upon the contents of the bladder.

"Spastic":

This term is applied to spasm of the bladder causing large volumes of urine to be passed sporadically. Urgency is a characteristic. This type may be due to the simple fact that the person cannot get to the toilet in time due to mobility problems. Do not always assume that urinary disease is present. Improvement of the person's mobility will improve the incontinence. Others in this category include spinal cord disease such as prolapsed intervertebral disc or spinal tumour and multiple sclerosis. These disorders are discussed in Chapter 14 - Central Nervous System.

Enuresis is a term which is reserved for incontinence in children. It is the involuntary passing of urine at night when asleep. The existence of incontinence during the day suggests a kidney or bladder condition. It is mainly a disorder found in boys and affects 10% of boys aged 4-11 years. There are estimated to be 500,000 cases in Britain between the age of 6 and 16. As a group they also have signs of decreased muscle tone, co-ordination problems and EEG abnormalities. It is considered to be a sleep disorder and so is treated by the antidepressant, imipramine. This is an attempt to alter depth of sleep and has little effect. There is the added danger of poisoning by overdose.

More effective are behavioural methods such as an alarm bell. This is connected to a mat under the sheet so that the bell sounds if the child wets the bed. Intranasal desmopressin[18], antidiuretic hormone, is used in some cases although the manipulation of pituitary hormones to treat bed-wetting seems a little like overkill. Enuresis is notoriously difficult to treat and is frequently related to psychological factors. It may be necessary to address the family as a whole as well as the child.

Alternative management:

In terms of Chinese medicine, enuresis is to do with the function of the Kidney, Spleen, Lungs and Bladder. There may be Deficiency of Kidney Yang, weakness of Spleen Qi or an affection of the Lung in its function of dominating Water passages. This can be considered as either a Before Heaven Qi or an After Heaven Qi problem. If the Before Heaven Qi is imbalanced then it may be that a factor in the parents or during pregnancy is more important. If the After Heaven Qi is imbalanced then you may consider more environmental factors such as diet and emotional issues in the family. As with all conditions of childhood, there can be complex familial issues at play. These are discussed more fully in Chapter 16 - Psychological Disorders and Chapter 19 - Children's Health.

- HYPERTENSION -

This is raised blood pressure and is a common situation in the Western world. It is invariably treated with drugs and generates anxiety in people and medical practitioners. You will definitely come across such cases and it is helpful to know how to manage the issues raised by this situation.

The blood pressure in the West and indeed many societies rises with age and this is a consequence of several factors regarding life-style. Excess intake of salt, stressful living patterns, overweight, lack of exercise and the presence of chronic degenerative disease all contribute to what is seen as a 'normal' pattern of rising blood pressure. In traditional societies such as South Sea Islanders and some nomadic groups there is no such rise and the same level is maintained throughout life[19].

In conventional thought, raised blood pressure is seen as leading to heart disease and stroke and so it is treated whenever it is diagnosed, there is no agreed level of normal so individual doctors

---

[18] In clinical trials only 31% of children are dry on such treatment. This is little better than placebo.
[19] A survey over 20 years of the blood pressure of nuns in a secluded monastic order revealed that their blood pressure did not change. This was in contradistinction to a control group whose blood pressure increased. Hypertension 1988 Oct; 12(4): 457-61.

differ, it tends to be diagnosed at relatively low levels and drugs are the mainstay of treatment. Treatment with drugs is considered to be for life. This is not only a lucrative option for the pharmaceutical industry, it also locks the person into a cycle of dependency and fear.

The blood pressure reading consists of two figures, e.g. 120/80. The top figure relates to cardiac systole, i.e. when the heart contracts, the bottom figure to cardiac diastole, i.e. when the heart relaxes. The diastolic reading is the important one since this is the pressure when in a state of relaxation. If it is high for persistent periods of time it indicates a general heightened state of tension in the system.

The figures I tend to use are those listed in Table 9.9. In conventional clinical practice there is great variation in the accepted figures and some doctors, whatever the age of the person, may diagnose hypertension when the diastolic figure is 90. The systolic pressure is less important in terms of diagnosing hypertension.[20]

BLOOD PRESSURE - UPPER LIMIT OF NORMAL[21]	AGE
120/90	20
160/95	50
170/105	75

TABLE 9.9: VARIATION OF BLOOD PRESSURE WITH AGE[22]

Blood pressure varies with many factors and so one reading means very little. It needs to be taken over several days and allowance made for factors such as exercise or stress. The correct size of cuff must be used for the size of the arm or false results will be obtained.

In conventional medicine, the majority of cases (90%) have no known cause and this is known as primary or essential (!) hypertension. There are relationships to genetic factors, overweight, alcohol intake, salt intake and stress levels[23]. Most of these may explain why blood pressure are consistently higher in the West than in traditional cultures.

Secondary hypertension is where there is demonstrable disease of the kidneys such as chronic glomerulonephritis and pyelonephritis, endocrine disorders such as Conn's syndrome and Cushing's syndrome, pre-eclamptic toxaemia of pregnancy and prescribed drugs - female sex hormones, carbenoxolone, vasopressin (see the treatment of enuresis in children) and occasionally with the mono-amine oxidase inhibitor type of antidepressants when the person also takes cheese, wine or some other contraindicated food.

Symptoms:

In conventional medicine, there are considered to be no symptoms unless the level of blood pressure is very high or if the person is "told that he has high blood pressure, then he worries about it and develops headaches, fatigue and poor memory."[24]

This is not true and most people only take their medication when they feel their blood pressure is high. The exact symptom picture will vary with the individual but it is common to see headache, dizziness, tinnitus, eye symptoms such as dry or red eyes, irritability or anger.

A severe variant is called malignant or accelerated hypertension. Malignant in this context indicates a progressive problem. There is no cancerous process. If it is not treated then 90% of this group die within one year. The levels of blood pressure are very high with severe headaches, red face and eyes, blurred vision, tremors, proteinuria and haematuria.

[20] The systolic figure is roughly 100 plus the person's age.
[21] Measurement is made in millimetres of mercury (mm Hg).
[22] "Davidson's Principles and Practice of Medicine", Edited by Macleod (Churchill Livingstone)
[23] It has been noted that the current level of blood pressure and the risk of high blood pressure are strongly related to the weight at birth and the weight of the placenta. This was a survey done in Preston, England. BMJ 1990; 301: 259-62.
[24] "Textbook of Medicine" by RJ Harrison, Third Edition (Hodder and Stoughton, 1984).

Complications[25]:

These must be differentiated into those which are due to the long-term effects of raised blood pressure and those which may occur in the short-term due to the actual level of blood pressure at the time.

COMPLICATIONS	SYMPTOMS TO LOOK FOR
Cardiac insufficiency	Palpitations, breathlessness, cough with pink frothy sputum, peripheral oedema
Accelerated or malignant hypertension	Very high blood pressure, blurred vision, red face, tremor, throbbing headaches
Cerebral haemorrhage (stroke)	There may the symptoms of accelerated hypertension prior to the event. Headaches, paralysis or weakness of limbs and face on one side of the body, loss of consciousness at the onset of the attack

TABLE 9.10: SHORT-TERM COMPLICATIONS OF HYPERTENSION

COMPLICATIONS	SYMPTOMS TO LOOK FOR
Heart attack	Central chest pain radiating to the arm, palpitations, vomiting, pallor
Stroke	Paralysis or weakness of limbs and face on one side of the body
Peripheral arterial disease	Cramping pain in the calves on exertion relieved by rest, cold feet, absent or diminished pulses in the feet
End-stage kidney disease	Proteinuria, tiredness, loin pain, anorexia, nausea, vomiting (see above)

TABLE 9.11: LONG-TERM COMPLICATIONS OF HYPERTENSION

Investigations:

In general, there are no investigations performed if the level of raised blood pressure is slight, there is no previous history suggestive that this is a case of secondary hypertension and the age of the person is over 40. If the blood pressure responds easily to treatment then this is confirmation that the diagnosis is almost certainly primary hypertension, i.e. of unknown cause.

In those cases where it is suspected that there is an underlying cause then investigations will be performed. These include chest X-ray, ECG, urinalysis, serum cholesterol, urea and electrolytes.[26]

Examination of the retina may show changes to the blood vessels typical of hypertension. These are graded into 4 levels indicating mild to severe damage.

Treatment:

The mainstay of treatment is with drugs but there are some moves towards a more holistic approach[27]. Certainly there will be general advice about reducing excess weight, stopping smoking,

---

[25] It is often stated that the treatment of blood pressure will lead to a reduction in problems later. Numerous trials have shown that such treatment is beneficial but *only* in terms of stroke. There is no change in mortality reduction from all causes and as conventional medical textbooks state, "... a very large number of people have to face the inconvenience, risks and side-effects of treatment to save one life."

[26] Urea and electrolytes (U and E's) is a common preliminary blood test to check on renal function and to monitor treatment such as diuretic therapy. The electrolytes include chloride, bicarbonate, sodium and potassium.

[27] There have been trials showing that non-pharmacological methods have a role to play in treating hypertension. These have not filtered into routine practice because they do not fit easily into the conventional medical model.
A trial using a type of Buddhist meditation (Dhammakaya) led to a reduction in serum cortisol, increases in serum total protein and reductions in blood pressure and heart rate. Physiol-Behav. 1991 Sep; 50(3): 543-8.
Another paper describes the non-drug measures for the treatment of hypertension and the existence of many well-controlled studies. It makes the point that if these are used widely then there may well be a fall in the incidence of complications from hypertension and halt the progression to moderate or

taking of regular exercise and reducing salt and alcohol intake. Salt intake in the West is around 14G per day which is over 4 times the amount compatible with health. There is some debate about the level of 'healthy' drinking of alcohol and there is advice about how many units[28] of alcohol are safe. My personal view is that since alcohol is a toxin, any intake is potentially a problem but some people may benefit from the relaxing effects. Most trials involving the calculation of these amounts have come to the conclusion that moderate drinking protects against certain diseases. This does not take account that some people do not drink alcohol for health reasons. The incidence of diseases related to drinking such as cirrhosis of the liver and some psychological disorders is directly related to the amount of alcohol drunk and the ease of availability in society.

An intake of alcohol less than 20 units for men and 13 units for women per week is considered to be without risk to health. Up to 36 units for men and 24 units for women per week is considered to be unlikely to lead to health problems. This seems to me to be a large amount which, in my experience, needs to be reduced if people are to maintain their health. 36 units of alcohol for a man is 18 pints of beer per week. This level of drinking is likely to damage the energy of the Spleen (digestion), Kidney and Liver. I consistently request people to perhaps drink only once per week to ensure as healthy state as possible. This is particularly true if there is any preceding Spleen or Kidney problems or in the presence of Damp accumulation (mucus).

The drugs used in the treatment of hypertension are summarised in Table 9.12. Combinations are commonly used in an attempt to reduce the incidence of side-effects and to increase the desired effect. The most common prescription seen is a combination of a diuretic and a betablocker. A vasodilator is added to these if there is an inadequate response. Other combinations are diuretic and ACE inhibitor, diuretic and centrally acting alpha agonist, diuretic and alpha-1 adrenergic blocker.

TREATMENT	TREATMENT LEVEL
Diuretic	1
Hypotensive agent Centrally acting alpha agonist, e.g. clonidine, methyldopa	2
Hypotensive agent • Calcium antagonist • Betablocker	3
Angiotensin-converting enzyme (ACE) inhibitor	4
Vasodilator • Alpha-1 adrenergic blocker, e.g. prazosin, indoramin • Alpha and betablocker, e.g. labetalol	5

TABLE 9.12: TREATMENT OF HYPERTENSION

Alternative management:

In terms of Chinese medicine, there are several energetic diagnoses which are associated with hypertension. Most of these are symptomatic and this is the reason why people go to the doctor. They are then diagnosed as suffering from hypertension. Few people have high blood pressure diagnosed in the asymptomatic phase.

The main syndromes are related to Kidney and Liver imbalances. Kidney Yin deficiency with Liver Yang Rising is a common one. Others include less deficient syndromes such as Stagnation of Liver Qi, Liver Fire Blazing. Spleen Qi or Yang deficiency with Damp Accumulation may also lead to high blood pressure.

The main groups of drugs are diuretics and hypotensive agents. Diuretics are cold in nature and make the Kidney let go of Yin (urine). Long-term they damage Kidney Qi and lead to Yin Deficiency. The predominant clinical picture will depend upon the original condition of the person.

The hypotensive drugs in general can be considered to have similar effects to betablockers. These are an excellent example of this group and are discussed in detail in Chapter 7 - Cardiovascular System.

---

severe hypertension. Cardiovasc-Drugs-They. 1989 Dec; 3(6): 847-52.
[28] One unit is half a pint of average strength beer, a single UK measure of spirits, one glass of sherry or one glass of wine. One unit contains the equivalent of 8G of absolute alcohol.

You can see from this that the effect on the person will depend upon the original condition. For example, if the cause of high blood pressure is Kidney Yin Deficiency with Liver Yang Rising, betablockers will reduce blood pressure as it destroys Yang. If, however, the cause of the problem is Spleen Qi Deficiency with Damp Accumulation, then betablockers will make the person ill. They may feel more tired, cold and lethargic. Therefore, with knowledge of the energetics it is possible to understand the response to drugs.

CASE

A man of 55 years came for treatment. He had been diagnosed with high blood pressure some 10 years previously and had been on medication ever since. This consisted of:

- Labetalol 200mg twice daily - alpha and betablocker
- Indapamide one daily - diuretic
- Allopurinol half a tablet daily - reduces uric acid levels in gout

He had a past medical history of prostatitis, cystitis and gout. His highest blood pressure had been 170/125 before he started his medication. He had low energy, irritability, loose bowels when tired. In terms of Chinese medicine, his diagnosis was Spleen and Kidney Yang Deficiency with DampHeat Accumulation. His past medical history revealed that the DampHeat would collect in the bladder and prostate and occasionally flare-up in the big toe. Allopurinol in its side-effects can *cause* high blood pressure. There are frequently occasions when you study combinations of prescribed drugs that they may interact or one may cause the original condition for which the person is receiving treatment.

He was very nervous about the prospect of reducing his tablets and it is important in such cases to wait until he is happy. He needs to gain confidence in the treatment and the ability of his body to effect changes. I treated him for 10 months before he started to discuss the question of reduction. He was then keen to try.

It is essential that any reduction is slow and to monitor blood pressure during the process. His blood pressure on his initial visits had been 130/95 to 150/100. This settled over the months of treatment and was 120/80 when he began to reduce his medication. He had stopped his allopurinol in the early weeks as it may cause high blood pressure.

He reduced his medication to 200mg morning and 150mg evening. This led to a rise in his blood pressure to 140/85. This is to be expected and it is important to wait for this to settle before continuing. He reduced his drugs by 50mg a day each time it was appropriate and waited for things to settle down in between. After some months, he felt he had more energy and was generally well.

He continued to reduce his medication until 4 months later he was able to stop them completely. It takes several further months to gain the full benefit of being without them.

The main cause of this man's blood pressure was a busy, stressful job with a history of overwork. With the treatment and discussions about relaxation and exercise, he was able to become more balanced in himself and the need for his drugs became less.

There is no problem with reducing blood pressure medication so long as the following issues are considered:

- The person taking the drugs must be happy about drug reduction
- An initial improvement in the person's condition must be seen
- Monitor blood pressure
- Slow reduction
- Wait for stabilisation
- Any rise in blood pressure after a reduction must not be more than about 30/20 and not accompanied by symptoms such as headaches, blurred vision, red eyes, dizziness, tinnitus

- KIDNEY STONES -

Stones in the urinary system usually form in the kidney. They do not cause symptoms unless there is an associated inflammatory condition or they move into the ureter. The changes in the form of disease are shown by the fact that bladder stones were common in the 18th Century. It was possible to earn a respectable living as a lithotomist - one who removes stones.

The stones are formed from the normal constituents of urine and usually occur first in the pelvis of the kidney. They may exist there for some time unnoticed and causing no symptoms. They are more likely in the following situations:

• hot climates where the urine is more concentrated
• high blood level of calcium, e.g. corticosteroid use, sarcoidosis, overconsumption of Vitamin D
• excessive intake of calcium
• with infective conditions of the urinary system
• increased blood levels of uric acid, e.g. gout, leukaemia - less than 5% of kidney stones are of this type

Symptoms:

There are three consequences of stones in the kidney. Firstly, they may asymptomatic. Stones do not lead to symptoms unless they move or if there is associated infection.

Secondly, the person may pass small amounts of 'gravel' which causes some pain for a brief period of time. The pain will be a much milder form of classical renal colic described below.

Thirdly, there may be severe symptoms of renal colic (also known as ureteric colic) which are due to spasms in the ureter as the stone is passing through the urinary system. The pain begins in the loin on the affected side and radiates round and down into the groin. It may also be felt in the thigh to the knee. The pain may come and go for several hours or days. Associated symptoms occur such as restlessness, vomiting, sweating and pallor. The stone may be small enough to be passed in the urine when there may be dysuria. Blood in the urine is common although it may only be discovered on urine testing.

Some people have stones which grow so big that they cannot pass into the ureter. These are usually associated with chronic urinary tract infections such as pyelonephritis. The stones act as a focus for organisms to live and organisms provide a focus around which stones form.

There may be associated infection in some and so there will be the added symptoms of fever, chills, dysuria, cloudy and strong smelling urine.

Investigations:

Urinalysis shows blood, protein, pus cells. Cystoscopy may be performed to enable catheterisation of the affected ureter to attempt removal of a blocked stone. Plain X-ray reveals the stone in 90% of cases as it usually contains calcium. Intravenous pyelogram will detect any blockage to urine flow.

Complications:

COMPLICATIONS	SYMPTOMS TO LOOK FOR
Acute pyelonephritis	Loin pain, fever, dysuria, frequent urination
Obstruction to urine flow in affected ureter	Increasing fever, severe pain in the loin, the person is ill

TABLE 9.13: COMPLICATIONS OF RENAL STONES

Treatment:

The person with kidney stones is advised to drink large amounts of fluid - in the order of 3 litres per day. Avoidance of calcium rich foods is recommended in cases due to excess calcium levels. Any infection will be treated with antibiotics.

Surgical treatment is reserved for those situations where the stone is too big to pass and is associated with chronic infection. In some, a stone is small enough to pass into the ureter but too large to complete its passage into the bladder. This situation may lead to urinary obstruction in that ureter with potentially dangerous consequences for the kidney.

Stones may be removed using a cystoscope, through an incision over the kidney (percutaneous nephroscopy) or by breaking them up using ultrasound (extracorporeal shock-wave lithotripsy). The latter situation is the most helpful because it is much less invasive and treatment can be administered to prevent a recurrence.

Alternative management:

The acute picture of renal colic will almost always be treated in hospital because of the degree of pain. The chronic condition is amenable to constitutional treatment by alternative medicine. If removal of the stone is required then breaking by ultrasound (see above) is the preferable method. Most people have no demonstrable biochemical abnormality and so advice can clearly follow principles of energetic medicine as there is no conventional advice which is clearly and logically indicated.

In terms of Chinese medicine, this condition usually corresponds to long-term Dampness and Heat which forms a stone from body fluids. This may obstruct the flow of Qi and interfere with urine flow.

- CANCER OF THE KIDNEY -

This makes up 10% of all cases of cancer. There are several types but the commonest is termed renal cell carcinoma.

Symptoms:

The classical presentation is of haematuria, loin pain and a palpable abdominal swelling. This, however, is only seen in 20% of cases. In 60% of people there is only haematuria. Painless haematuria, therefore, must always be taken seriously and consideration made of the origin of the bleeding.

Investigations:

Diagnosis is made by performing intravenous urography, computerised axial tomography and ultrasound.

Treatment:

At the time of diagnosis, 50% of people with cancer of the kidney have evidence of spread to local or distant sites. Secondaries occur in the adrenal glands, lymph glands, lung and long bones. The comments I made in Chapter 6 - Cancer with regard to treatment are relevant here.

- CANCER OF THE BLADDER -

This is twice as common in men than women. It presents with similar symptoms to cancer of the kidney.

Symptoms:

The main presentation is of haematuria, frequency of urination and dysuria without evidence of infecting organisms. These symptoms reflect a degree of bladder irritation from the cancer. The cancer takes the form of warty growths on the bladder lining. They tend to be localised and grow slowly - 80%. If there is distant spread then this tends to be to the lymph nodes, lung and bone.

Investigations:

Diagnosis is made by cystoscopy and biopsy. Computerised axial tomography of the chest and abdomen together with bone scans are an integral part of the staging process.

Treatment:

This is by local removal via cystoscopy with regular check-ups. If there is recurrence, intra-bladder chemotherapy wash-outs will be used.

- MALE GENITAL DISORDERS -

BENIGN ENLARGEMENT OF THE PROSTATE

This is more common over the age of 60 years and is rare before 40 years. The prostate gland enlarges which obstructs the flow of urine as it leaves the bladder. The cause is unknown in conventional medicine but it is noticed that it is rarer in those of African or Asian races and never seen in eunuchs. Despite this latter situation, I have never known removal of the testes to advocated as a preventative measure! - compare this with the suggested treatments of gynaecological symptoms.

Symptoms:

The classical clinical features are those of *urinary outflow obstruction*. They are frequency of urination, difficulty in beginning to urinate, nocturia, urgency, poor urinary stream and dribbling at the end of urination. People may develop acute retention of urine. Treatment with diuretics may precipitate this event.

Some people may have impaired kidney function and there will the signs and symptoms of chronic kidney disease (see chronic pyelonephritis and glomerulonephritis) with anaemia.

Differential diagnosis:

There are several causes of obstruction to the flow of urine and they include:

*   cancer of the prostate (see below)
*   urethral narrowing due to gonorrhoea (stricture)
*   neurological disorders - see Chapter 14 - Central Nervous System especially multiple sclerosis, intervertebral disc prolapse

Investigations:

Rectal examination is performed to feel the size and shape of the prostate. A benign enlargement is smooth. Urine culture is done to determine if urinary infection is present. Kidney function tests of serum urea and creatinine give an idea of renal function. Further tests of the kidney include plain X-ray, intravenous urography and ultrasound. Cystoscopy is always done. The main aim of these investigations is to determine if there is damage to the upper urinary tracts by the back pressure of urine as a result of the obstruction to flow.

Treatment.

The primary treatment is by the operation of prostatectomy which is done either by a urethral or abdominal approach. The former is the more common one as it has a lower mortality rate, results in less ill-health post-operatively and hospital stays are shorter. It is common for people to have bowel difficulties after the operation. This is long-term and takes the form of a weakness in evacuation.

In terms of Chinese medicine there are several syndromes which may be seen. The commonest ones are Deficiency of the Spleen and Kidney and DampHeat accumulation in the Lower Jiao.

CANCER OF THE PROSTATE

This makes up 7% of all cancer in men. The incidence of prostatic cancer increases with age until at the age of 80 some 80% of men have evidence of some malignant cells in the prostate. Most of these are minor and only discovered by chance or at post-mortem examination.

Symptoms:

The symptoms are similar to benign enlargement of the prostate which are detailed above. However, since the underlying process is malignant the symptoms appear more quickly and are progressive over a period of weeks and months.

The cancer spreads to lymph glands, pelvis, lumbar spine, femur, thoracic spine, ribs, lung and liver in decreasing order of frequency.

Investigations:

These are the same as performed in benign enlargement with the addition of a needle biopsy of the prostate. On rectal examination there is a hard, irregular prostate. An ultrasound scan can reveal the size of the prostatic enlargement. A biopsy will be performed to determine the exact nature of the cells and to confirm malignancy. If secondaries are present the serum acid phosphatase level will be increased. Isotope bone scans and X-rays of bone may be performed to detect secondaries.

Treatment.

Prostatectomy is performed if the cancer has not spread. If secondaries are present the testes will be removed (orchidectomy) combined with hormonal treatment. This is by means of oestrogens or antiandrogens.

ORCHITIS

This is inflammation of the testis and is mainly secondary to mumps in post-pubertal men. It rarely leads to sterility despite the popular belief that it does and it never interferes with sexual function.

Symptoms:

There is the onset of fever with chills, headache and lower abdominal pain. The affected testis is painful and tender. The symptoms subside after 5 days.

Treatment:

Cases resolve spontaneously and so analgesics are the only treatment required.

EPIDIDYMITIS

This is inflammation of the epididymis. It is almost invariably a consequence of an infection in the urinary tract and this may be gonorrhoea or non-specific urethritis. There may be associated cystitis or prostatitis.

Symptoms:

There is pain and swelling of the affected side with redness of the overlying scrotum. There is malaise and low grade fever.

Treatment:

This is invariably with antibiotics although it is a chronic disease, and like prostatitis, relapses easily.

TORSION OF THE TESTIS

This is twisting of the testis within the scrotum. It is serious because the blood supply to the testis is obstructed.

Symptoms:

It occurs in males under the age of 18 years. There is an extremely rapid onset of severe pain in the affected testis which becomes swollen. The symptoms rapidly worsen. There may be previous episodes of testicular pain.

Treatment:

This is a surgical emergency and if the problem is not corrected within 4 hours the testis dies.

IMPOTENCE

This is an inability of the penis to become erect and this can be total or partial. Conventionally, it is divided into organic, i.e. structural causes and functional, i.e. psychological causes. This underlines the division between mind and body taken by conventional medicine. In practice, there is often a combination of influences with few cases due to purely physical disease.

It may occur due to disease of the nervous system perhaps secondary to diabetes mellitus or a spinal cord problem and in severe endocrine disease such as under- or overactivity of the thyroid gland. The other thing to consider is peripheral arterial disease leading to poor blood circulation in the lower part of the body. All these situations are rare but may be blamed as an acceptable physical reason. This commonly tends to be true for conditions in men where emotional factors may be difficult to face.

Psychological factors are extremely important and there is often the added factor of 'performance anxiety' where the man worries whether he can produce an erection at the appropriate time. Erections during sleep would seem to confirm that the problem is psychological rather than physical.

A common situation is the effect of prescribed drugs which may cause impotence. Alcohol and cannabis are the well-known 'recreational' drugs to lead to inability to produce an erection. The prescribed drugs which may do this are listed in Table 9.14.

Adrenergic neurone blocker	Anticholinergics	Antidepressants
Hypotensive drugs	Anti-Parkinsonism drugs	Barbiturates
Benzodiazepines	Betablockers	Cimetidine/ranitidine
Cancer chemotherapy	Diuretics	Immunosuppressants
Lithium	Opiates	Phenothiazines
Vasodilators		

TABLE 9.14: PRESCRIBED DRUGS WHICH MAY CAUSE IMPOTENCE

In terms of Chinese medicine, impotence usually corresponds to Kidney Yang Deficiency with or without damage to the Qi of the Heart and Spleen.

PREMATURE EJACULATION

This is very common although people may find it difficult to discuss sexual problems with anyone. It is difficult to define but is ejaculation by the male before the 'appropriate' time. Kinsey in his well-documented report on sexual matters in the USA reported that 75% of men ejaculate within 2 minutes of penile insertion. In severe cases of premature ejaculation, this can occur before insertion of the penis. It is very much seen as due to psychological factors. These must be addressed if there is to be any improvement in the symptom,

In terms of Chinese medicine, this symptom is seen as part of the picture of Deficient Yin and Excess of Yang, Sinking of Qi, or Disharmony between Kidney and Heart. The principle here is that there is an excess of Yang compared to Yin so that the fluid of semen is lost prematurely.

INFERTILITY

Male factors in infertility are discussed together with female factors in Chapter 18 - Gynaecology.

- REVIEW OF SYMPTOMS -

PAIN

Pain in the loin or low back pain are common indicators of kidney disease. Conventional medical texts often consider low back pain to be a condition of the back whereas energetic medicine may see this as a Kidney imbalance. In my experience, virtually all cases of chronic low back pain are associated with a weakness of Kidney energy and treating only the back will not lead to long-term relief. I discuss this in more detail in Chapter 14 - Central Nervous System.

Pain from the ureter is felt radiating from the loin round to the inguinal region and sometimes into the thigh to the knee. This is in the distribution of the first and second lumbar nerves.

URINARY DISTURBANCES

Frequency may be seen during the day or if at night is known as nocturia. It can be an early symptom of many urinary conditions or of systemic conditions such as diabetes (mellitus or insipidus).

The normal urinary volume is 800-2400 ml in 24 hours. It varies according to intake and other losses such as sweat and respiration. Polyuria is an increased urine volume and is not necessarily the same as urinary frequency which is passing urine more often.

Dysuria is used to describe pain or discomfort when urinating. This can be felt either in the bladder in cystitis or in the urethra. It may be severe with gonorrhoea.

Urinary disturbances such as urgency, frequency, poor flow, terminal dribbling are due to obstruction to the flow of urine and implies a problem with the urethra, bladder neck or prostate in men.

HAEMATURIA

This is blood in the urine and the precise colour depends upon the amount of blood present. A trace of blood will not be apparent in the urine unless urinalysis is performed. Larger amounts may be seen as a smoky appearance in the urine and eventually reddish urine occurs. Blood in the urine at the beginning of urination indicates that the source is distal to the bladder, blood mixed with urine indicates the source is any part other than the urethra.

OEDEMA

Swelling of the tissues by fluid was discussed in Chapter 7 - Cardiovascular System. Kidney disease may lead to oedema which is typically seen in the eyelids and upper part of the body although eventually it will be widespread.

- HOW TO RECOGNISE A SERIOUS CONDITION OF THE URINARY SYSTEM -

It is important to know how to recognise if a symptom arises from a serious situation. You can use Table 9.15 below as a guide to refer to when faced with a person who has one or more of these symptoms. I make no mention of disease labels in the column on the right as I would not expect you to be able to diagnose conventionally. Seriousness can be assessed merely by reference to symptom pictures.

SYMPTOM	COMMENTS
PAIN IN LOIN	Severe
PAIN IN ABDOMEN	Severe Persistent With abdominal rigidity With guarding With rebound tenderness
PAIN IN URETHRA	Not serious
ANURIA	Always
OLIGURIA	Severe Persistent Without clear reason such as hot climate, decreased fluid intake
ENURESIS	Severe especially if with incontinence in the day
FREQUENT URINATION	Severe Progressive Short history
DRIBBLING	Severe Progressive Short history
URGENCY	Severe Progressive Short history
PAIN IN THE TESTIS	Rapid onset of severe pain under the age of 18 years
SWELLING OF THE TESTIS	Progressive No signs/symptoms of a urinary tract infection[29]

TABLE 9.15: HOW TO RECOGNISE SERIOUS CONDITIONS IN URINARY SYSTEM DISEASE

SUMMARY

The conventional view of the kidney is of a physical sieve.

The alternative view of the kidney reveals the idea of energy which is the root of all the other organs. Therefore, the strength of the kidneys is very important in health and connected to vital aspects of life such as constitution, longevity and reproduction.

Many people have symptoms of kidney disease but are not so severely affected that disease labels such pyelonephritis or glomerulonephritis can be applied

---

[29] This is the presentation of cancer of the testis.

10 MUSCULOSKELETAL SYSTEM

OBJECTIVES:

At the end of this Chapter you will be able to:
Describe the differences between the alternative and conventional views of the musculoskeletal system.
List the symptoms attributable to disturbances of the musculoskeletal system.
State when a symptom(s) would indicate a serious underlying condition.
Describe the main symptoms of diseases covered in this Chapter.
Explain the relevant management by an alternative practitioner of each disorder.

- INTRODUCTION -

The musculoskeletal system is that part of the body which is responsible for movement and structure. It is deeper than the skin, yet more superficial than the organs of the body. Disease at this level, therefore, tends to be some of the most superficial with which practitioners have to deal. An important proviso here is that some conditions of the musculoskeletal system are generalised in nature and reflect deep internal disturbances. These are the disorders named as the autoimmune diseases.

Autoimmune disorders are those which are characterised by the presence of antibodies attacking the body's own tissues. There are many and varied types including those discussed in this Chapter. Others such as diabetes mellitus, Addison's disease and thyroid disease are discussed in Chapter 15 - Endocrine System. Pernicious anaemia which is caused by an immune attack on the stomach is mentioned in Chapter 7 - Cardiovascular System. In terms of seriousness, these disorders clearly indicate a deep imbalance in the body. The blood is disturbed[1] as revealed by the presence of antibodies, the body is attacking itself which could be termed "suicide by immune reaction" and the diseases affect deep, internal organs as well as the surface of the body.

They are becoming commoner with time which is an indication that the health of the general population is becoming worse. It is interesting here to consider diseases of this type in relation to other disturbances of the immune system. I am using this term here in its narrower conventional sense when it is used to describe disturbances in reactions on the level of the antigen-antibody. Such diseases are summarised in Table 10.1 with mild disease at the top and severe disease at the bottom.

DISEASE	COMMENTS
Allergy, e.g. hay fever, asthma	Over-reaction to an external factor, e.g. pollen, dust
Autoimmune diseases	Over-reaction to an internal factor, e.g. kidney tissue in glomerulonephritis, connective tissue in rheumatoid arthritis
Cancer	Lack of reactivity to abnormal cells leading eventually to their appearance as tumours
AIDS	Complete collapse of the immune system resulting in severe infections by organisms not normally pathogenic

TABLE 10.1: DISTURBANCES OF THE IMMUNE SYSTEM

Whenever any system is imbalanced, the first reaction is one of overproduction or overactivity. An example of this is thyroid disease. The first signs of disease are those of hyperthyroidism. After some years, with or without treatment, the natural history of the disease is for hypothyroidism to become evident. As the energy in the system declines there is replacement of over-reaction by an exhaustion. In the case of immune system diseases as listed in Table 10.1, over-activity is represented by allergy and autoimmune disease. These are situations where the immune system is too active. It attacks external or internal factors strongly and produces symptoms by so doing. It is clearly more harmful to attack internal tissues and so the autoimmune diseases are more serious than the allergic.

If the person's energy is more imbalanced and correspondingly weaker, there is not enough energy to produce strong reactions. Cancer is a situation where abnormal cells, which are constantly produced, are not recognised as such. They grow to produce clinically detectable tumours. AIDS is the end-state where there is no reactivity and strange organisms can invade the body with no or little response. Interestingly, when people with cancer improve by alternative medical methods, they often report the appearance of symptoms such as joint swelling and stiffness suggestive of an inflammatory arthritis. Allergic reactions may also develop.

Such connections are easily made in terms of alternative medicine. In conventional medicine there have been some moves to try and understand these relationships. The relatively recent speciality of psychoneuroimmunology is an attempt to do this.

In Chinese medicine, Blood is considered to be responsible for moistening, cooling and the nourishment of muscles and joints. Damage to the Blood may be manifest by symptoms such as muscle pain, stiffness, joint swelling and pain which may be labelled arthritis by a conventional practitioner. It has been known for many years that overuse of a joint and injury may lead to the development of osteoarthritis (see below). Recently, it has been observed that over-exercise, particularly to extremes by athletes, results in impaired functioning of the immune system, increased susceptibility to viral infections and general symptoms of debility.[2] As mentioned in Chapter 7 - Cardiovascular System, there is a close relationship between emotions and Blood. Stressful activity, overwork, worry and emotional turmoil all contribute to harming the Blood and to the development of autoimmune disorders. Meditation and relaxation are known to be powerful methods to improve immune system function.[3] Similarly, excessive muscular activity particularly when associated with sweating will increase the risk of Blood disturbances and the appearance of musculoskeletal diseases.

---

[1] Comparisons can be made here with ideas of Blood (in the energetic sense) which were introduced in Chapter 7 - Cardiovascular System.

[2] Recent trials have shown that overtraining damages the immune system. These findings confirm the observations of Chinese medicine over the past 3000 years that the Blood is important in maintaining health.

[3] I have already referred to the effect of Buddhist meditation on circulating corticosteroid levels. Also see "Mind as Healer, Mind as Slayer" by Pelletier (Allen and Unwin, 1972) particularly Chapter 6 - Meditation and Chapter 7 - Autogenic Training and Visualisation.

The common symptoms of disease of this system include pains, stiffness and swelling in the joints and muscles, weakness of the muscles, muscle wasting in severe cases and joint deformities. They are extremely common especially in climates which are cold and damp. In the UK they make up a significant proportion of the workload of an alternative medicine clinic.

- BASIC ANATOMY AND PHYSIOLOGY -

There are several basic facts of anatomy and physiology which it is useful to know. I consider that most courses in these subjects are over detailed and reflect orthodox thinking rather than the particular needs of the alternative practitioner. I have listed the objectives which I consider useful to achieve as a preliminary to study of disease of the musculoskeletal system. These are detailed in Table 10.2.

As a preliminary to study of musculoskeletal disease you are able to:
List the structures comprising the musculoskeletal system
Describe the functions of the musculoskeletal system
Discuss the mechanism of muscular contraction and its relationship to nervous tissue

TABLE 10.2: OBJECTIVES FOR ANATOMY AND PHYSIOLOGY AS PREREQUISITE FOR STUDY OF DISEASE OF THE MUSCULOSKELETAL SYSTEM

- CLASSIFICATION OF MUSCULOSKELETAL DISEASE -

The main differentiation in all disease must be based upon the clinical picture. In musculoskeletal diseases this is between those where inflammation is a predominant feature and those where it is not. This is summarised in Table 10.3

INFLAMMATORY	NON-INFLAMMATORY[4]
Autoimmune disease	Osteoarthritis
• Rheumatoid arthritis	Other musculoskeletal conditions
• Systemic lupus erythematosus	• Tennis elbow/golfer's elbow
• Polyarteritis nodosa	• Bursitis
• Scleroderma	• Nerve compression
• Ankylosing spondylitis	• Repetitive strain injury
• Systemic sclerosis	• Frozen shoulder
• Dermatomyositis	
• Polymyalgia rheumatica	
Gout	

TABLE 10.3: CLASSIFICATION OF MUSCULOSKELETAL DISEASE

- AUTOIMMUNE DISEASES -

This is a term which is applied to a whole range of diseases where the immune system breaks down and begins to attack the body's own tissues. The actual site of the problem then determines the name of the disease. In this section I want to mainly consider those diseases which affect the musculoskeletal system[5]. Other examples which are studied in their relevant Chapter include hypothyroidism, hyperthyroidism, ulcerative colitis, pernicious anaemia. In energetic terms these are very deep serious conditions and can be considered to be immune system self-destruction. The equivalent on an emotional or mental level would be suicide.

I have listed most of the autoimmune disorders below. These are the ones you will see in the clinic. I have covered treatment in detail in the section dealing with rheumatoid arthritis. I would ask you to refer to this when studying the others as I have not unnecessarily repeated information later.

---

[4] Inflammation is either not evident or plays a minor part in the disease.
[5] Autoimmune diseases of the musculoskeletal system affect the connective tissue substance (collagen) of the body. They are, therefore, named collagenoses.

The treatments of most of the autoimmune disorders are similar except that in diseases other than rheumatoid arthritis, corticosteroids are used early and in very high dosages.

I have summarised alternative management at end of the section dealing with autoimmune disease. My comments there can be equally applied to all the similar diseases.

RHEUMATOID ARTHRITIS

This is a chronic, inflammatory, destructive and deforming polyarthritis. It is systemic in nature and so affects a wide range of tissues. It affects 3% of people in the West and three times more women than men. It usually begins at about 30-40 years of age. It is worse in damp and cold climates.

The cause is unknown according to conventional medicine although it is known that it is autoimmune in nature. There is a continual search for an infective origin and this theory recurs from time to time.

Symptoms:

There is the development of joint pain, stiffness and swelling. There are the classical appearances of inflammation, i.e. pain, redness, swelling, heat and loss of function.

Pain is brought on by movement at first then appears after resting. Early morning stiffness of joints occurs later. The main joints affected are the small joints of the fingers and toes. Proximal interphalangeal and metacarpophalangeal joints of the hands and the equivalent joints in the feet are primarily affected in a symmetrical pattern. The distal interphalangeal joints are not usually involved. Other joints affected are the wrists, elbows, shoulders, knees and ankles. The hip is involved in severe cases. Pain and stiffness are common in the neck and there may be symptoms in the temporomandibular and sternoclavicular joints.

There is a progression of pain, muscle spasm and joint destruction. Muscle pain is widespread with concomitant weakness and wasting. Common symptoms in the extremities are weakness, tingling and numbness as a result of a combination of nerve entrapment, tendonitis and inflammation of the nerves themselves. As the tendons are increasingly affected by the inflammatory process, they may rupture adding to the deformity and disability. Eventually there is joint instability, limited joint movement and deformities. Subcutaneous nodules occur in 20% of people, mainly at pressure sites such as the elbow around the olecranon.

Rheumatoid arthritis is a generalised disease and so there are associated symptoms of anorexia, weight loss and lethargy. Raynaud's phenomenon is common. The lymph glands are enlarged generally.

The eyes may be dry and red and secretions in general are reduced. There may be dry mouth. Sjögren's syndrome is the term applied to such symptoms.

Bone density decreases and osteoporosis may become evident on X-ray or bone scan. The blood shows evidence of anaemia which is of the type seen in chronic disease.

Prognosis:

After 10 years of the disease the following are seen:

•   complete remission - 25%
•   moderately impaired - 40%
•   severely disabled - 25%
•   severely crippled - 10%

These figures show the severity of the disease but remember that it is the conventional prognosis. If people are seen in the early stages and treated by means of alternative medicine, the prognosis will be less serious.

Investigations:

The diagnosis is usually clinically obvious but blood tests will be used to support this. Rheumatoid factor is found in 70% of people with rheumatoid arthritis. It is interesting to note that rheumatoid factor may also be found in people with no evidence of joint problems. A full blood count will reveal anaemia. X-rays will show joint destruction in the later stages of the disease.

Treatment:

There is no cure in terms of conventional medicine. The aim is to reduce, as much as possible, the degree of inflammation in the hope that this minimises the long-term damage. This is attempted by means of drugs. In the acute phase the person is told to rest and the joints may be splinted. Physiotherapy is initiated once the inflammation has subsided to some extent. This is to help preserve muscle strength and bulk.

The treatment of rheumatoid arthritis is separated into various stages depending upon the strength of the drug used. The medications available are listed in Table 10.4

TREATMENT	TREATMENT LEVEL
Aspirin, non-steroidal anti-inflammatory agents	1
Sulphasalazine	2
Gold, chloroquine, penicillamine	3
Corticosteroids	4
Immunosuppressants	5

TABLE 10.4: DRUGS USED IN THE TREATMENT OF RHEUMATOID ARTHRITIS

Aspirin is the drug of choice to treat inflammation but only 50% of people can tolerate it because of the side-effects. It is given in high dosage of 2 tablets every 4-6 hours.

Non-steroidal anti-inflammatory agents are related to aspirin and are commonly prescribed for all types of joint pains. They are acidic in nature, as is aspirin and all have similar side-effects. They burn the stomach leading to indigestion, poor appetite, nausea and vomiting. In severe cases they may cause upper gastrointestinal tract bleeding. There are several people who die each year from such problems. This whole group of drugs is widely used for rheumatoid arthritis and for any general musculoskeletal problem even with little or no evidence of inflammation.

If the inflammatory process fails to be controlled with these drugs then more powerful agents are used. All of these take between 6 weeks and 6 months to act and produce their full effect. Their use should be monitored closely by the prescribing practitioner.

Sulphasalazine is a combination of aspirin and a sulphonamide antibiotic. It is also used in the treatment of ulcerative colitis. It may lead to blood disorders of many types. These include agranulocytosis, aplastic anaemia, anaemia, leucopenia and thrombocytopenia.

Gold is one of the few treatments to survive from the alchemical days of medicine. It is the survivor of substances such as mercury, lead, arsenic and so forth. It is given either orally or injected and it takes several months for any alteration in symptoms to take place. It may cause kidney damage.

Penicillamine may lead to kidney damage or autoimmune diseases (!!) such as systemic lupus erythematosus and myasthenia gravis.

Chloroquine is a derivative of quinine - the malarial treatment. It may damage the eyes when used for long periods of time. It is less commonly used than the others in this group.

Corticosteroids are frequently given for this disease. They are symptomatic in that they reduce the degree of inflammation. They do nothing to arrest the underlying cause which is, in any case, unknown in conventional medicine. The usual formulation is prednisolone. This is the common prescription for all these autoimmune diseases. The dosage[6] may be defined as:

- low dose - 1mg daily
- medium dose - 5 mg daily
- high dose - 10mg or more daily

In the case of an acute onset of disease, particularly with the conditions of systemic lupus erythematosus or polyarteritis nodosa, there may be 100mg per day given in the early stages. This will be reduced as the symptoms are controlled but long-term administration of 10mg or more daily is not unusual.

They are powerful drugs and physiologically arise from the adrenal glands. Their prescription, therefore, leads to a suppression of adrenal activity. With long-term use, sudden withdrawal is dangerous as the adrenal glands will not be able to supply sufficient corticosteroids to maintain life. This appearance is of Addison's disease which is discussed in Chapter 15 - Endocrine System. It is

---

[6] In the case of other corticosteroids which may be prescribed it is important to check the dosages which compare to those given here.

normally said that reduction must take place no quicker than 1mg per month. Therefore, if someone is taking 10mg per day it will take almost one year to get them off prednisolone if there are no large flare-ups with which to contend. In practice, it may be quicker than this but care is needed because the adrenal glands have to recover their function.

Surgery is used in several situations. In the acute phase, the synovial membrane may be removed (synovectomy) from the joint. This is only done if the disease is unresponsive to drugs. A similar effect may be obtained by placing radioactive isotopes into the joints for some weeks. In the later stages of the disease, joint replacement may be an option for the hips, knees, elbows and fingers. Of these, the hip is the most amenable to replacement.

Rehabilitation has a major place to play in the conventional treatment of rheumatoid arthritis. Many people have great problems with joints after some years of the disease. Modification of the home, the use of walking aids and specially designed tools all have a part to play in easing difficulties with mobility.

SYSTEMIC LUPUS ERYTHEMATOSUS (SLE)

This is a systemic disease which affects most of the connective tissue of the whole body. It is particularly common in the US and Far East. Women are affected nine times more than men. It usually first presents in teenage years or twenties. There is often a past history of migraine and depression.

Symptoms:

The initial presentation is of fever with joint pain, swelling, redness and heat. Malaise and tiredness is marked. It may be indistinguishable from an acute onset of rheumatoid arthritis. It is common for the skin to be affected. There is redness of the face and cheeks in a butterfly distribution. Urticaria, sensitivity reactions to light and purpuric spots may all be seen. Alopecia is present in over half of people.

Systemic symptoms such as anorexia and weight loss are common. Multiple organ systems are involved in the inflammatory process leading to the appearances in Table 10.5.

ORGAN INVOLVED/DISEASE	SYMPTOMS TO LOOK FOR
Raynaud's phenomenon	Coldness of fingers and hands, precipitated by cold, classical appearance of whiteness, blueness and then redness
Pericarditis	Sharp chest pain, palpitations
Pleurisy	Sharp chest pain in axillary or scapular area worse for breathing
Myocarditis	Chest pain, palpitations, tiredness
Pneumonitis	Cough, breathlessness
Glomerulonephritis (in over half of people)	Loin pain, oedema, high blood pressure

TABLE 10.5: ASSOCIATED SYMPTOMS OF SYSTEMIC LUPUS ERYTHEMATOSUS

The presence of kidney disease indicates the worst prognosis. There may be psychological symptoms such as depression or even dementia.

Investigations:

The ESR is typically very high. Rheumatoid factor is positive in half of people. Kidney biopsy reveals a typical appearance.

Treatment:

Corticosteroids are given to damp down the immune reaction especially in the acute phase. Aspirin and non-steroidal anti-inflammatory agents are given for symptomatic relief. These drugs may cause skin sensitivity to light which is one of the symptoms of the original disease. In severe cases immunosuppressants may be used.

About 5% of people with SLE die within 5 years of diagnosis. For most people there is a chronic course of symptoms which come and go but are usually present. They are controlled by corticosteroids to a variable degree but side-effects are universal because of the dosages employed. There is less joint destruction than occurs in rheumatoid arthritis.

POLYARTERITIS NODOSA

This usually affects middle-aged men and is quite uncommon. There is widespread involvement of small arteries so that blood flow is diminished to many organs.

Symptoms:

There is the acute onset of fever with rapid heart rate, malaise, pains in the muscles and joints. Weight loss is common. It is virtually indistinguishable from an acute onset of rheumatoid arthritis. Later, as kidney damage develops, there is high blood pressure and abnormal kidney function tests. There may be heart and lung involvement with breathlessness, palpitations, oedema and chest pain. Numbness and tingling are experienced in those with central nervous system involvement. It is the kidney disease which is the most important prognostic indicator. Kidney disease is the usual cause of death.

Investigations:

The ESR is raised markedly but biopsy of liver or kidney is the usual method of definitive diagnosis.

Treatment:

This is with corticosteroids often combined with immunosuppressants such as azathioprine. Most people with this condition survive less than 5 years after diagnosis.

SCLERODERMA

In this type of autoimmune disease, the skin is affected to become swollen and hardened. The lungs, oesophagus, heart muscle and kidneys are also involved.

Symptoms:

The main manifestations are on the skin. Three times more women are affected than men and it usually begins at a young age. The skin is affected by thickened, waxy patches which may enlarge with time or come and go. If they disappear then this area is darker than surrounding skin. If large areas develop then restriction of movement may occur with severe skin thickening, pains in the muscles and joint stiffness.

Treatment:

There is nothing, conventionally, which will change the long-term of the disease although corticosteroids may be given for symptomatic relief.

ANKYLOSING SPONDYLITIS

This is an inflammation affecting the spinal column. 90% of cases occur in males and the common age of onset is 20-40 years.

Symptoms:

The classical presentation is of pain and stiffness in the back. The sacroiliac joints are a common first site for such symptoms. As there is an inflammation there may be fever and malaise also. The whole vertebral column is affected. The symptoms increase in severity until the whole spine becomes stiff and rigid. Joints may also be involved in the process especially in the lower limbs and become swollen and stiff. Breathing may be painful and shallow due to the chest wall being affected. Inflammation of the iris (iritis) is seen in 20% of people with this condition giving rise to redness in the eye.

Examination of the spine reveals loss of the normal lumbar curve and an exaggerated kyphosis of the thoracic spine.

Investigations:

The ESR is raised. X-rays of the spine almost always show abnormalities. Early radiological examination shows thickening of bone and erosion of sacro-iliac joints. Later there is fusion of the sacro-iliac joints with calcification in the spinal ligaments.

Treatment:

Corticosteroids may be given but it is generally accepted that they make no difference to the outcome and will only result in the addition of side-effects to the clinical picture. Symptomatic treatment with aspirin and non-steroidal anti-inflammatory agents is given. Sulphasalazine may be prescribed long-term. This drug is discussed above with regard to rheumatoid arthritis. Radiotherapy may be administered to the spine to reduce the inflammation. Physiotherapy is used to try and reduce the degree of stiffness and impaired function.

SYSTEMIC SCLEROSIS

This is an autoimmune disease which mainly affects the skin. It is three times more common in women than men. It tends to begin under the age of 50 years.

Symptoms:

Multiple organs and tissues are affected in this disease. The skin becomes hardened and swollen. There is subsequent restriction of movement particularly in the hands and fingers. In the face, there is fixing of the expression and sharpening of the nose. Muscular aches and pains are common.

Raynaud's phenomenon occurs in around three quarters of people with systemic sclerosis. These symptoms may develop some years before the diagnosis of systemic sclerosis is made.

Oesophageal involvement leads to heartburn, dysphagia and indigestion. Diarrhoea and abdominal distension also occurs. Affection of the lungs causes breathlessness. Palpitations reveal cardiac involvement. Dry eyes due to Sjögren's syndrome are usual. This is a common feature of many autoimmune diseases.

As with all the autoimmune disorders, the kidneys are affected in severe cases. This will lead to frequent urination, loin pain and tiredness.

Investigations:

The ESR is raised since it is a non-specific indicator of inflammation. Rheumatoid factor is positive in 30% of cases. Antinuclear antibodies are more commonly positive. Anaemia is usual and is due to multiple factors.

Treatment:

This is only symptomatic. No treatment, even corticosteroids or other immunosuppressants, makes any difference to the course of the disease. The disease tends to be severe in its manifestations and only half of people with systemic sclerosis are alive 5 years after diagnosis.

DERMATOMYOSITIS

As its name suggests, this disease affects skin and muscle. It is characterised by muscle weakness and there are inflammatory changes in the muscle and skin. It is related to polymyositis which primarily leads to muscle symptoms.

Symptoms:

There is weakness and wasting of the muscles especially of those around the shoulders, hips and pelvis. The muscles are painful and tender. Joint pains, swelling and stiffness are common. This may resemble the appearances of rheumatoid arthritis but long-term joint destruction does not occur. Difficulty in swallowing and speaking are seen in over half of people. The symptoms of Raynaud's phenomenon and Sjögren's disease are frequent accompaniments.

Skin rashes are common. These include reddish/blue discolouration over the exposed areas. Redness of the eyelids is classically seen. These appearances with muscle weakness indicate that dermatomyositis is the diagnosis. Malignant disease is a common development especially of the lung in men and ovaries in women.

Investigations:

Serum creatine phosphokinase is raised and indicates that muscles are involved. Electromyography (EMG) shows typical changes. Muscle biopsy will give the definitive diagnosis.

The ESR is raised. There is an anaemia and the white cell count is raised. Test for rheumatoid factor is often positive.

Treatment:

This is by means of corticosteroids although it has little effect in chronic cases. Immunosuppressant drugs such as azathioprine or methotrexate may be given in addition.

POLYMYALGIA RHEUMATICA

This is an affection of the muscles and the inflammatory process may also involve the temporal artery - temporal or cranial arteritis. It is this complication which is potentially hazardous to sight.

Polymyalgia rheumatica usually first develops around 60-70 years of age and three times more commonly in women than men.

Symptoms:

There is the sudden onset of pain and stiffness in the muscles, particularly of the shoulders, hips and pelvis. The neck and lumbar spine is a common site for pain and stiffness. The symptoms are typically worse in the mornings on getting out of bed. There may be systemic symptoms such as weight loss, anorexia, malaise, tiredness. Fever is common but mild.

There may be an associated headache which is localised to the temple. There is tenderness in this area and the temporal artery may be thickened and tender. In severe cases there may be no pulsation felt over the cranial artery. It is this complication which is hazardous as it may lead to sudden and irreversible blindness.

Investigation:

The ESR is very high at around 100mm per hour. Anaemia is common. Serum alkaline phosphatase is raised. Temporal artery biopsy is done in some cases but the diagnosis is usually obvious clinically.

Treatment:

This is by means of corticosteroids which reduces the inflammation and ESR. This treatment is continued for at least 2 years and may be resumed if there are relapses. After 4 years the disease has disappeared in virtually everyone. Corticosteroids are given to everyone with polymyalgia rheumatica as there is a slight risk of blindness. If there is temporal arteritis then this risk is greatly increased.

ALTERNATIVE MANAGEMENT OF AUTOIMMUNE DISEASE

As I mentioned in the Introduction, there is a close relationship between the musculoskeletal system and the functioning of Blood in its energetic sense. The other organ which is closely involved is the Kidney as it dominates bone, produces Bone Marrow and is at the root of all the body's energies. These connections are made in Chapter 9 - Urinary System. This is an interesting association in that the main treatment for these conditions is with corticosteroids which anatomically come from the adrenal glands situated on top of the kidneys. In terms of Chinese medicine, such diseases are often Bi Syndrome (usually of the Hot type) with mainly underlying Kidney Yang Deficiency and Blood Deficiency. There may be other organ imbalances to consider in addition.

There now follow some cases which describe people with a variety of the autoimmune diseases mentioned above. The general approach to such disease will become evident and I include comments about corticosteroids at the same time. All these diseases tend to be severe and difficult to treat. Diagnosis will be hampered by the almost invariable presence of corticosteroids or other powerful drugs. You would expect treatment to be prolonged.

CASE 1

A woman of 30 years presented for treatment with generalised pains in the joints. She had been involved in a road traffic accident some 3 months previously when she had sustained marked bruising over her right hypochondrium and abdominal wall from the safety belt. Some four weeks after the accident, she developed pains in the chest which were worse when breathing, stiffness in the muscles and joints, hot swellings of the joints, nausea, fever, night sweats and general malaise and tiredness.

Her symptoms worsened to the point where she could hardly move and she had to be admitted to hospital. After some days a diagnosis of polyarteritis nodosa was made and she was given:

*   Prednisolone 100mg daily
*   Azathioprine 125mg daily

Her symptoms quickly improved and at the time of her consultation with me she had some residual tightness and discomfort in the chest, weak legs, hot and swollen wrists. Her appetite was normal now and she slept well. Her dosage of prednisolone had been reduced to 60mg daily. She came for treatment because she wanted relief of her symptoms and to come off her drugs. She had been specifically told by her consultant that the drugs had no side-effects. She had met people who had taken corticosteroids long-term and realised that she was likely to develop problems, particularly at the dosage she was prescribed.

The dosage of corticosteroids reflects the strength of inflammation in this case. As she had been on the medication for some 2 months now it was not sensible to reduce quickly. I impressed on her that the appropriate time to start drug reduction would be when she started to improve. If she reduced them too soon then the original clinical picture would return.

In terms of Chinese medicine, her diagnosis was DampHeat Stagnation which was confirmed by a pulse quality of full and slippery. Her tongue was pale and swollen which is contradictory as it would be expected to be red with a thick, yellow greasy coat. This was because of the effect of the corticosteroids which I shall discuss later. The accident was clearly the trigger because of damage to the Blood, particularly Liver Blood given the site of the injury. A predisposing cause was the oral contraceptive which tends to lead to Blood disturbances particularly Stagnation. This is discussed fully in Chapter 18 - Gynaecology. Also, she had a history of a kidney 'infection' when aged 7 years necessitating hospital admission. Prior to and after the car accident she was under a lot of emotional strain at home.

I gave her an acupuncture treatment and 5 packets of herbs to release the Stagnation and protect the Blood. She returned some 2 weeks later. She told me that after her last visit she had decided to stop the prescribed drugs and flushed them down the toilet! She had started to feel better and decided to take charge. She felt very shaky and nauseous for a week but this then settled. She now had very few symptoms with some aching in her neck and wrists. Her general weakness had subsided and there were no swellings.

Over the course of the next few months, I concentrated on correcting her underlying Kidney and Blood imbalances. After 6 months of treatment she was well with no problems.

This case illustrates several important points. Her initial reaction to the injury illustrated a pre-existing susceptibility at a fairly deep level. However, the strong nature of her symptoms, the acute onset and her rapid response to treatment reveal a basically strong constitution. This was responsible for her clearly taking charge of her medication. Two months of medication is not long enough to lead to significant suppression of adrenal function and if the alternative treatment is correct there will be little in the way of a flare-up.

This brings me onto the question of the energetic action of corticosteroids. There is some discussion in alternative circles as to whether they are Cold or Hot in nature as they are commonly used for inflammatory conditions. The key is to look at what happens if the body does not produce its own supply or if long-term prescribed corticosteroids are withdrawn rapidly. The clinical appearance is that of Addison's disease which is described in Chapter 15 - Endocrine System. There is low blood pressure, low temperature, general slowing of the body functions and eventually coma and death. This corresponds to a collapse of Yang picture in Chinese medicine and so corticosteroids would be the counterpart of a Rescue Yang formula.

They are Hot in nature and primarily affect the Lung, Spleen and Kidney Yang. They are strongly moving and release Stagnation syndromes. such as Bi Syndrome. They will rescue the Yang Deficiency with Water Overflowing of severe cardiac insufficiency. In the long-term they will lead to depletion of Blood and Yin especially of the Liver and Kidney (see Case 2 below). In the acute phase, because the Heat is due to Stagnation, the clinical symptoms and signs of Heat will disappear. This is why this woman's tongue was pale rather than the expected red with a thick yellow coat. In long-term use Heat will be much more evident as the fluids become damaged.

Since these drugs are Hot and strongly moving, they will tend to disperse the Yang of the Lung, Spleen and Kidney. This explains the typical side-effects of oedema, especially of the upper and middle parts of the body. The Lung is responsible for the water passages through its dispersing and descending function and the Spleen transforms and transports. Interference with these two organs leads the appearance of oedema.

There is increased appetite due to Stomach Heat, there is wasting of the limbs due to the damage to body fluids and muscles, diabetes mellitus can develop as the Yin is consumed, heating of the Heart can lead to mental disturbances and psychotic manifestations in some. The effect on Lung Yang is why there is relief from wheezing in asthma but long-term use may lead to Yang Collapse. Long-term, of course, there will be Kidney Yin and Yang Deficiency as this organ is weakened.

The strongest effects are with oral corticosteroids but there is similar results with all prescriptions - inhaled, enemas, nasal, topical on the skin, eye drops.

CASE 2

This case is more revealing of the long-term results of corticosteroid prescriptions. A woman of 56 years came for treatment. She had been diagnosed as having systemic lupus erythematosus some 38 years previously. Her current medication was:

• Prednisolone 10mg and 7.5mg daily on alternate days

Her symptoms began after an episode of low back pain and she rapidly developed a similar clinical appearance to those described in Case 1 above. She was one of the first people to receive corticosteroids in the UK in the late 1950's and she had remained on them ever since. Whenever she tried to reduce them there would be a flare-up of joint pain, redness, swelling and heat.

Her main symptoms now were pain and cracking in the joints which was worse after exercise, pain in the epigastrium with acidity in the chest, diarrhoea several times each day, nocturia four times each night, dryness of skin, hair, mouth and eyes. She had bleeding gums and teeth which would suddenly become loose and drop out. She had palpitations. Occasionally, she would experience hot feelings on the surface of the body with severe icy coldness inside. At these times she would feel exhausted and these had occurred every few weeks over the past 10 years or so.

In terms of Chinese medicine she had marked Blood and Yin Deficiency of Liver and Kidney, Heat in the Stomach and Yang Deficiency of the Spleen and Kidney. There was some evidence of DampHeat Stagnation in the joints but this only became obvious when she reduced her corticosteroids. Her tongue was very red, thin and dry which revealed the damage to body fluids as caused by the prescribed drugs. This case shows much more clearly the Hot nature of corticosteroids and their long-term effect.

It is sometimes said that there is little point treating such people as their energy is too severely depleted. Whilst it is true that this woman was greatly weakened by the drugs, it is rarely the case that nothing can be done. No attempt must be made to reduce the corticosteroids since her energy is weak and unless improvement begins, it is in danger of collapsing especially if reduction is rapid. The attacks of heat on the exterior and cold on the interior is typical of a condition called True Cold False Heat where lack of Fire internally leads to Yang floating to the surface. It is indicative of a severe Yang deficiency.

I treated her with acupuncture and herbs trying to strengthen her Qi and Blood gently to begin with. She improved gradually and more so than I originally expected. She has a strong spirit and despite her long years of corticosteroid therapy was remarkably well. Many people in a similar situation are very ill with more problems. Her digestion improved as did her nocturnal urination. Her general energy picked up and she would occasionally develop discharge of green mucus from the nose with mild fever and sweating. This is indicative that her energy is improving to the point where it can 'throw out' internal toxins.

She continued treatments for some months and was able to reduce her corticosteroid medication. She would experience some tiredness when this happened and mild flare-ups of joint pain and swelling. Her treatment continues some 18 months later and she is now taking occasional analgesics only. Her general health is much improved. If she could have had alternative treatment 38 years previously then she would have been saved the debilitating effects of a long-term corticosteroid prescription. This is the point I made in Chapter 2 - Philosophy. It is not appropriate to continue powerful, acute treatments for a long time. They need to be replaced by more gentle, balanced methods.

CASE 3

A man of 22 years came for treatment who had started to develop joint pains at the age of 8 years. His main problems were in his knees, elbows, shoulders and hips. He had marked stiffness in these areas which was worse if he sat still for a long time. He felt better for movement. He had recent X-rays which showed evidence of ankylosing spondylitis. He had attacks of eye problems with redness, soreness and general dryness. His vision was generally weak with floaters in the field of vision. He had some hot, burning pains in his stomach which would radiate up to the throat and wake him at night with burning pain. His general energy was weak and he would sleep for an hour or so every afternoon.

In terms of Chinese medicine, his diagnosis was Blood Deficiency, Heat in the Liver and Stomach with underlying Kidney Yang Deficiency. This was a result of long-term emotional difficulties. His treatment consisted of acupuncture and herbs. I advised him to keep away from foods which are exceptionally heating such as coffee, alcohol, spicy food, citrus fruit and to take gentle regular exercise. He made a steady improvement and was able to stop his non-steroidal anti-inflammatory drugs.

People with ankylosing spondylitis are fortunate in that they are rarely given corticosteroids. The case is clearer because it is not obscured by these powerful drugs and the case is clearer. It is easier to treat therefore. It is much better to see people early in their disease. If you see people who have developed great stiffness and rigidity it is more difficult to obtain great improvement.

CASE 4

A woman of 25 years came for treatment with generalised joint pains. She had started some 5 years earlier after great emotional shocks in the family. All her joints were painful, stiff, swollen, aching but not especially hot. She was much better in hot weather and a holiday in the Mediterranean sun would completely relieve her symptoms. She had cold hands and feet and felt tired all the time. Her sleep was disturbed by her joint problems. She sweated easily during the day. Her conventional diagnosis was rheumatoid arthritis and her current medication was:

- Sulphasalazine 500mg twice daily
- Piroxicam 20mg daily - non-steroidal anti-inflammatory agent

In terms of Chinese medicine, this woman was diagnosed as suffering from Kidney Yang Deficiency and ColdDamp Bi Syndrome. The diagnosis of Kidney Yang Deficiency is a common one in cases of rheumatoid arthritis and reflects the association between Kidney and Bone. This is the explanation behind the oft-noted observation that rheumatoid arthritis is much improved with heat. If the joints are hot and swollen this may seem to be a contradiction. It is not if you understand that the interior of the body will be warmed leading to increased Yang function. This will lead to less heat and swelling in the joints. If the person spends some time in a hot climate then the joint symptoms may disappear completely.

The drug sulphasalazine is a combination of aspirin (acetylsalicylic acid) and a sulphonamide antibiotic. It can be considered, therefore, to have the same energetic action as non-steroidal anti-inflammatory agents (of which piroxicam is an example). These drugs correspond to a category of herbs which relieve conditions due to WindDamp. They are warm in nature and move the Blood to relieve obstruction and thence pain. Long-term, especially if used alone and in high doses, i.e. as pharmaceutical medicines, they will lead to Blood and Yin Deficiency with signs of heat. They will also disperse and weaken the Qi. They will primarily affect the Liver and Kidney.

As mentioned in Chapter 9 - Urinary System, the non-steroidal anti-inflammatory agents are responsible for a significant proportion of kidney problems due to their propensity to cause analgesic nephropathy. Interestingly, Blood Deficiency is responsible for symptoms of joint pain and stiffness and so long-term prescription of these drugs will lead to arthritis-like syndromes. It has been observed that the use of such drugs in osteoarthritis (see below) can lead to the worsening of the condition.[7]

- GOUT -

This is an inflammatory arthritis which, in conventional medicine, is due to an excess of uric acid in the blood. Crystals are formed in joints which leads to the severe symptoms of this condition. Uric acid is a breakdown product of purine. Increased levels occur due to drugs such as frusemide and thiazide diuretics or dietary factors. Foods with a high protein content, e.g. meat and alcoholic drinks increase uric acid levels. Middle-aged men are more commonly affected.

Symptoms:

This condition is extremely painful and most of us have an image of an elderly, irritable man with a heavily bandaged foot suffering from gout. The pain of gout is so severe in most cases that any contact is excruciating. The commonest joint affected is the first metatarsophalangeal joint but others may include ankles, hands, knees and elbows in an assymmetrical pattern. There is usually an associated fever.

In chronic cases, there may be joint deformity due to damage from crystal deposits. Collections of uric acid may be found in the cartilage of the ears - tophi.

Investigations:

The serum uric acid level is raised as are the ESR and white cell count.

Treatment:

This is by means of drugs to reduce the inflammation such as aspirin and non-steroidal anti-inflammatory agents. Dietary advice is given to reduce the amount of uric acid in the blood and drugs may be administered to do the same. Such medication is long-term and those commonly used are sulphinpyrazone, probenecid and allopurinol.

Alternative management:

This is essentially the same as for the general inflammatory conditions described above. Gout usually affects one or few joints and in terms of Chinese medicine corresponds to DampHeat Accumulation

---

[7] The use of non-steroidal anti-inflammatory agents accelerates joint deterioration. Lancet 1989; Sep.2, Page 519. With an understanding of their energetic action as described on this Page it can be seen as being due to a general depletion of the Blood so that the joints and muscles are nourished less.

which affects the Spleen and Liver (hence its usual site over the Liver and Spleen channels in the foot). It is important to take diet into consideration and to avoid or reduce foods which generate Damp and Heat. These include excessive sweet food, greasy food, spices, alcohol, red meat, citrus fruit and whitebait.

- OSTEOARTHRITIS -

This is a degeneration of the joint cartilage with growth of new bone and connective tissue within the joint. Inflammatory changes are minor and secondary to this process. 80% of people over the age of 65 years have evidence of osteoarthritis yet only 25% have symptoms. The evidence takes the form of X-rays. It is more common in women than men. There are more symptoms if the weather is cold and damp.

The risk of this condition is increased if the joint is affected by a previous fracture, in cases of overuse such as professional sports people or manual labourers or if there has been previous damage to the joint, e.g. inflammatory arthritis, trauma.

Symptoms

This disease mainly affects the spine, load-bearing joints of hips and knees and the first metacarpophalangeal joint. There is the gradual onset of joint pain with aching. Pain is worse for movement and better for rest. Stiffness is common and may be worse after resting for some time or in the mornings.

There is cracking in the joint and the muscles surrounding the joint may be tender. These muscles may waste in long-term cases. There may be joint swelling due to increased amounts of fluid in the joint - effusion.

Bony swellings appear on the hands over the distal interphalangeal joints. In some cases they are red, hot, swollen and painful but this inflammation settles to leave hard swellings.

Investigations:

There are typical appearances on X-ray of narrowing of the joint space, bone formation (osteophytes) at the edges of the joint, thickening of the adjacent bone and the presence of loose debris in the joint. Blood tests are normal.

Treatment:

There are many treatments available for osteoarthritis yet none are completely satisfactory in terms of symptom relief. General advice will include reducing excess weight, change of occupation and physiotherapy.

Prescribed drug use is common. Aspirin and non-steroidal anti-inflammatory agents are given despite the lack of any degree of inflammation in most cases. Corticosteroids are applied locally by injection rather than systemically. Repeated use weakens the joint and may lead to further joint damage and deterioration. This is particularly true in weight bearing joints. Surgery is offered as a last resort if there is great discomfort and disability.

Alternative treatment:

In terms of Chinese medicine, osteoarthritis usually corresponds to Bi Syndrome (frequently Cold and/or Damp). There is frequently an underlying syndrome such as Blood Deficiency. This is why such symptoms appear in people who have overused their joints through physical activity. The Blood is weakened and so cannot nourish the muscles and joints.

Treatment may be effective in some people if just the joint is treated. In others it is important to nourish the Blood at the same time. Physical therapies such as massage are helpful as an adjunct to such treatment. I find a combination of massage and acupuncture to be particularly effective. General advice to take regular *gentle* exercise and for a healthy whole food diet is important. Reduction of weight, if excessive, is useful to take the strain off affected joints particularly in the lower part of the body.

CASE

A woman of 55 years came for treatment of her painful knees. She has been a nurse for many years and her job involved a lot of lifting. Her knee X-rays revealed osteoarthritic changes to the joint. She had stiffness and pain in the knees which prevented her from walking long distances. She had particular problems on walking up or down stairs. The symptoms had been worsening for the past five years and treatment with non-steroidal anti-inflammatory agents had given her little relief. Her basic constitution was sound and treatment of her knees with massage and acupuncture led to relief from much of the pain and stiffness. At the end of treatment she had no limitation of activity and would have minor symptoms only if she walked long distances.

- OTHER MUSCULOSKELETAL CONDITIONS -

There are a wide range of conditions of the musculoskeletal system which are usually labelled as being inflammatory, i.e. they have the suffix of -itis but do not fit comfortably into a categorisation of rheumatoid or osteoarthritis. There are myriad terms used such as rheumatism, fibrositis and so forth which are often used imprecisely in cases of muscular and joint aches and pains. Investigations are invariably normal and treatments such as physiotherapy, prescribed drugs and exercise are of variable effectiveness. Injected corticosteroid preparations may be given but it is common to find that people have chronic problems. At times their activity may be severely limited. It is not possible to list all the conditions which exist but I do mention below the most common.

Achilles tendonitis
Carpal tunnel syndrome
Fibrositis
Frozen shoulder
Golfer's elbow
Morton's metatarsalgia
Olecranon bursitis (student's elbow)
Osgood-Schlatter's disease
Plantar fasciitis
Prepatellar bursitis (housemaid's/clergyman's knee)
Repetitive strain injury
Sacroiliac strain
Tennis elbow
Trigger finger

TABLE 10.6: COMMON MUSCULOSKELETAL CONDITIONS

TENNIS ELBOW/GOLFER'S ELBOW

This is a tendonitis due to overactivity which is usually not sport related despite its terminology. Tennis elbow affects the lateral epicondyle of the humerus and golfer's elbow the medial epicondyle. Any repetitive activity may lead to its development and they are common in housewives, manual workers and so forth. The common activity is a twisting action of the forearm as for example using a screwdriver or opening jars. I have seen tennis elbow in herbalists due to their having to open dozens of jars each day containing herbs.

Symptoms:

There is frequently pain up and down the arm and the muscles around the shoulder may be affected. There may be weakness which leads to difficulty opening jars or carrying objects. The muscles and tendon over the affected epicondyle are acutely tender.

Treatment:

Non-steroidal anti-inflammatory agents may be used but corticosteroid injections are common.

Alternative management:

As stated above with regards to osteoarthritis, the key to treating this condition is to assess the condition of the energy and Blood. If it is a sole occurrence in an otherwise healthy person, treatment of only the elbow may be sufficient to relieve it. If there are aches and pains in other areas or there is evidence of Deficiency of Blood generally[8] perhaps with insomnia, palpitations, anxiety or worry then local treatment must be combined with constitutional remedies. This is a common situation in women who may have Blood Deficiency or in people who have over exercised.

In those who have received corticosteroid injections, treatment tends to be prolonged with more aggravations along the way. This is because these drugs weaken the tendon and so it takes time to overcome this.

BURSITIS

A bursa is a small sac or pouch lined with synovial membrane. They are present around joints. Inflammation in a bursa may arise because of repetitive injury as in housemaid's knee, clergyman's knee, student's elbow and so forth or can be part of a more widespread disorder such as rheumatoid arthritis.

Symptoms:

The affected area is swollen, hot, tender and perhaps reddened. Movement will be limited. There may be an association with a recurrent type of activity.

Treatment:

Injection of corticosteroid locally is the usual method of treatment.

NERVE COMPRESSION

The classical example of this is carpal tunnel syndrome. The clinical appearance has similarities with that of repetitive strain injury (RSI) described below. A case of RSI below gives a good example of the approach to these situations.

Symptoms:

There is tingling and pins and needles in the hands, wrists and occasionally into the arm. Despite its supposed cause in conventional medicine, i.e. pressure on the median nerve in the wrist, there are often symptoms up the arm. Weakness of the muscles of the hands and forearms is common. In severe cases there is wasting.

Treatment:

This is directed at the area in the wrist where the nerve passes through a fibrous tunnel. Local corticosteroid injections are common but surgery is used in long-standing cases. This necessitates a long incision from the anterior aspect of the wrist into the palm of the hand. In my experience, the conventional treatments are of variable effectiveness and many people may have the symptoms after treatment with the addition of a scar.

---

[8] See Anaemia in Chapter 7 - Cardiovascular System for a discussion of the symptoms of Blood Deficiency as this term is understood in alternative medicine.

REPETITIVE STRAIN INJURY (RSI)

This is a common problem amongst people whose work entails a repetitive action. It tends to be under diagnosed although there has been interest recently in the problems of keyboard operators.

Symptoms:

There is tingling, pins and needles and even numbness in the affected areas. This is usually the hands and forearms. The symptoms occur after prolonged activity such as typing, writing and so forth. There is weakness also which can interfere with function to a great degree. People find that they are able to do less and less before symptoms appear. In some cases, normal activity is impossible.

Treatment:

This is by means of physiotherapy and non-steroidal anti-inflammatory agents but these are of variable effectiveness. It is important to consider the work situation especially with regard to length of continuous activity, posture, height of chairs and work surfaces and so on.

CASE

This is a good example of how to deal in general with musculoskeletal problems of this type. A woman of 28 years came for treatment of her repetitive strain injury. She is a teacher and for the past 3 years has had symptoms in her upper limbs. These developed after writing a lot of reports for school. She had variable degrees of trouble over the past 3 years but the symptoms had been constant for the 8 months prior to coming to see me.

She had burning and stabbing pains with tingling over the shoulders, into the arms to the hands. They came on after using her hands and arms and she recently found that minor degrees of activity could precipitate symptoms. She also had visual floaters, insomnia and pre-menstrual breast soreness with irritability. She was occasionally constipated with abdominal cramps. She was taking a non-steroidal anti-inflammatory agent daily with little change in symptoms.

In terms of Chinese medicine, this is a case of Liver Blood Deficiency and you could treat her arms for ever with little result. She needed constitutional treatment and I gave her herbs to strengthen her Liver Blood. After 5 bags of herbs, a quick response, she had much less pain in her shoulders and arms. Her sleep was still disturbed but she felt better in herself. After several months of treatment she was able to use her arms and hands with no discomfort although prolonged exercise would cause minor degrees of tingling.

This case reveals why treatments such as physiotherapy and local corticosteroid injections are of variable effectiveness, particularly in chronic conditions. It is essential to consider the underlying state since the symptoms will be relieved only when this has improved. I find that physiotherapy is most effective in acute injuries as it is strongly moving in terms of Qi and Blood. For chronic conditions however it is much preferable to use treatments which take the constitution into account. People with a chronic condition due to weakness of Qi and Blood may, in fact, be made worse by physiotherapy (or indeed local acupuncture treatment). This is because the energetic pathways on the surface are opened without there being adequate supplies of Qi and Blood in the interior. This also explains why some cases of migraine (Chapter 14 - Central Nervous System) are made worse by local treatment of the energetic pathways.

FROZEN SHOULDER

This, as its name suggests, is a 'freezing' of the shoulder joint. It is common in people who have restricted activity generally or perhaps after a stroke when the affected side cannot be moved. It is usually one-sided

Symptoms:

There is pain and stiffness in the affected shoulder. There is marked limitation of movement and this causes problems with dressing, brushing hair and the like. The limited movement may be in one direction, e.g. extension, flexion, abduction and so on. This is of significance in Chinese medicine as it indicates the channels mainly affected.

Treatment:

Prevention is helpful so exercise of the shoulder in cases of reduced activity is helpful. In established cases, physiotherapy, non-steroidal anti-inflammatory agents and local corticosteroid injections are used with variable effectiveness.

- OSTEOPOROSIS -

This is a decrease in the density of bone which occurs as part of the ageing process. It is a problem with the substance of bone rather than the calcium structure. Calcium supplements, therefore, have no part to play in either its prevention or its treatment. It is more common with lack of activity, low body weight, smoking, corticosteroid medication and in women after the menopause.

Symptoms:

There are usually no symptoms and the diagnosis is made by X-ray or bone scan. In conventional practice, the diagnosis may be made on the presence of joint pains and stiffness. These are *not* symptoms of osteoporosis. The prescription of hormone replacement therapy (oestrogen with or without progesterone) may lead to the disappearance of such symptoms. This is merely because such hormones have a corticosteroid effect of relieving inflammation.

In some people there may be fractures and so there are manifest symptoms. The lumbar and thoracic vertebrae, the neck of femur, upper end of humerus and lower end of radius are the commonest sites. With vertebral collapse there may be pain, backache, loss of stature and kyphosis.

Investigations:

X-rays reveal a less dense bony structure. Bone scans with radioactive isotopes show the same changes. There are raised levels of alkaline phosphatase.

Treatment:

There is little treatment which is available once osteoporosis has developed. Some people spontaneously improve. Fractures are treated if and when they occur.

Prevention is a fashionable topic at the moment with increasing prescriptions given of hormone replacement therapy. The issues around this are discussed in full in Chapter 18 - Gynaecology.

Alternative management:

The main problem here for alternative practitioners is the large number of women who are being prescribed hormone replacement therapy. There should be specific indications for its use. In practice it is given in many situations for which it is difficult to see any reason. Its correct use can be summarised as treating symptoms during the menopause and to prevent osteoporosis. Issues dealing with the menopause are dealt with in Chapter 18 - Gynaecology. Osteoporosis and the fear of its development may be used by conventional practitioners to 'persuade' women to take HRT. I would stress that osteoporosis is part of the normal ageing process. It tends to be more severe in some situations. However, to prescribe a powerful drug to everyone on the basis that they may develop a disease is potentially hazardous. This takes no regard of the time, money and effort spent on prescriptions, monitoring its use and dealing with the side-effects.

Women who smoke, have a family history of osteoporosis, are of a light build, under-exercise and have received corticosteroids are at more risk. Most of these factors can be addressed by changing life-style. In terms of Chinese medicine, the condition of bone is related to the function of the Kidney. As the Kidney function fades later in life, the bone may be affected. It would make sense, therefore, to protect Kidney function early in life and to strengthen this organ as much as possible.

- HOW TO RECOGNISE A SERIOUS CONDITION OF THE MUSCULOSKELETAL SYSTEM -

The main point to make here about the symptoms of the musculoskeletal system is that, in themselves, they are rarely hazardous to life. However, there may be a process which is potentially damaging and it is important to know these, unusual, situations.

Any symptom which is severe, acute and with strong systemic features needs to concern you. The other situation is the case of a single joint which acutely becomes hot, swollen and painful. This may indicate an infective arthritis which rapidly damages the joint.

- SUMMARY -

Musculoskeletal conditions are extremely common and form a large part of the caseload of an alternative medicine clinic.

The most effective treatment will be a combination of physical therapy such as massage, gentle exercise and strengthening methods such as acupuncture, homoeopathy and herbs.

Autoimmune disease is characterised by systemic involvement as well as joint and muscle symptoms. These are deep diseases and treatment is usually prolonged.

11 DERMATOLOGY

OBJECTIVES:

At the end of this Chapter you will be able to:
Describe the differences between the alternative and conventional views of the skin.
List the symptoms attributable to disturbances of the skin.
State when a symptom(s) would indicate a serious underlying condition.
Describe the main symptoms of diseases covered in this Chapter.
Explain the relevant management by an alternative practitioner of each disorder.

- INTRODUCTION -

When I was about to go to University to study medicine, my general practitioner told me to specialise in dermatology if I had the opportunity. He said that he had missed such a chance himself and regretted it ever since. When I asked him why, he replied that it was because there are plenty of people with skin problems, lots of private practice and no-one ever gets better. At the time I was quite shocked by his apparently cynical attitude. Later, with the benefit of experience I saw that this was, indeed, the conventional view. Rashes may come and they may go but in the end they are usually chronic in nature. The conventional treatments help to some extent but no-one pretends that it is a cure.

It was when I was in general practice myself that I saw the effect of alternative medical treatments. A young boy with eczema and asthma had been treated by me with conventional medication with little relief - a common story. After some months, his mother brought him to see me and he was the best he had ever been. He had received acupuncture over the intervening period with steady improvements. After my training in acupuncture, but especially in Chinese herbal medicine, it is clear that treatments exist which are powerful yet gentle and effective and this is especially so for skin diseases.

Skin disease is variable in its response to any form of treatment. This is because it may be either a problem which is merely on the surface of the body or it may reflect a deeper underlying imbalance. In cases where the skin rash is superficial, perhaps only affecting the palms or hands, the response to treatment can be dramatic and rapid. This is in line with Hering's Law of Cure where disorders on the lowermost and outermost parts of the body are the least severe. In cases where there is a marked internal imbalance, treatment may be long and involved. However, it is rewarding for the individual, if they persist with treatment, as relief of skin symptoms can have important effects in areas such as employment, confidence, physical activity and so on.

- BASIC ANATOMY AND PHYSIOLOGY -

There are several basic facts of anatomy and physiology which it is useful to know. I consider that most courses in these subjects are over detailed and reflect orthodox thinking rather than the particular needs of the alternative practitioner. I have listed the objectives which I consider useful to achieve as a preliminary to study of dermatology. These are detailed in Table 11.1.

As a preliminary to study of dermatological disease you are able to:
Describe the structure and functions of the skin.

TABLE 11.1: OBJECTIVES FOR ANATOMY AND PHYSIOLOGY AS PREREQUISITE FOR STUDY OF
DERMATOLOGICAL DISEASE

The skin is sometimes thought of as being an inert protective covering which does little more than line the outside of the body. There could be nothing further from the truth. Skin is a living dynamic organ with interesting connections with the interior of the body. Anyone with skin disease knows how quickly it can react to adverse situations. Lesions may appear over the course of a few hours (and disappear with equal rapidity). These are not the actions of an inert object.

The energetic view of the skin is that it is connected to the Lung - see Chapter 8 - Respiratory System. The Lung dominates Water passages and so is responsible for moisture reaching the surface of the body. Its energy is dispersing and descending and so passes out to the extremities of the body. The Blood is necessary for moistening, cooling and nourishing so imbalances in the Blood may lead to dryness, scaling and itching. Internal factors such as Heat, Dampness, Wind and so forth may manifest on the skin. The skin, therefore, may be an excellent indicator of internal imbalances.

In conventional medicine, it is frequently realised that skin disease may indicate internal disease. However, without a view of energetic connections it is impossible to see these symptoms as part of a coherent whole. In addition, treatment is frequently only applied to the surface of the body and then in the form of medicaments to suppress inflammation. This is invariably by means of corticosteroids. The inflammation may then pass deep into the body and cause a worsening of the internal imbalance. A good example of this is the use of corticosteroid medications for eczema. Removal of the skin rash by this suppressive action frequently results in the appearance of lung disease such as asthma or bronchitis.

The essence of alternative medicine is that it sees the underlying disharmony, balances this and therefore resolve the skin symptoms. As this happens the skin symptoms may get worse for a short time but the end results are often excellent. The conventional approach is to treat from the outside and although there may be short-term relief, the long-term result is invariably chronic problems - external or internal.

- DEFINITION OF TERMS -

It is helpful to review the somewhat specialist terminology applied to dermatology. The ideal thing to do is obtain an illustrated guide to skin disease[1] so that you get a clear idea of appearance.

Atrophy - thinning of the skin often accompanied by wrinkling
Bulla - large blister filled with clear fluid
Crusts - dried secretions
Cyst - a lump containing fluid which may be thin or thick
Ecchymosis - small bruise more than 3mm in diameter
Erosion - break in the continuity of a surface but shallow than an ulcer
Erythema - redness
Excoriation - marks caused by scratching or damage to the skin
Exfoliation - scaling or peeling of superficial skin layers
Lichenification - thickening of skin with increase in appearance of skin markings
Macule - small, flat, discoloured, round spot
Maculopapule - a combination of a papule and a macule
Nodule - palpable solid area which may or may not be raised more than 5-10mm diameter
Papule - small, raised, round spot less than 10mm in diameter
Petechiae - small bruises less than 3mm in diameter
Plaque - a group of confluent papules
Pruritus - itching
Purpura - bleeding into the skin
Pustule - small blister filled with yellowish fluid (pus)
Scale - dry flake of skin
Sclerosis - hardening of an area of skin
Ulcer - break in the continuity of surface tissue. This may be skin or mucous membrane.
Vesicle - small blister filled with clear fluid
Wheal - localised area of oedema surrounded by redness

TABLE 11.2: TERMINOLOGY OF SKIN DISEASE

- CLASSIFICATION OF SKIN DISEASE -

In conventional medicine, skin disease is classified according to its causation or listed in any order if this is unknown. In terms of conventional medicine, the key differentiation is between infective and non-infective skin rashes. The former will receive antibiotics or antifungal agents whilst the latter will, more often than not, receive corticosteroid preparations. Any skin condition of an infective type will become rapidly much worse if corticosteroids are given. Conversely, antibiotic and antifungal preparations have a propensity to cause allergic reactions in people with sensitive skin. The pharmaceutical industry has attempted to get round this problem by combining corticosteroids and antibiotics or antifungal agents in the same preparation. This is hardly subtle medicine but it does cover all the options. This practise can, in fact, be very dangerous since it may mask serious infection if the organism is not responsive to the drug given.

The lists in Table 11:3 are not in any particular order of severity. They will vary according to each individual. There is a summary of the skin diseases at the end of this Chapter where they are listed according to their appearance.

---

[1] Examples include, "A Colour Atlas of Physical Signs in General Medicine" by Zatouroff (Wolfe Medical Publications, 1976). "Dermatology - An Illustrated Guide" by Fry (Butterworths, 1984).

INFECTIVE	NON-INFECTIVE
Staphyloccal infections • Boils Streptococcal infections • Erysipelas • Impetigo Fungal infections • Tinea pedis • Tinea corporis • Tinea capitis • Pityriasis versicolor (Tinea versicolor) • Candidiasis Infestations • Scabies • Head lice	Eczema Psoriasis Acne vulgaris Acne rosacea Urticaria Alopecia Vitiligo Tumours of the skin • Warts • Basal cell carcinoma • Squamous cell carcinoma • Malignant melanoma • Kaposi's sarcoma

TABLE 11.3: CLASSIFICATION OF SKIN DISEASE

- ECZEMA -

This is an inflammation of the skin and is known as dermatitis. By convention, dermatitis is applied to those cases which are the result of coming into contact with specific irritants - contact dermatitis. The term eczema, is used for those cases which occur without contact and are more to do with internal factors.

There is a relationship between eczema and asthma in that they frequently co-exist in the same person and there may be a family history of both conditions. Other diseases in the family may include migraine and hay fever. Atopy is the term applied to a state of sensitivity to factors such as pollen, foods and so forth.

Symptoms:

There are many individual forms of eczema and so the following description is a general one. The main symptoms are dryness and itching. The skin may be red, thickened and in some cases may weep a clear fluid. In this latter situation, there may also be vesicles (small blisters) in affected areas. The itching may be so severe that the patient scratches until the skin bleeds. The areas most affected are the flexor surfaces of the elbow and knee but in severe cases the whole skin is involved. The skin may never look normal in between affected patches with thickening and dryness.

In children, it may start at any age with common triggers being vaccination and the introduction of cow's milk. It is important to enquire about events in the life of the child which may have precipitated the illness. It may start on the face, cheek and scalp but invariably there is involvement of the wrists, ankles, and antecubital and popliteal fossae. Some cases seem to settle down after some years and the rule of 7 years[2] (8 for boys) is a factor. That is, girls may recover at 7 or 14 years of age and 8 or 16 for boys. Almost 50% of cases go on to develop asthma and hay fever. If the eczema is severe then asthma is more likely to develop later.

---

[2] It is considered in Chinese medicine that males go through cycles of 8 years and females 7 years. This is further discussed in relation to the cycles of menstruation and fertility in Chapter 18 - Gynaecology.

It is important to take into account factors such as occupation. Hairdressing, engineering and any work which involves contact with irritant substances carry a risk of precipitating eczema. Items which may exacerbate or precipitate eczema include:

- wool[3]
- petroleum products[4], oils
- cleaning agents used to remove grease and oil from the skin
- metals such as nickel in watches and jewellery
- chemicals contained in deodorants, sprays, perfumes
- 'biological' washing powders, detergents, soaps
- rubber

If a skin problem is caused by contact there will be a typical area of distribution. It may be on the palms of the hands or in a site where jewellery or a watch has been worn. There will be a clear-cut area with scaling, itchiness and redness.

Dietary factors are important in some, notably dairy products and food additives. Many dietary ingredients may be implicated and individual cases will vary in their sensitivity to these. Eczema has a hereditary component and a child has a 60% chance of developing the disease if both parents are affected.

Treatment:

The conventional treatment of all skin diseases is variable in its effectiveness, to say the least. The mainstay of treatment is with corticosteroid applications. This suppresses the inflammation in the skin. Useful general advice includes bathing using a simple, non-perfumed soap. Emulsifying ointment is helpful to moisturise the skin but care should be exercised with those based upon lanolin (wool fat) or hydrocarbons (paraffin and the like). Allergic reactions are common with both these types and will cause symptoms indistinguishable from the original condition.

Tar based preparations are an old form of treatment which includes sulphur applications. Homoeopaths know that sulphur is one of the strongest suppressors of skin conditions and the tar applications utilise this effect.

Corticosteroids are central to the conventional management of eczema and many other skin conditions. They are mainly administered as local applications. Oral administration may be given in severe cases. Although the milder forms should be prescribed if at all possible and care should be taken in putting such products on the face. In clinical practice you will see departures from these rules. They have a suppressive effect and will not cure. Removal of the creams will lead to a flare-up of the rash which may be many times worse than the original. The degree of flare-up is dependent upon the condition of the patient, the strength of the corticosteroid application, the original condition and the duration of treatment.

There are 4 potency levels for corticosteroid applications as summarised in Table 11.4.

POTENCY	EXAMPLES
Mildly potent	Alcomethasone, fluocinolone 1:10 (0.0025%), hydrocortisone, methylprednisolone
Moderately potent	Clobetasone, desoxymethasone 0.05%, fluocinolone 1:4 (0.00625%), fluocortolone, flurandrenolone
Potent	Beclomethasone, betamethasone, budesonide, desoxymethasone 0.25%, diflucortolone, fluclorolone, fluocinolone 0.025%, fluocinonide, hydrocortisone 17-butyrate, triamcinolone
Very potent	Clobetasol, diflucortolone 0.3%, halcinonide

TABLE 11.4: STRENGTH OF CORTICOSTEROID APPLICATIONS

The use of corticosteroids leads to an increased risk of infection or sudden spreading of the

---

[3] Lanolin, wool fat, is a common component of creams and ointments may cause a contact dermatitis which is indistinguishable in its appearance from the original condition.
[4] Petroleum products may cause allergic reactions in the skin and it is helpful to enquire what applications the patient is using.

skin symptoms if infection is already present. For this reason, there are many applications which contain a mixture of a corticosteroid with an antibacterial or an antifungal agent. This may, in some instances, lead to their prescription when the precise diagnosis is unknown. There can be confusion between an eczema and some fungal rashes. The application of a mixture of drugs may be used to avoid adverse effects. The problem with such a practice is that it confuses the clinical picture, there is no precise diagnosis and the application of antibacterial and antifungal agents on to the skin is associated with a high risk of allergic reactions. This will result in symptoms which are identical to the original condition.

Alternative management:

In terms of Chinese medicine, this is due to a combination of Wind, Heat and Dampness depending upon the actual appearance of the rash. Underlying Blood Deficiency is common as is Lung Deficiency due to its function of dominating skin. Spleen Qi Deficiency is usually involved in cases with Damp Accumulation.

CASE ONE

A woman of 27 years came for treatment of her eczema. This was generalised, flaky and mainly on her face, arms and popliteal fossae. It was worse in the heat and she scratched it until it bled. This would relieve the itching. She had eczema as a child until the age of 7 years when it disappeared. It recurred 2 years ago and had been worse in the past 18 months. The eczema was always worse in the sun. She was using mild potency corticosteroid applications.

She often had a feeling of not being able to get enough air into the lungs. There was no wheezing or cough. She would be short of breath occasionally when this sensation was severe.

Her diagnosis in terms of Chinese medicine was Blood Deficiency and Kidney Yang Deficiency Not Grasping Lung Qi. The connection between the Lung and Kidney in energetic medicine is noted in Chapter 9 - Urinary System. After some months of treatment she felt more able to cope with her symptoms and less depressed. Her general energy was better. Her skin had improved to the point where there was only some problem in patches and mainly in the skin creases. Her circulation had improved. The skin problem was moving distally now and was mainly on the legs and arms. This is in line with Hering's Law of Cure.

Her skin would always be much better whenever she went away into the country or to the Alps for skiing. The eczema would return within 12 hours of her return to London. The things to think about in such a situation are diet, water, stress levels and air quality. As the Lung dominates skin, the purity of air and the function of the Lung are closely associated with skin symptoms.

After 6 months of treatment, her skin was generally good. She had occasional patches of dryness. She would have some flare-up with emotional stress but she was much more in touch with her feelings. Her insight was good and she was much more aware of her reactions.

CASE TWO

A woman of 56 years came for treatment of her eczema. She had developed a skin condition some 10 years earlier. The skin of her feet and hands were dry, scaly, itchy and weeping. The soles of her feet were particularly affected and were hot, red, sore, weeping and peeling. These areas were extremely itchy. Nothing ever made any difference to her skin condition. She had used hydrocortisone cream twice daily for 2-3 years. She had stopped this for one week before her visit to me.

In terms of Chinese medicine, this was diagnosed as DampHeat in the skin. I gave her 5 bags of herbs and she noticed an improvement within 2 days of taking them. At her second visit some 4 weeks later, she now had no symptoms. Her hands were normal and her feet were slightly discoloured only. There was no weeping, scaling or itching. She came into the clinic with a new pair of shoes - the first for many years! The speed of her response reveals that the pathology was already at the extremity of the physical body - the soles and palms. With alternative medicine this should be fairly easy to treat. This is not the case with psoriasis which is notoriously more stubborn or in those cases as Case 1 where the skin is generally affected.

CASE THREE

A boy of 10 months came for treatment of a skin rash. He had developed chickenpox when he was 2 weeks old (at the same time as his mother). At the age of 3 months he had a diptheria, whooping cough, tetanus and polio vaccination. He felt hot after this and then developed a dry, scaly area on his scalp. This goes by the name of 'cradle cap'. His scalp would occasionally weep also. He had a repeated vaccination at 5 months and at 7 months. After the last one he developed a fever and wheezing which was diagnosed as a 'chest infection'. He received antibiotics.

This episode was followed by skin problems. He developed a dry, itchy, flaking rash over his face, neck, scrotum, umbilical area and behind one knee. This had improved with a dairy-free diet but only slightly. He always had loose bowel motions and a phlegmy cough.

His diagnosis in terms of Chinese medicine was Spleen Qi Deficiency, Lung Qi Deficiency and DampHeat Accumulation. This is a typical story after vaccination and reveals the powerful force for disease of this procedure. His health was clearly already compromised as he had chickenpox at the age of 2 weeks. Since chickenpox is an attack of DampHeat, it shows why he now has such a condition and an associated Spleen Deficiency. I regard it as indefensible to vaccinate a child with such a compromised immune system particularly to repeat a second and third vaccination after a reaction.

His improvement after a dairy-free diet points to a Spleen involvement. Dairy products produce Damp (mucus) particularly in the presence of Spleen problems. Their removal will take the strain off the digestion. I gave him Chinese herbs and within 1 month his bowels had started to improve. He had an attack of cough and phlegm during that first month when his bowels had become noticeably worse. After 4 months of treatment, his bowels were normal, he was energetic and his skin was almost normal. He had some dry, reddish patches on his feet but this was the only abnormality.

It is clear from the above that it is important to take all aspects of the person into account. In conventional medicine it is just the skin which is treated. When you are treating a person with eczema there may be a sudden worsening of the skin problem. Such an event should make you think of emotional stress, dietary indiscretion, changes in climate or a reaction to a recent vaccination. These are the classical factors which lead to acute flare-ups.

It can be difficult managing people who also take conventional medication, i.e. local corticosteroid applications. Withdrawal must be slow or a flare-up is likely and you may lose the case. People find it difficult to return if their original symptoms are gradually worsening. This is especially true if areas such as the face are involved. Ask also about other applications since allergies are common to substances with lanolin (wool fat) or those based on petroleum. I find it preferable to advise people to use simple moisturisers in the form of oils or creams. Try to avoid applications with chemical additives.

With the correct treatment, eczema can be rewarding for the person involved and the practitioner. Improvement of a skin condition can lead to great changes in people's lives as they have more confidence. Treatment can be prolonged in the cases of internal imbalances and in such cases it is more important to address factors such as diet, stress levels, work environment and so forth.

A note is applicable here about the use of Chinese herbs for skin disease. There is some discussion about them being toxic to the liver and kidneys. This is true to the extent that all medicinal substances in a material dose have a toxic potential, some more so than others. The problems which people have developed have been the result of taking *large* doses of Chinese herbs.

In China, where people are generally of a stronger constitution, large doses are regularly given. If these are then used in the West, people may develop problems. Treatment must be adapted to correspond to the constitution of the person. It is not satisfactory to assume that what is correct for one person is automatically correct for another. The *principles* of Chinese medicine have stood the test of time. It is their *application* which must be attended to.

I have treated people who have taken strong herbal formulae for an extended period and they have been severely weakened by this. Herbs which get rid of things from the body, i.e. detoxify, are those which tend to be the strongest. However, it is not just toxins which are removed. Qi and Blood will also be removed by this process. If the person is depleted in Qi and Blood there is the potential for harm. Sadly, some practitioners do not seem to realise this and so we see cases of liver and kidney disease. The difference here between conventional and Chinese medicine is that with the former, side-effects are an accepted and unavoidable part of treatment. With the latter, side-effects are the result of the misapplication of the treatment.

- PSORIASIS -

This is one of a group of skin diseases which are characterised by scaling. It is of unknown cause in conventional medicine. It is uncommon before the age of 15 years and it as common in men as women. It is chiefly a cosmetic nuisance because of its appearance and degree of scaling. The standard treatments of tar or dithranol add to this as they are messy and time-consuming. The skin becomes overactive and so it thickens, more scales become apparent and there is redness and heat of the affected area. Around 1 in 10 people with psoriasis have symptoms of joint disease.

Symptoms:

Areas of skin become thickened, red and scaly. This usually occurs over the extensor surfaces of the elbow and knee. The patches vary in size from small, almost pin-head size to large areas of the body. I was taught at medical school that psoriasis is never itchy and that itchy skin rashes are almost certainly eczema. This is not true and people with psoriasis may itch. The scales on the surface of the rash are white or silvery. There may be severe scaling in some people and this can cause embarrassing cosmetic problems . The nails may be pitted, thickened and discoloured. In some cases they separate from the underlying nail bed. The scalp is also a relatively common site to be affected.

The appearance of the skin lesions can take different forms in different people. Some have tiny, pinpoint areas (guttate psoriasis), others have thickened, reddish areas overlain with silvery scales (plaque psoriasis) whilst others develop pustules containing sterile yellowish material (pustular psoriasis).

It is a characteristic of all skin disease that damage to an area of skin may result in the appearance of skin symptoms at that site. This is known as the Koebner phenomenon. Scratching or rubbing may lead to the typical scaly rash appearing in that area.

Some people may be severely affected with generalised disease. In this case, there may be difficulties due to loss of heat from the body. Very severe cases may require hospital treatment. The disease is worsened or precipitated by emotional stress[5], associated tonsillitis, treatment with lithium carbonate[6] and betablockers.

Treatment:

TREATMENT	TREATMENT LEVEL	COMMENTS
Ultraviolet light	1	Psoriasis commonly improves in strong sunlight
Coal tar	1	An old treatment which relies upon the sulphur contained in tar. Stains the skin. Messy application. May cause a rash due its irritant effects
Dithranol	1	A synthetic alternative to tar with the same problems
Low dose tetracycline (antibiotic) orally	2	Long-term in some cases of pustular psoriasis
Corticosteroid applications	3	Conventionally this is not useful and may create problems In the long-term. In common usage, nevertheless
Corticosteroid orally	4	See above
Etretinate	5	Causes foetal damage and so not for pregnant women. Effective contraception must be used. Toxic to the liver.
Immunosuppressants, e.g. methotrexate[7], azathioprine	6	Only used in severe or life-threatening disease. The main problem is damage to the bone marrow and thence blood cell production

TABLE 11.5: CONVENTIONAL TREATMENTS OF PSORIASIS

---

[5] A study found that the use of stress reduction techniques such as meditation and imaging led to a marked improvement in cases of psoriasis. Acta Derm.Venereol-Suppl-Stockh. 1991; 156: 37-43.
[6] Lithium compounds are used in the treatment of manic depression.
[7] This may cause liver fibrosis and patients require a liver biopsy before treatment commences and then yearly.

Alternative management:

In terms of Chinese medicine, this is due to Wind and Damp complicating cases of Blood Deficiency. Other syndromes to consider are Heat in the Intestines and Stomach which explains the usual distribution over the Yangming channels.

CASE

A woman of 32 years came for treatment of a scaly skin rash on the skin over her shins from the knees to the ankles. This had developed some 7 years previously. This was itchy especially in the heat and it felt generally hot. Her scalp was affected when the rash was severe. She suffered from constipation and only had a bowel movement once per week. This had been the case from the age of 5 years. She had strong symptoms of pre-menstrual tension particularly with irritability. In terms of Chinese medicine, a diagnosis was made of Heat in the Intestines with Liver Blood Deficiency and Liver Qi Stagnation.

I treated her with Chinese herbs as well as giving her advice about relaxation, avoiding heating foods such as spices, alcohol and coffee. It took 2 months of treatment before there was a slight change in her skin and 6 months before a significant change. After 1 year of treatment her skin was almost normal, her bowels were fine and she felt more relaxed generally as well as having fewer problems before a period.

This is typical of psoriasis in that it is slow to respond and it is important for people to persevere. Stress is a common trigger and so relaxation is very important.

- ACNE VULGARIS -

This is common acne and experienced by most adolescents of both sexes although males are more severely affected. The cause of the problem is not understood in conventional medicine. There are various theories about sebaceous gland secretions (sebum) despite the fact that sebum is unchanged even when the symptoms clear in their early twenties.

Symptoms:

The conventional idea is that sebum blocks the sweat glands and leads to blackheads and then inflammation. Pustules develop which may leave scars. The face is the usual site but in severe cases the chest and upper back are affected. Some people develop large spots which may be uncomfortable. The main issue, particularly at this age, is a cosmetic one and almost everyone has some spots at some time during puberty. For some people it becomes more than this with large areas of skin affected by multiple pustules. There may be areas of redness which affect similar sites.

Treatment:

TREATMENT	TREATMENT LEVEL	COMMENTS
Antiseptic washes, e.g. hexachlorophene Abrasive agents	1	These are fairly innocuous and at the level of simple hygiene. There are many available and of variable effectiveness
Ultraviolet light	1	Many skin diseases improve on exposure to sunlight
Antibiotics, topical	2	This now at entering the levels of medicinal effects. Topical drugs are suppressive but less so than those below
Antibiotics, oral	3	Long-term use has the effect of reducing inflammation.
Retinoic acid	4	Vitamin A derivative. It causes liver damage, foetal abnormalities and bone changes
Cyproterone	5	Anti-androgen. It is occasionally given for acne vulgaris.
Oral contraception (females only)	5	Female sex hormones are in Chapter 18 -Gynaecology

TABLE 11.6: TREATMENT OF ACNE VULGARIS

Alternative management:

In terms of Chinese medicine, this is due to the Accumulation of Heat in the Lung, Spleen and Stomach. There is almost always an element of Qi Stagnation which may manifest as Liver symptoms of irritability, headaches and the like.

CASE

A woman of 33 years came for treatment. She had indigestion, diarrhoea each day and abdominal bloating. She was generally tired and felt irritable and depressed. She had a constant runny nose. She frequently had headaches across her forehead. She had been diagnosed as having polycystic ovaries some 2 years previously.

Her skin was badly affected by large pustular swellings on the face. These would appear at any time but particularly before a period. These had begun when she was 13 years old. Her current medication was:

- Cyproterone 50mg daily for 10 days after end of her period
- Cyproterone 2mg with oestrogen for the 3 weeks commencing on the first day of her period

Cyproterone is a drug which blocks androgen - the male hormones. It is used in high doses of 50mg daily mainly for male sexual offenders. I had never seen it used before.

In terms of Chinese medicine, the diagnosis was Spleen Qi Deficiency with Liver Qi Stagnation. This was clearly a severe case because of the powerful drugs used and the presence of other indications of Stagnation such as the ovarian cysts. The aim of treatment in this case is to strengthen the Spleen whilst relieving the Qi Stagnation. After some time of treatment then it would be possible to reduce the drugs. She was very nervous about reducing them because of the severity of the facial eruptions. They would be like boils on the face before her period, large and quite painful.

After some months of treatment, her bowel function was much improved and her remaining skin eruptions subsided. It is important to reduce the cyproterone slowly although the second formulation with the addition of oestrogen must be stopped suddenly to prevent any possibility of breakthrough bleeding (see Chapter 18 - Gynaecology for a discussion on withdrawal of female sex hormones).

She reduced the 50mg dose down to 25mg and a large red skin eruption appeared under the skin at the side of her nose. This settled with treatment. She then saw her consultant who stopped all her drugs suddenly because she had been having headaches with visual disturbances. The drugs are very strong and he was worried that they were giving her side-effects. This takes any question of drug withdrawal out of her hands. On the one hand this was a sudden withdrawal and will probably lead to severe consequences. Conversely, at least it was possible to treat without the interference of the drugs.

Her skin flared-up quite badly with large pustules on her face and chin, irritability, severe pre-menstrual symptoms and depression. She was treated for several weeks before these started to settle. After some months she felt well, her skin would occasionally flare-up before a period but much less than before and her digestion was much stronger. Some 2 years later she is well and happy.

The difficulty with such a case is the degree of heavy drug suppression. It takes time to sort out what is going on and each time the drug is reduced there will be a release of symptoms. This needs to be resolved before moving on. The root of the case can be difficult to see and this will vary according to each person. It is essential to take each level in turn as it presents itself. In this way, progress will be slow but sure and the person will, in the end, be much healthier.

- ACNE ROSACEA -

This is quite a different disease to the above despite their common use of the term acne. It is a chronic rash seen on the face. It affects women more than men.

Symptoms:

There is a redness of the cheeks, nose and sometimes chin in a 'butterfly' distribution. There are broad patches over the cheeks like the wings of a butterfly with a narrow connecting strip across the nose. There are papules and pimples which can be severe at times. There may be swelling of the affected skin. Redness of the eyelids and eyes are seen about a half of patients. These appearances may take the form of blepharitis, conjunctivitis, keratitis, episcleritis or iritis.

There may be general flushing of the face in response to stressful situations, hot climate, hot drinks, spicy food and alcohol. There may be associated upper gastrointestinal symptoms such as indigestion.

Treatment:

General advice will be given to avoid factors which cause flushing.

TREATMENT	TREATMENT LEVEL	COMMENTS
Tetracycline	1	Long-term prescription - compare acne vulgaris
Metronidazole	2	Long-term prescription of a more hazardous antibiotic
Corticosteroid - topical	3	It is unusual to see oral corticosteroids
Retinoic acid derivative	4	Very powerful. It causes liver damage, foetal abnormalities and bone changes

TABLE 11.7: TREATMENT OF ACNE ROSACEA

Alternative management:

In terms of Chinese medicine, this is considered to be due to Stagnant Blood Accumulation due to injury of the Lungs by Stomach Fire.

- URTICARIA -

This is a rash which is similar in appearance to that seen due to contact with the stinging nettle (Urtica urens). In conventional medicine the cause is generally unknown. The common things to think about are allergic reactions to drugs and chemicals. Skin and laboratory tests are unreliable

Symptoms:

In the acute phase, there is the appearance of wheals which are localised swellings of the skin surrounded by redness. They are itchy. Around the lips and eyes there may be oedema. The attack may last for minutes or hours and the skin then returns to normal. There are many possible causes of such a reaction. It is essentially allergic in nature although many cases are of unknown cause.

Dermatographia is a variant of urticaria where scratching the skin produces the typical wheal reaction. It is possible to gently scratch a name or symbol on the skin and soon there will be oedematous swellings following that shape. Other triggers of such appearances include cold weather, water and sunlight.

Internal causes of this condition are varied and include prescribed drugs especially aspirin and non-steroidal anti-inflammatory agents, opiates, antibiotics, injections of radiological examination dyes, foods, parasitic infestation, blood transfusion and so forth. The list is actually endless as any substance may produce an allergic reaction in the susceptible individual. The above are merely the commoner ones or those recognised.

If the attacks continue for more than 6 weeks or if the symptoms are continuous for this length of time, the term chronic urticaria is used. It is less likely in such cases that a trigger will be found.

Attacks in these cases may last for up to a day but some people are more or less constantly affected. It is more likely that oedema of the eyes or lips will be a feature.

Treatment:

Any known cause is removed but in many people the urticaria arises for ill-definable reasons.

TREATMENT	TREATMENT LEVEL	COMMENTS
Antihistamine - oral	1	Drowsiness is the common symptom and so is usually given at night. Tranquillisers may also be used.
Cimetidine/ranitidine	2	These drugs are more commonly seen in the treatment of peptic ulcers. They interfere with the production of histamine which is also involved in gastric acid secretion
Corticosteroid - oral	3	May be used in chronic cases
Adrenaline - subcutaneous	4	In severe cases where there is anaphylaxis[8]

TABLE 11.8: TREATMENT OF URTICARIA

Alternative management:

In terms of Chinese medicine, this is due to several causes. There may be Damp in the superficial tissues complicated by WindHeat or WindCold. DampHeat Accumulation in the Stomach and Intestines or disturbance of the Chong and Ren due to irregular life-style may also lead to these symptoms.

- ALOPECIA -

This is loss of hair and may be of any degree from partial to total. It may be localised or generalised. In severe cases, there is loss of all body hair including eyebrows and eyelashes. It may be part of a skin disease such as tinea capitis or systemic lupus erythematosus. Radiation to the scalp causes permanent loss of hair to the specific area affected. Alopecia areata is a specific type of hair loss which is described below.

Symptoms:

This may be localised or complete and usually affects just the scalp. There may be acute loss of hair. Patches of baldness typically have distinct margins. It is common and occurs as often in men as women. It is related to stressful situations and events. The risk of recurrence is increased in accordance to the degree of hair loss. Thus, the more hair which is lost then the more likely is any recurrence.

Treatment:

There is no effective treatment in conventional medicine for alopecia areata although many things may be used. Systemic corticosteroids may be given but they have a high incidence of side-effects. Local applications of corticosteroids in high-potency are often given. Triamcinolone, a type of corticosteroid, may be injected into the scalp but it has to be repeated every 4-6 weeks. It may cause blindness and lead to long-term effects systemically due to its absorption. Minoxidil is an anti-hypertensive drug which has side-effects that include overgrowth of hair. It is sometimes used for cases of alopecia as a local application. Irritant substances may be applied to the scalp in an attempt to make hair grow but the usual outcome is persistence of baldness with the addition of itching, soreness and weeping.

The management of alopecia due to skin disease will be to treat the underlying disease.

---

[8] Anaphylaxis is a severe allergic reaction characterised by wheezing, breathlessness, cyanosis, low blood pressure, nausea, vomiting and diarrhoea. It is a life-threatening situation.

Alternative management:

In terms of Chinese medicine, the function of the Kidney and Blood is related to head hair. This is why alopecia comes on after a shock as the Kidney is particularly susceptible to fear and fright. Treatment is easier the sooner you see people after the commencement of symptoms. If the alopecia is long-term then treatment will necessarily be more difficult and prolonged.

CASE

A girl of 15 years came for treatment of her hair. She had suffered with alopecia areata for the past 7 months. This was one month after starting new school. She was generally anxious about lots of things including exams and school. She had fears of dogs and the dark. Her sleep had never been good and she often had a lot of unpleasant dreams. She would wake at intervals through the night. She had palpitations frequently. The cause was a previous accident and problems at school.

In terms of Chinese medicine, the diagnosis was Kidney Yang Deficiency, Liver Blood Deficiency and Spleen Qi Deficiency. I gave her Chinese herbs to strengthen her Qi and Blood. The first thing her mother noticed was that she was much happier. Her hair became stronger and less fell out. She was energetic and after some 3 months her hair was fine.

She had a bout of alopecia some years before and this had recovered. At this recent stressful time she had suffered a recurrence. It would probably get better on its own again but the point of treatment is to make sure that it happens quicker, that she is stronger than before and to reduce any likelihood of a later relapse. It is true that most of us have the ability to recover by ourselves but treatment can aid this process and provide us with more strength than originally.

- VITILIGO -

This is depigmentation of the skin. It is a common occurrence and indicates an autoimmune process. It is seen in about 1% of the population and is mainly a cosmetic nuisance. There is depigmentation of the skin of the face, neck and knuckle areas. The significance of this condition is that is it associated with underlying diabetes mellitus, pernicious anaemia, Addison's disease, myxoedema and hyperthyroidism.

Some one third of cases may repigment spontaneously. In most people the affected areas extend gradually. Treatment may be given in the form of local corticosteroid applications but with little response.

Alternative management:

In terms of Chinese medicine, this corresponds to an invasion of Wind and Dampness. It is known as "white Wind". There must be an internal disharmony to allow for this invasion, particularly in the case of a systemic autoimmune disease.

- SKIN INFESTATIONS AND INFECTIONS -

STAPHYLOCOCCAL INFECTIONS

A staphylococcus is a bacterium which is associated with localised inflammation and the formation of pus. This usually takes the form of boils or abscesses but in people with weak energy it may descend into deeper levels and cause pneumonia, septicaemia and so forth.

BOILS

Bacterial conditions of this type, particularly if recurrent, may be associated with underlying disease. This may merely be a vague sensation of tiredness and being 'run down'. The underlying medical condition to consider is diabetes mellitus especially in recurrent boils, multiple boils and carbuncles[9].

---

[9] A carbuncle is a collection or group of boils.

Symptoms:

The hair follicle becomes infected with staphylococcal organisms and there is the appearance of localised inflammation with pus formation. This is the characteristic 'spot'. Its technical name is furuncle. It only occurs on skin where hair is found. They are commonest on the neck, axilla, buttocks and thighs. If they become multiple in number they may form a carbuncle.

Investigations:

Swabs may be taken of sites such as the nose, axillae and perineum. Hospital workers are routinely checked to detect the presence of such bacteria.

Treatment:

Oral antibiotics are invariably given to people with boils. These are of little use unless it is at an early stage, there is surrounding redness and there are constitutional symptoms such as malaise and perhaps fever. The use of antibiotics may lead to a reduction in size of the boil but the end result will be that the pus becomes surrounded by a thick wall and increases the likelihood of a recurrence. The body is now prevented from discharging the pus onto a surface which is the natural way of ridding the body of the problem. If the boil has formed pus then the correct conventional treatment is drainage. The boil is lanced and the purulent material allowed to discharge. The routine use of antibiotics in this inappropriate manner can only result in erosion of people's health and the occurrence of "sterile" boils.

If boils are recurrent, emphasis is placed on the use of antiseptic washes and bathing. In my experience there are of variable effectiveness as the boil is a manifestation of an inner imbalance. Concentrating on the skin is treating the wrong place, disturbing the natural bacterial balance of the skin and increases the likelihood of recurrence.

Alternative management:

In terms of Chinese medicine, this is described as being due to invasion of Summer Heat. This is unusual in the climate of the UK. The more likely diagnosis is excessive intake of heating and greasy food leading to Heat in the internal organs. This causes the accumulation of Poison or DampHeat which manifests on the skin.

It is worth making a point here about treating people with conditions which are associated with organisms. Of course, we only develop these if we are susceptible. It would still be advisable to ensure that contact is controlled as far as possible. The people who are most likely to be susceptible are babies, pregnant women and those who take drugs which deplete the immune system. Sensible precautions to reduce contact are welcome but avoid alienating people since most disorders are difficult to "catch". If items such as towels or couch covers are in contact with infected areas then these must be adequately cleaned before allowing contact with another person. This is particularly true of the more infectious diseases of herpes infections, erysipelas and impetigo. Anything which perforates the skin must be sterilised.

STREPTOCOCCAL INFECTIONS

The streptococcus is associated with inflammation which is spreading in nature. It is connected to a wide variety of disorders which include acute tonsillitis, scarlet fever, erysipelas, puerperal fever and wound infections (traumatic or operative). The spreading nature is evident if wounds are infected by the spread into the surrounding tissues. In the case of tonsillitis there may be spread into the general circulation to produce rash (scarlet fever), heart symptoms (rheumatic fever) or kidneys (acute proliferative glomerulonephritis, nephritic syndrome, Bright's disease).

ERYSIPELAS

This is streptococcal infection of the skin. It can occur at any age but is most severe in the very young and the very old. It often affects the face since the bacteria can live in the nostrils. Legs may be affected in areas of varicose ulceration or in infants around the umbilical cord where it will spread onto the trunk. Circumcision wounds may also be affected.

Symptoms:

These develop quickly with shivering and fever. There is painful swelling of the superficial tissues in the affected area with redness and soreness. The condition spreads rapidly outwards from the first area affected. Blisters may develop in the centre of the area because of the degree of inflammatory oedema. There are systemic symptoms of toxaemia such as fever, restlessness, insomnia and possibly delirium. The relevant groups of lymph nodes will be enlarged. Oedema may be present in recurrent cases.

Treatment:

Penicillin is always given to eradicate the streptococci and reduce the inflammation.

Alternative management:

In terms of Chinese medicine, this is due to an invasion of Wind and Fire.

IMPETIGO

This is a superficial skin infection which is streptococcal in some cases. Staphylococci may be involved in others.

Symptoms:

The typical appearance is of superficial vesicles which rupture to leave a yellowish crusting area. It mainly affects the face, especially around the chin and angle of the mouth, and is commonest in children. It may spread in some cases but is usually fairly localised.

Treatment:

It can be spread by close contact and via towels, flannels and so forth. The main treatment is by means of antiseptic washes. Oral antibiotics are only required if there is widespread disease.

Alternative management:

In terms of Chinese medicine, this is due to Heat in the Lung channel and Damp in the Stomach channel which explains it typical distribution. The Stomach channel crosses the cheek close to the angle of the jaw.

- FUNGAL INFECTIONS -

RINGWORM

This, despite its name, is a fungal infection. It is given different terms depending upon the site affected. The infection is spread from animals, humans or the environment.

TINEA PEDIS

This is when the feet are affected. There is inflammation which can be severe and secondary infection may develop. It is spread in swimming baths, saunas and showers. This association has led it to be termed 'athletes foot'. Several members of the same family may be affected.

Symptoms:

The main areas affected are in between the toes and the soles of the feet. There is redness, scaling, weeping and occasionally blistering. It may spread to the hands, groins (tinea cruris) and perianal area.

Treatment:

The older type of treatments include local application of potassium permanganate solution which is dark purple in colour and correspondingly unpopular. Antifungal agents are commonly used. Griseofulvin is given orally for about 3 months. Local applications are with the imidazoles, clotrimazole or miconazole.

Alternative management:

In terms of Chinese medicine, this is due to DampHeat in the Stomach and Spleen draining downwards into the feet and manifesting on the skin.

TINEA CORPORIS

This is increasingly common as a result of the wide use of topical corticosteroids. It is ringworm affecting the body.

Symptoms:

Patches of redness and scaling are seen on the body. There may also be papules and pustules in some cases. The areas are itchy. These are the symptoms of eczema. The main points of differentiation are that people with eczema may have generalised skin symptoms such as dryness and itching and the typical distribution whereas with ringworm it tends to be more fixed in one site. Eczema tends to worsen and improve in a cyclical nature.

Treatment:

In general, this is treated as tinea pedis above. If the nails are affected then systemic treatment with griseofulvin is given for at least 9 months for finger nails and 2 years for toe nails. Itraconazole may also be used. This condition is notoriously resistant to treatment. In some cases the nails will be removed.

Alternative management:

In terms of Chinese medicine, this is due to invasion of DampHeat into the skin.

TINEA CAPITIS

This is rare now.

Symptoms:

There are patches of scalp affected by scaling and hair loss. It is much more likely to occur in children. In some there is associated inflammation with weeping and crusting. This more severe type may result in permanent hair loss.

Treatment:

The disease spreads from animals and so the source of infection is treated. This is by means of systemic anti-fungal treatments. Griseofulvin is an older drug which has been largely replaced by itraconazole. Treatment is given for up to 3 months.

Alternative management:

This is due to invasion of Wind and may develop as either a white or a yellow appearance.

PITYRIASIS VERSICOLOR (TINEA VERSICOLOR)

This is caused by a yeast and is common in tropical climates. It has become commoner in more temperate climates in recent years. There is scaling and confluent macules on the trunk, upper arms and neck. They may be hyper- or hypopigmented, usually the latter.

Treatment:

This is by means of the local application of the antifungal agents miconazole, clotrimazole or econazole. In severe cases there may be oral ketoconazole given.

Alternative management:

In terms of Chinese medicine, this is described as "white skin Wind". It is due to invasion of Wind into the skin.

CANDIDIASIS

This is a yeast type of fungus which may cause symptoms in many areas of the body. In this situation it leads to skin symptoms. The fungus, Candida albicans, is present in many people with no symptoms. Symptoms occur when the immune system is depleted and these include diabetes mellitus, pregnancy and drugs such as female sex hormones, antibiotics, corticosteroids, cancer chemotherapy. I discuss candidiasis in relation to gynaecological symptoms in Chapter 18 - Gynaecology and bowel symptoms in Chapter 13 -Gastrointestinal System.

Symptoms:

Moist areas of the body are more commonly affected, e.g. skin folds, groin, axilla, napkin area in babies. There is the appearance of a skin rash which bears some similarities to eczema. There is redness, soreness, some scaling although this is slight if there is any wetness and itching.
        The nails may be affected (paronychia) and is commoner in situations where the hands are frequently wet. There is redness and soreness of the cuticle and eventually deformity of the nail.

Treatment:

It is important to keep the affected area clean and dry. Specific treatment is given by means of antifungal agents. They may be given locally, e.g. nystatin or an imidazole such as miconazole or clotrimazole. Oral drugs may be given, e.g. trizoles such as fluconazole, itraconazole. Some cases may be given a combination corticosteroid and antifungal to reduce inflammation as well as kill the fungus. Ketoconazole is used for cases which are extremely severe and life-threatening since it causes potentially serious liver damage.

Alternative management of fungal infections:

This is essentially as that described under eczema. The appearance is the same and the fungus only attacks the skin because of an underlying susceptibility. To treat the skin with antifungal agents is to run the risk of suppressing the imbalance deeper into the body. Constitutional treatment is necessary and this may have to be prolonged to change nail disease.

SCABIES

This is a disease which is classed as an infestation since it is caused by a tiny parasite which burrows under the skin. It is possible to have the disease and be infectious but to experience no symptoms for the first 4 weeks or so. It is contracted, in susceptible people, by close contact. It is an occupational hazard of teachers, nurses and casualty officers. Usually the contact has to be very close and so sexual partners and family are affected.

Symptoms:

The common sites affected are in between the fingers, wrists, elbows, ankles, genitals and breasts. Linear burrows are seen under the skin surface with a blister at one end. This will contain the parasite which can be removed by a needle. Eggs and faeces may be present along the burrow. There is intense itching and so the consequent scratching may destroy the burrow and blister before examination. It is important to have a high index of suspicion if symptoms are restricted to the wrists and webs of fingers.

Treatment:

The aim of treatment is to kill the parasites. This is done with the application of gamma-benzene hexachloride (lindane) or malathion. It is applied to all areas apart from the face after a bath and left on for 24 hours. Then it is washed off. Clean clothes are put on at each time. It may irritate the skin. Lindane and malathion, in common with all pesticides, can damage the nervous system.

Alternative management:

In terms of Chinese medicine, this is considered to be due to an invasion of parasites complicated by Wind, Heat and Damp. It is appropriate to treat by a combination of internal and external remedies.

HEAD LICE

Lice may be present on the head, body or pubic area. Head lice are the ones common in the UK.

Symptoms:

There is itching of the scalp and neck area. There may be evidence of excoriation and impetigo may be superimposed on the damaged skin. Eggs ('nits') will be seen sticking to the hairs. Spread is by close contact and so schoolchildren and family members are frequently affected.

Treatment:

This is by means of gamma-benzene hexachloride (lindane) or malathion which kill the parasites and its eggs. Malathion is the one usually used now as the parasite is usually resistant to lindane. All the family will be treated. Treatment is made easier by cutting the hair.

- TUMOURS OF THE SKIN -

WARTS

These are tumours which are associated with a virus. They may be spread to susceptible people by contact. This usually occurs from public bathing places such as swimming baths. Once they have appeared, they may disappear spontaneously within 6 months. Up to 30% of cases may do this.

Symptoms:

Warts are papular growths on the surface of the skin and may appear in a short period of time. They may be seen in any area but the hands, knees and feet are the commonest sites. In some cases the warts may be flatter and more elongated. These are known as plane warts. On the feet they are termed verrucas and on the soles turn inward due to pressure. They are evident there as flattened, hard areas with a darkish centre. They may give rise to discomfort when walking.

As mentioned in relation to psoriasis, damage to the skin in any skin disease may lead to the appearance of symptoms at that site. This also occurs with warts where damage done to warts by scratching, rubbing or conventional treatments often leads to the appearance of more warts in the surrounding area.

Treatment:

Warts may disappear spontaneously and so it is often preferable to leave well alone. People may request treatment due to cosmetic considerations or because skin problems are often poorly tolerated in our society. Conventional treatments are aimed at burning the wart with chemicals, carbon dioxide snow or liquid nitrogen. The warts may be surgically removed in some instances.

When warts disappear naturally they leave no scars. The treatments above damage the skin and may leave scars which, in some cases particularly on the feet, may be painful.

Alternative management:

In terms of Chinese medicine, the exact cause depends upon the appearance of the warts. They are usually considered to be due to Liver and Blood Deficiency. Flat warts are related to Liver Fire and Invasion of Wind and Heat.

A time-honoured way of removing warts is to have them 'charmed'. This may be by means of rubbing them with potato peel, broad bean pod or one of several items of food and bury this in the garden. As the object rots then the wart disappears. One method I advised was to draw a circle the same size as the wart. This was to be repeated each day but drawing a slightly smaller circle. After several weeks when the circle had reduced in size to a dot this was to be rubbed out. The warts should then disappear. I was waiting with bated breath to see if it worked but I never saw the person again! Either the warts had completely disappeared or the person thought it was too strange to return to visit. I would place wart charming in the same category as visualisation. As I discussed in Chapter 6 - Cancer, this can be a powerful force for health and has proven beneficial effects on the immune system.

GENITAL WARTS

These are often associated with sexually transmitted disease. They may be penile, vulval or anal in site.

Symptoms:

Genital warts are more fleshy in their appearance than the simple warts above. They appear quite moist. In women it is the vulva which is usually affected. In men the warts are found around the glans penis. Both sexes may be affected by anal warts.

There is an association with a whole range of disorders including sexually transmitted disease, cervical dysplasia, pelvic inflammatory disease and so on.

Treatment:

They are treated by the application of mildly burning chemicals or by surgery.

MALIGNANT TUMOURS OF THE SKIN

Tumours of the skin are common as it is in constant contact with ultraviolet light, chemicals and external influences and is continually actively regenerating. I shall discuss here four malignant tumours of skin which are the most important clinically.

BASAL CELL CARCINOMA

This also known as 'rodent ulcer' and is found mainly on the head and neck. Its frequency is increased with more exposure to sunlight, particularly in a hot climate, and in fair skinned races. Other causes include medical irradiation and arsenic medication[10].

Symptoms:

There is the development of a papule which grows slowly. Its centre starts to degenerate and an ulcer is eventually formed. A common first complaint is of a 'sore' which will not heal. As they grow commonly on the face it may be cut whilst shaving and this may be the first sign. The cancer tends to invade locally, hence its name 'rodent ulcer'. Secondary spread is extremely rare.

Treatment:

This is by means of radiotherapy or local excision.

SQUAMOUS CELL CARCINOMA

This is a more invasive type of malignancy which can spread to distant sites. It is more frequent in skin which has been damaged in the past to the point of scarring, perhaps by chemicals. Sunlight increases the likelihood of such a cancer.

Symptoms:

The tumour appears as a hardened lump usually on the ear or lip. There is thickening of surrounding tissue. It may ulcerate.

Treatment:

This is by local excision. Radiotherapy may also be applied.

MALIGNANT MELANOMA

This is much more frequent with the increase in sunbathing and the desire for suntans. It is more common in fair-skinned races. Melanoma is a mole which is a benign, pigmented lesion found in many people. It becomes a problem only if it undergoes malignant change

Symptoms:

If a mole changes in size, shape or colour then malignancy must be suspected. There may be symptoms of itching or bleeding.

Treatment:

The outcome, conventionally, depends upon the size of the tumour at the time of diagnosis and the site on the body. If it is less than 1mm thick, histologically, then the 5-years survival rate is more than 90% and less than 50% if more than 3_ mm thick. The prognosis is better on the trunk than the face and the limbs than the trunk.

---

[10] Arsenic was formerly used to treat syphilis and parasitic infestations.

Local excision is the treatment of choice with a wide area of skin taken from around the melanoma. Secondaries are treated with a combination of radiotherapy and chemotherapy which, even conventionally, makes no difference to the outcome.

KAPOSI'S SARCOMA

This is more common now as it is one of the malignancies seen in people with AIDS.

Symptoms:

The original symptom is of a discoloured area which resembles a bruise. This becomes darker and develops into a lump. They may be multiple in site. They may also occur in the gastrointestinal tract, liver and lymph glands.

Treatment:

In people with AIDS they are frequently rapidly progressive which reflects their weakened energetic state. Classically, treatment is by means of radiotherapy and chemotherapy but this can only be considered to be symptomatic in such cases. The treatment, of course, will make people weaker and more ill.

Alternative management:

The discussion in Chapter 6 - Cancer with regard to malignant disease is relevant here. Most people will probably opt for conventional treatment. People with secondaries from malignant melanoma may present for alternative medical treatment but usually at a severe stage. In terms of energetic medicine, these cancers should be the easiest to produce improvement as they are on the most superficial physical organ. Certainly in discussion with practitioners who treat cancer by alternative methods it seems this is true. This is, of course, at variance with the conventional prognosis, particularly of malignant melanoma.

- HOW TO RECOGNISE SERIOUS CONDITIONS OF THE SKIN -

Skin diseases are common in our society and the symptoms listed below are extremely common. It is important to know how to recognise if a symptom arises from a serious situation. You can use Table 11.9 below as a guide to refer to when faced with a patient who has one or more of these symptoms. I make no mention of disease labels in the column on the right as I would not expect you to be able to diagnose conventionally. Seriousness can be assessed merely by reference to symptom pictures.

SYMPTOMS	WHEN TO WORRY
Vesicles	Haemorrhagic
Bullae	Large
Redness, weeping	Severe Large areas of skin surface
Lumps, nodules	Short history Recent change Progressive Bleeding

TABLE 11.9: HOW TO RECOGNISE SERIOUS CONDITIONS IN DERMATOLOGY

- SUMMARY -

At this point, it is helpful to summarise the diseases in this Chapter. Table 11.10 is a list of skin diseases ordered according to their appearance. This will be more helpful if you obtain an illustrated guide to skin disease as mentioned in the Introduction to this Chapter.

SYMPTOM	DISEASE LABEL
Crusting	Impetigo
Dryness	Eczema
Exfoliation	Psoriasis
Itching	Eczema, psoriasis, urticaria, tinea, candidiasis, scabies, head lice
Lumps, nodules	Warts, tumours
Plaque	Psoriasis (some types)
Pustule	Psoriasis (some types), acne vulgaris, boils
Scaling	Psoriasis, tinea, candidiasis
Redness	Eczema, psoriasis, acne rosacea, erysipelas, tinea, candidiasis
Thickening of the skin	Eczema, psoriasis
Ulcer	Tumours
Vesicles (blisters)	Eczema, erysipelas, impetigo, tinea, scabies
Weeping	Eczema, impetigo, tinea, candidiasis
Wheal	Urticaria

TABLE 11.10: SKIN DISEASES LISTED ACCORDING THEIR APPEARANCES

Skin disease is very common and conventional treatment is relatively ineffective.

Conventional treatments suppress the skin lesions resulting in internal disease at the worst or variable control of the skin symptoms at best.

Alternative treatment of skin disease may result in a worsening before improvement particularly if it has been suppressed. This has cosmetic considerations.

Although the skin is the outermost level of the physical body, it does reflect internal imbalances. If the skin problem is associated with a marked internal imbalance the treatment may take a long time to achieve results.

If the skin problem is relatively superficial, i.e. on the palms or soles and there is little in the way of an internal imbalance, response can be rapid and dramatic.

INDEX

Main entries are in bold type.